Handbook of Laboratory Animal Science *Second Edition*

Volume II

Animal Models

Edited by

Jann Hau and Gerald L. Van Hoosier, Jr.

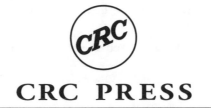

CRC PRESS

Boca Raton   London   New York   Washington, D.C.

Senior Editor: John Sulzycki
Project Editor: Gail Renard
Project Coordinator: Pat Roberson
Cover Designer: Dawn Boyd-Snider
Marketing Manager: Nadja English

Library of Congress Cataloging-in-Publication Data

Handbook of laboratory animal science / edited by Jann Hau, Gerald L. Van Hoosier, Jr.—2nd ed.
    p. cm.
    Includes bibliographical references and index.
    Contents: v. 1. Essential principles and practices — v. 2. Animal models.
    ISBN 0-8493-1086-5 (v. 1 : alk. paper) — ISBN 0-8493-1084-9 (v. 2 : alk. paper)
    1. Laboratory animals. 2. Animal experimentation. 3. Animal models in research.
    I. Hau, Jann. II. Van Hoosier, G. L.

QL55 .H36 2002
599' .07'24—dc21   2002031315

Visit the CRC Press Web site at www.crcpress.com

No claim to original U.S. Government works
International Standard Book Number 0-8493-1084-9
Library of Congress Card Number 2002031315
Printed in the United States of America 1 2 3 4 5 6 7 8 9 0
Printed on acid-free paper

Preface

The *Handbook of Laboratory Animal Science, Second Edition: Animal Models, Volume II* is dedicated to the use of laboratory animals as models for humans. This book explains in great detail the comparative considerations underlying the choice of animal species and strains in different research disciplines. Volume II consists of chapters written by experts in their respective fields and covers a range of scientific areas in which animals play a crucial role as models for humans. Unlike many other publications, this book is not exclusively restricted to laboratory animal models for the study of human diseases. It takes a wider approach, which is in accordance with modern interpretation of the animal model concept.

Most of our knowledge of human biology is derived from animal studies, and fortunately, the conservative nature of animal evolution often renders reliable extrapolation of findings between species the rule rather than the exception. However, we found that there is a great need for a handbook on the choice of animal species and strains, and on the development and application of models in different areas of biomedical research. The book consequently focuses on the relevant comparative aspects in the many different contexts in which animals are used as well as on the spontaneous genetic mutants and the genetically modified animal models available within different research areas.

The authors have strived to include the most recent information available as well as generally recognized facts to make the book relevant, practical, and attractive to other specialists. Reporting from the cutting edge of a scientific discipline involves including some, but obviously not all, of the most recently reported findings. This selection will invariably make some scientists feel that their results have been neglected, and for this we apologize. We welcome comments from readers and colleagues that may assist us in keeping the text up-to-date and in correcting errors.

Both Volumes I and II of the *Handbook of Laboratory Animal Science* are, in many ways, very technical books. We hope that our readers will find them useful, whether they be postgraduate students who are not familiar with laboratory animals and their use as research tools, veterinarians who specialize in laboratory animal science and welfare, or experienced scientists who are looking for an overview and reference text of the large and heterogeneous field that is laboratory animal science.

Jann Hau
Uppsala University
Uppsala, Sweden

Gerald Van Hoosier
University of Washington
Seattle, Washington

About the Editors

Jann Hau is Professor of Comparative Medicine at the University of Uppsala in Sweden. Dr. Hau graduated in experimental biology from University of Odense in Denmark after medical and biology studies in 1977, and specialized in laboratory animal science. Following research fellowships at University of Odense, he did his doctorate (Dr. Med.) at this university. In 1983, he joined the Department of Pathology at The Royal Veterinary and Agricultural University (RVAU) in Copenhagen as Associate Professor and Head of the Laboratory Animal Science Unit. He was later Head of the Department of Pathology and Dean of the Faculty of Animal Husbandry and Veterinary Science at the RVAU.

In 1991, he moved to the Royal Veterinary College (RVC) in London as Professor in the London University Chair in Laboratory Animal Science and Welfare. At the RVC, he was responsible for the undergraduate and postgraduate teaching in laboratory animal science and welfare, which included a specialist Master of Science course in Laboratory Animal Science that attracted a number of postgraduate students from many parts of the world.

In 1996, Dr. Hau was appointed Professor in Comparative Medicine in Uppsala and Head of a new Department of Comparative Medicine. Following amalgamations of departments at the medical faculty, Comparative Medicine is presently integrated with the Department of Physiology, of which Dr. Hau is presently Head. In Uppsala, he has established a number of courses for undergraduate and postgraduate students, including specialist education programs.

Dr. Hau has organized several international meetings and courses on laboratory animal science. He is the editor-in-chief of the *Scandinavian Journal of Laboratory Animal Science* and editor of the laboratory animals' section of the UFAW journal *Animal Welfare*. He is a member of a number of laboratory animal science organizations and former president of the Scandinavian Society of Laboratory Animal Science and the Federation of European Laboratory Animal Science Associations.

Dr. Hau has supervised many postgraduate Master's and Ph.D. students and published several hundred scientific papers and chapters in books. Together with Dr. P. Svendsen, he wrote the first Danish textbook on laboratory animals and animal experiments published in 1981, 1985, and 1989, and they co-edited the first edition of the *CRC Handbook of Laboratory Animal Science*, published in 1994.

Dr. Hau's current research interests include development of refined laboratory animal models for studies of biological mechanisms in reproductive biology and infections as well as development of methods to assess stress and welfare in animals. His research activities also include projects focused on ways to replace, reduce, and refine the use of animals in antibody production.

Gerald L. Van Hoosier, Jr., is Professor of Comparative Medicine in the School of Medicine at the University of Washington in Seattle, Washington. Dr. Van Hoosier graduated from the College of Veterinary Medicine at Texas A&M University at College Station, Texas, in 1957 and subsequently obtained postdoctoral training in virology and epidemiology at Berkeley, California, and in pathology at Baylor College of Medicine in Houston, Texas. From 1957 to 1962, he served as a Commissioned Officer in the U.S. Public Health Service assigned to the biologics program at the National Institutes of Health in Bethesda, Maryland, where he focused on the development and safety evaluation of poliomyelitis and measles vaccines. Following 5 years in the Public Health Service, Dr. Van Hoosier joined the faculty of the Division of Experimental Biology at Baylor College of Medicine in Houston, Texas, and did research on the role of viruses in the etiology of cancer. In 1969, he moved to Pullman, Washington, where he was a faculty member in the Department of Veterinary Pathology in the School of Veterinary Medicine and Director of Laboratory Animal Resources at Washington State University. He introduced a course on laboratory animals into the third year of the veterinary school curriculum, taught a graduate course on the pathology of laboratory animals, and began the development of a series of audio tutorials in collaboration with the American College of Laboratory Animal Medicine. In 1975, Dr. Van Hoosier was invited to develop an experimental animal program at the University of Washington. He obtained a training grant for veterinarians from the National Institutes of Health and established the Department of Comparative Medicine, which offers a Master's degree. He served as the department chairman and Attending Veterinarian until 1995.

After becoming a Diplomate of the American College of Laboratory Animal Medicine in 1968, he served as President in 1977–1978. Other professional activities have included serving as Chairman of the Board of Trustees of the American Association for Accreditation of Laboratory Animal Care in 1981–1982, President of the American Association of Laboratory Animal Science in 1992, and a member of the Governing Board of the International Council for Laboratory Animal Science from 1995 to 1999. In addition to approximately 100 scientific papers, Dr. Van Hoosier was a co-editor of *Laboratory Hamsters*, one of a series of texts by the American College of Laboratory Animal Medicine and served as editor of *Laboratory Animal Science* from 1995 to 1999. He is currently a member of the Editorial Council of the *Baltic Journal of Laboratory Animal Science* and *Animales de Experimentacion*.

He is the recipient of the Griffin Award from the American Association of Laboratory Animal Science and a Distinguished Alumni Award from the College of Veterinary Medicine at Texas A&M University.

Contributors

Abbas Ardehali
Division of Cardiothoracic Surgery
UCLA Medical Center
School of Medicine
Los Angeles, California

Karsten Buschard
Bartholin Institute
Copenhagen, Denmark

Anthony M. Carter
Department of Physiology and
  Pharmacology
University of Southern Denmark
Odense, Denmark

Christi M. Cavaliere
Section of Plastic Surgery
University of Michigan
Ann Arbor, Michigan

Ryan P. Frank
Department of Orthopedic Surgery
University of Michigan
Ann Arbor, Michigan

Cynthia E. Glover
Department of Comparative Medicine
University of Washington
Seattle, Washington

Kurt D. Hankenson
Departments of Orthopedic Surgery and the Unit
  for Laboratory Animal Medicine
University of Michigan
Ann Arbor, Michigan

Jann Hau
University of Uppsala
Uppsala, Sweden

Henrik Elvang Jensen
Laboratory of Veterinary Pathology
Royal Veterinary and Agricultural University
Frederiksberg, Denmark

Jörgen Jönsson
Institute of Odontology
Huddinge University Hospital
Karolinska Institute
Stockholm, Sweden

Björn Klinge
Institute of Odontology
Huddinge University Hospital
Karolinska Institute
Stockholm, Sweden

Otto Meyer
Danish Veterinary and Food Administration
Soborg, Denmark

Jesper Mogensen
Cognitive Neuroscience
Department of Psychology
University of Copenhagen
Copenhagen, Denmark

Robert Murison
Department of Biological and Medical
  Psychology
University of Bergen
Bergen, Norway

Jørgen Rygaard
Bartholin Institute
Copenhagen, Denmark

Ove Svendsen
Department of Pharmacology and
  Pathobiology
Royal Veterinary and Agricultural University
Frederiksberg, Denmark

Rikke Thon
Taconic M & B
Lille Skensved, Denmark

Gerald L. Van Hoosier, Jr.
University of Washington
Seattle, Washington

David Whiting
Division of Cardiothoracic Surgery
UCLA Medical Center
School of Medicine
Los Angeles, California

Table of Contents

Animal Models

Jann Hau

CONTENTS

INTRODUCTION

Most of our basic knowledge of human biochemistry, physiology, endocrinology, and pharmacology has been derived from initial studies of mechanisms in animal models.[1] Throughout history, scientists have performed experiments on animals with the aim of obtaining knowledge of animal and human biological structure and function (see, e.g., Held;[2] Loew[3]). Often such studies have not been and are not possible in the human. This may be due to ethical or religious considerations, but often practical, economic, and scientific reasons make initial studies in animals the best solution to studies of a biological phenomenon.

Laboratory animal science may be defined as the study of the scientific, ethical, and legal use of animals in biomedical research, that is, a multidisciplinary field encompassing biological and pathobiological specialties for the optimal scientific use of animals as models for humans or other species.

Basic laboratory animal science is concerned with the quality of animals as sentient tools in biomedical research. It encompasses comparative biology of laboratory animals, technical aspects of breeding, housing and husbandry, anesthesia, euthanasia, and experimental techniques. Laboratory animal medicine is a veterinary specialty, focusing on the diagnosis, treatment, and prevention of diseases in animals used as subjects in biomedical activities. High-quality animals and animal care ensure the highest possible health and welfare status of the animals and are prerequisites for good science and public acceptance of the use of animals in research.

Volume I of this handbook is an introduction to basic laboratory animal science, whereas the present volume focuses on applied laboratory animal science, which is the use of animals as models for humans — or in some instances as models for other species.

THE CONCEPT OF ANIMAL MODELS

A model is an object of imitation, something that accurately resembles something else, a person or thing that is the likeness or image of another.[4] Prometheus, who has been deigned by poets to have first formed Man, formed a model from water and earth and then stole fire from the sun to animate the model.[5] An animal model is thus an animated object of imitation in the image of humans (or other species), used to investigate biological or pathobiological phenomena.

A laboratory animal model describes a biological phenomenon that the species has in common with the target species.[6] A more accurate definition has been given by Held on the basis of Wessler's original definition:[7] "a living organism in which normative biology or behavior can be studied, or in which a spontaneous or induced pathological process can be investigated, and in which the phenomenon in one or more respects resembles the same phenomenon in humans or other species of animal." What is generally understood by the term "animal model" is modeling of humans. It is not the image of the used animal that is the focus of research but the analogy of the physiological behavior of this animal to our own (or another) species. It would thus be more correct to refer to animals as "human models" in this context. Laboratory animal science, comparative medicine, and animal experiments are indeed much more about humans than about any other animal species.[8]

The significance and validity with respect to usefulness in terms of "extrapolatability" of results generated in an animal model depend on the selection of a suitable animal model. A good knowledge of comparative anatomy and physiology is an obvious advantage when developing an animal model. Animal models may be found throughout the animal kingdom, and knowledge about human physiology has been achieved in species far removed from the human in terms of evolutionary development. A good example is the importance of the fruit fly for the original studies of basic genetics. Animal models are used in virtually every field of biomedical research, as reflected in the chapters of this book.

CLASSIFICATION OF ANIMAL MODELS

A plethora of animal models has been used and is being used and developed for studies of biological structure and function in the human. The models may be *exploratory,* aiming to understand a biological mechanism, whether this is a mechanism operative in fundamental normal biology or a mechanism associated with an abnormal biological function. Models may also be developed and applied as so-called *explanatory* models, aiming to understand a more or less complex biological problem. Explanatory models need not necessarily be reliant on the use animals but may also be physical or mathematical model systems developed to unravel complex mechanisms. A third important group of animal models is employed as *predictive* models. These models are used with the aim of discovering and quantifying the impact of a treatment, whether this is to cure a disease or to assess toxicity of a chemical compound. The anatomy or morphology of the model structure of relevance to the studies may be of importance in all three of these model systems. The extent of resemblance of the biological structure in the animal with the corresponding structure in humans has been termed *fidelity*. A high-fidelity model with close resemblance to the human case may seem an obvious advantage when developing certain models. What is often more important, however, is the discriminating ability of the models, in particular the predictive models. When using models, for instance to assess the carcinogenicity of a substance, it is of the essence that at least one of the model species chosen responds in a manner that is predictive of the human response to this substance. Thus the similarity between humans and model species with respect to relevant biological mechanism is often more important than the fidelity of the model. Often the two go hand in hand, and high-fidelity models offer the best opportunity to study a particular biological function.

An animal model may be considered homologous if the symptoms shown by the animal and the course of the condition are identical to those of humans.[9] Models fulfilling these requirements are relatively few, but an example is well-defined lesion syndromes in, for instance, neuroscience.[10] An animal model is considered isomorphic if the animal symptoms are similar but the cause of the symptoms differs between human and model. However, most models are neither homologous nor isomorphic but may rather be termed "partial." These models do not mimic the entire human disease but may be used to study certain aspects or treatments of the human disease.[10]

CLASSIFICATION OF DISEASE MODELS

The majority of laboratory animal models are developed and used to study the cause, nature, and cure of human disorders. They may conveniently be categorized in one of the following five groups, of which the three first are the most important, as given in numerical order:

1. Induced (experimental) disease models
2. Spontaneous (genetic) disease models
3. Transgenic disease models
4. Negative disease models
5. Orphan disease models

Induced (Experimental) Disease Models

As the name implies, *induced models* are healthy animals in which the condition to be investigated is experimentally induced, for instance, the induction of diabetes mellitus with encephalomyocarditis virus,[11] allergy against cow's milk through immunization with minute doses of protein,[12] or partial hepatectomy to study liver regeneration.[13] The induced-model group is the only category that theoretically allows a free choice of species. Although one might be tempted to presume that extrapolation from an animal species to the human is the better the closer this species resembles humans (high fidelity), phylogenetic closeness, as fulfilled by primate models, is not a guarantee for validity of extrapolation, as the unsuccessful chimpanzee models in acquired immunodeficiency syndrome (AIDS) research have demonstrated.[14] It is just as decisive that the pathology and outcome of an induced disease or disorder in the model species resembles the respective lesions of the target species. Feline immunodeficiency virus infection in cats may therefore for many studies be a better model for human AIDS than is human immunodeficiency virus infection in simians. Although mice and rats have many biological characteristics in common, they do not necessarily serve equally well as models of human disease. For example, schistosomiasis (*mansoni*) infection may be studied in experimentally infected mice but not in rats, whose immune system is able to fight the infection effectively.[15]

Most induced models are partial or isomorphic because the etiology of a disease experimentally induced in an animal is often different from that of the corresponding disease in the human. Few induced models completely mimic the etiology, course, and pathology of the target disease in the human.

Spontaneous Animal Disease Models

These models of human disease use naturally occurring genetic variants (mutants). Many hundreds of strains and stocks with inherited disorders modeling similar conditions in humans have been characterized and conserved (see, e.g., http://www.jax.org). A famous example of a spontaneous mutant model is the nude mouse,[16] which was a turning point in the study of heterotransplanted tumors and, for instance, enabled the first description of natural killer cells. Other famous spontaneous models include Snell's dwarf mice, without a functional pituitary,[17] and the curly-tail mouse, in which fetuses develop a whole range of neural-tube defects.[18] Many of the mutants are available in inbred strains, with corresponding coisogenic or congenic strains. This is very useful because the influence of just one affected gene or locus may then be studied against a reference strain with similar genetic background as the mutant (see also Volume I, Chapter 9).

An extensive literature is available on spontaneous models, and the majority of these are mice and rat models, although a wide range of mutants in many different species has been described. A good example of the amount of information available is the publication of Migaki,[19] which references >200 diseases in animals exclusively caused by inborn errors of metabolism.

The spontaneous models are often isomorphic, displaying phenotypic similarity between the disease in the animal and the corresponding disease in the human — this is called *face validity*; for instance, type I diabetes in humans and insulin-requiring diabetes in the BB rat. This phenotypic similarity often extends to similar reactions to treatment in the model animal and the human patient, and spontaneous models have been important in the development of treatment regimens for human diseases.

However, if the object of a project is to study the genetic causes and etiology of a particular disease, then comparable genomic segments involved in the etiology of the disorder — *construct validity* — is normally a requirement. It should be remembered, however, that an impaired gene or sequence of genes very often results in activation of other genes and mobilization of compensating metabolic processes. These compensatory mechanisms may of course differ between humans and the animal model species.

Transgenic Disease Models

The rapid developments in genetic engineering and embryo manipulation technology during the past decade have made transgenic disease models perhaps the most important category of animal disease models. A multitude of animal models for important diseases have been developed since this technology became available, and the number of models seems to be increasing quickly. Mice are by far the most important animals for transgenic research purposes, but farm animals and fish are also receiving considerable interest.

Many physiological functions are polygenic and controlled by more than one gene, and it will require considerable research activities to identify the contribution of multiple genes to normal as well as abnormal biological mechanisms. The insertion of DNA into the genome of animals or the deletion of specific genes gives rise to sometimes unpredictable outcomes in terms of scientific results as well as in terms of animal well-being in the first generations of animals produced. Thereafter, transgenic lines can be selected and bred or cloned to avoid or select for a specific genotype. It is not an accurate science, although the methodology is constantly improving with the aim of eliminating unwanted effects. The embryo manipulation procedures themselves do not appear to affect the welfare of offspring in the mouse,[20] and the large-offspring syndrome observed in farm animals has so far not been reported in rodents (see Volume I, Chapter 18 for welfare aspects associated with transgenic animals).

Mutations induced by the use of mutagens such as ethyl-nitroso-urea represent another approach to the generation of new mutants, which may serve as models of human disorders. In many aspects, these mutants may be similar to spontaneous mutants and to the ones generated by transgenic embryo manipulation. The maintenance of a line raises similar issues for chemically induced genetic mutants as for animals that have been genetically modified through embryo manipulation.

The recent completion of the maps of the genomes of mouse and human will increase the research activities in genomics and proteomics; and using high-density microarray DNA chip technology in human patients as well as in animals, it will be possible to investigate which genes are switched on or off in different diseases.[21]

With both the human and the mouse genome maps available, this new technology is expected to rapidly increase knowledge on the genetic background and etiology of important diseases. This paves the way for a range of new homologous animal models with homology between animal and human (construct validity) for genotype as well as for phenotype. This development may result in a change in animal use from models for the identification of causative genes to models for studying the effects of changes in genetic pathways, gene–gene interactions and gene–environment interactions.[22]

Negative Animal Models

Negative model is the term used for species, strains, or breeds in which a certain disease does not develop, for instance, gonococcal infection in rabbits after an experimental treatment that induces the disease in other animals. Models of infectious diseases are often restricted to a limited number of susceptible species, and the remaining unresponsive species may be regarded as negative models for this particular human pathogenic organism. Negative models thus include animals that demonstrate a lack of reactivity to a particular stimulus. Their main application is in studies on the mechanism of resistance that seek to gain insight into its physiological basis.

Orphan Animal Models

Orphan model disease is the term that has been used to describe a functional disorder that occurs naturally in a non-human species but has not yet been described in humans and that is recognized when a similar human disease is later identified. Examples include Marek's disease, Papillomatosis, bovine spongiform encephalopathy, Visna virus in sheep, and feline leukemia virus. When humans are discovered to suffer from a disease similar to one that has already been described in animals, the literature already generated in veterinary medicine may be very useful.

EXTRAPOLATION FROM ANIMALS TO HUMANS

When experimental results have been generated in an animal model, they have to be validated with respect to their applicability to the target species, which normally is the human. The term "extrapolation" is often used to describe how data obtained from animal studies reliably can be used to apply to the human. However, extrapolation is generally not performed in its mathematical sense, in which data fit a certain function that may be described graphically and the graph extends beyond the highest or lowest sets of data to describe a situation outside the window of observation. Establishing toxicity data in animals and using these to determine safe levels of exposure for people is perhaps what comes closest to mathematical extrapolation in animal studies. However, most studies of animal structure and function are never extrapolated to be applicable for describing the corresponding features in the human; this is not relevant. What laboratory animal experimentation is about is very similar to other types of experiments. Scientists aim to obtain answers to specific questions. Hypotheses are tested, and the answers are obtained, analyzed, and published. As an example of this, one might question the possible health hazards of a new synthetic steroid and ask a number of relevant questions to be answered in animal studies before deciding on the substance's potential usefulness as a human hormonal contraceptive. For instance, does it exist in the same form in humans and animals? How does it affect the estrus cycle in rodents? How does it affect endogenous hormone levels in rodents and other species? How soon after withdrawal do the animals revert to normal cyclicity? Does it interfere with pregnancy in rodents and primates? Does it affect fetal development in rodents and primates? Is the frequency of fetal malformations in mice affected? Are puberty, the ovarian cycle, and pregnancy in rodent and dog offspring of mothers treated with the substance affected? And so on. Analyzing the data from experiments of this nature would give information on the potential of the new synthetic steroid as a hormonal contraceptive in the human.

A recent survey by a large multinational pharmaceutical company analyzed data compiled from 150 compounds for the concordance between adverse findings in human clinical data and data that had been generated in the preclinical tests in animals.[23] The concordance rate was found to be 71% for rodent and non-rodent species, with non-rodents alone being predictive for 63% of human toxicity (HT), and rodents alone, for 43%. High concordance rates were found, such as for cardiovascular HTs (80%), hematological HTs (91%), and gastrointestinal HTs (85%). Lower concordance rates were observed, such as for the neurological group, because it is difficult to identify symptoms like headache and dizziness in the animals studied. The only gastrointestinal HT that did not correlate with animal studies was, not surprisingly, nausea. One of the conclusions reached in this study was that the choice of species used might be subject to more thoughtful consideration. By tradition, studies are often carried out using rats and dogs, without an open-minded consideration of whether alternative species might be more appropriate for testing a specific compound.

Although the predictive value of animal studies may seem high if they are conducted thoroughly and have included several species, uncritical reliance on the results of animal tests can be danger-ously misleading and has resulted in damages to human health in several cases, including those of some drugs developed by large pharmaceutical companies. What is noxious or ineffective in non-human species can be innoxious or effective in humans and vice versa; for instance, penicillin is fatal for guinea pigs but generally well tolerated by humans; and aspirin is teratogenic in cats, dogs, guinea pigs, rats, mice, and monkeys but obviously not in pregnant women, despite frequent consumption.[24] Thalidomide, which crippled 10,000 children, does not cause birth defects in rats[25] or many other species[26] but does so in primates. A close phylogenetical relationship or anatomical similarity is not a guarantee of identical biochemical mechanisms and parallel physiological response, although such is the case in many instances.

The validity of extrapolation may be further complicated by the question, "To which humans?" As desirable as it often is to obtain results from a genetically defined and uniform animal model, the humans to whom the results are extrapolated are genetically highly variable, with cultural, dietary, and environmental differences. This may be of minor importance for many disease models but can become significant for pharmacological and toxicological models.

It is not possible to give reliable general rules for the validity of extrapolation from one species to another. This has to be assessed individually for each experiment and can often only be verified after first trials in the target species. An extensive and useful overview on the problem of predictive anthropomorphization, especially in the field of toxicology research, is *Principles of Animal Extrap-olation* by Calabrese.[27] The rationale behind extrapolating results to other species is based on the extensive homology and evolutionary similarity between morphological structures and physiolog-ical processes among different animal species and between animals and humans.[28]

MODEL BODY SIZE AND SCALING

The use of laboratory animals as models for humans is often based on the premise that animals are more or less similar with respect to many biological characteristics and thus can be compared with humans. However, there is one striking difference between mouse and human, and that is body size. In proportion to their body size, mammals generally have very similar organ sizes expressed as percentage of body weight. Take the heart for instance, which often constitutes 5 or 6 g per kilogram of body weight; or blood, which is often approximately 7% of total body weight.

It is well known that the metabolic rate of small animals is much higher than that of large animals. It has also been demonstrated that capillary density in animals smaller than rabbits increases dramatically with decreasing body weight.[29] However, considering that most animals are similar in having heart weights just above 0.5% of their body weight and a blood volume corresponding to 7% of the body weight, it becomes obvious that to supply the tissues of small animals with sufficient oxygen for their high metabolic rate, it is not sufficient to increase the stroke volume. The stroke volume is limited by the size of the heart, and heart frequency is the only parameter to increase, which results in heart rates well over 500 per minute in the smallest mammals. Other physiological variables, like respiration and food intake, are similarly affected by the high metabolic rate of small mammals.

This means that scaling must be an object for some consideration when one calculates dosages of drugs and other compounds administered to animals in experiments. If the object is to achieve equal concentrations of a substance in the body fluids of animals of different body size, then the doses should be calculated in simple proportion to the animals' body weights. If the object is to achieve a given concentration in a particular organ over a certain time period, the calculation of dosage becomes more complicated, and other factors, including the physicochemical properties of the drug, become important. Drugs and toxins exert their effect on an organism not per se but because of the way that they are metabolized, the way that they and their metabolites are distributed and bound in the body tissues, and how and when they are finally excreted.

However, metabolism or detoxification and excretion of a drug are not directly correlated with body size but, more accurately, to metabolic rate of the animal (see Schmidt-Nielsen[29,30] for more details). Kleiber[31] in 1932 was the first to demonstrate that in a log–log plot of mammalian body weight to metabolism, the graph forms a straight line with a slope of 0.75.

The metabolic rate of an animal as expressed by oxygen consumption per gram body weight per hour is related to body weight in the following manner:

$$M = 3.8 \times BW^{-0.25}$$

where M is the metabolic rate (oxygen consumption in milliliters per gram of body weight per hour) and BW is body weight in grams. This equation may be used to calculate dosages for animals of different body weights if the dose for one animal (or human) is known:[32]

$$Dose_1/Dose_2 = BW_1^{-0.25}/BW_2^{-0.25}$$

$$Dose_1 = Dose_2 \times BW_1^{-0.25}/BW_2^{-0.25}$$

The equations should be considered as assistance for calculating dosages, but caution should be exerted with respect to too broad a generalization of their use, and the 0.50 power of body weight should be employed when dealing with animals with body weights of <100 g.[33] Some species react with particular sensitivity toward certain drugs, and marked variations in the reaction of animals within a species occur with respect to strain, pigmentation, nutritional state, time of day, stress level, type of bedding, ambient temperature, and so on.[32]

CONCLUSION

The choice or selection of animal model depends on a number of factors relating to the hypothesis to be tested but also on more practical aspects associated with the project and with project staff and experimental facilities. The usefulness of a laboratory animal model should be judged on how well it answers the specific questions it is being used to answer, rather than on how well it mimics the human disease.[34]

Often, a number of different models may advantageously be used to scrutinize a biological phenomenon; and for major human diseases, like diabetes, a whole range of well-described induced models is available, as are spontaneous models in both mouse and rat strains.

Most of the regulating authorities require two species in toxicology screening, one of which has to be non-rodent. This does not imply that excessive numbers of animals will be used, because an uncritical use of one-species models may mean that experimental data retrospectively turn out to be invalid for extrapolation, representing a waste of animals. The appropriateness of any laboratory animal model will eventually be judged by its capacity to explain and predict the observed effects in the target species.[35]

The free choice of species when developing animal models is more or less restricted to the induced models making use of clinically healthy animals, in which a condition deviating from normality is experimentally induced. Although all laboratory animal species are in principle available for model development, it has been a clear trend during the past 30 years that the most popular species, the house mouse and the Norwegian rat, are increasing in popularity at the expense of farm animal species and pet species.[36] The completion of the map of the mouse genome and the dominating position of mice in transgenic research seem to indicate that the dominance of the mouse as the most popular model for humans will increase further in the future.

REFERENCES

1. Coffey, D.S. and Isaacs, J.T., Requirements for an idealized animal model in prostatic cancer, in *Models for Prostate Cancer,* Murphy, G.P., Ed., Alan R. Liss, New York, 1980, 379.

2. Held, J.R., Muhlbock Memorial Lecture: considerations in the provision and characterization of animal models, in *Animal Quality and Models in Biomedical Research, 7th ICLAS Symposium Utrecht 1979,* Spiegel, A., Erichsen, S., and Solleveld, H.A., Eds., Gustav Fisher Verlag, 1980.

3. Loew, F.M., Scholarship and clinical service; comparative and laboratory animal medicine, in *Frontiers in Laboratory Animal Science. Proceedings of Joint International Conference of ICLAS, Scand-LAS and FinLAS, Helsinki 1995,* Nevalainen, T., Hau, J., and Sarviharju, M., Eds., *Scand. J. Lab. Anim. Sci.,* 23(Suppl. 1), 13, 1996.

4. *Oxford English Dictionary,* compact ed., Oxford University Press, Oxford, United Kingdom, 1971.

5. De Foe, *Systema Magicum,* 30, 1727, 1849.

6. Hau, J., Andersen, L.L.I., Rye Nielsen, B., and Poulsen, O.M., Laboratory animal models, in *Proceedings from the 19th ScandLAS Annual Symposium, Scand. J. Lab. Anim. Sci.,* 16 (Suppl. 1), 7, 1989.

7. Wessler, S., Introduction: what is a model?, in *Animal Models of Thrombosis and Hemorrhagic Diseases,* National Institutes of Health, Bethesda, MD, 1976, xi.

8. Salén, J., Animal models, principles and problems, in *Handbook of Laboratory Animal Science, Vol. II, Animal Models,* Svendsen, P. and Hau, J., Eds., CRC Press, Boca Raton, FL, 1994, chap. 1.

9. Kornetsky, C., Animal models: promises and problems, in *Animal Models in Psychiatry and Neurology,* Hanin, I. and Usdin, E., Eds., Pergamon Press, Oxford, United Kingdom, 1977, 1.

10. Mogensen, J. and Holm, S., Basic research and animal models in neuroscience — the necessity of "co-evolution," *Scand. J. Lab. Anim. Sci.,* 16(Suppl. 1), 51, 1989.

11. Hau, J. and Buschard, K., Effect of encephalomyocarditis (EMC) virus on murine foetal and placental growth monitored by quantification of maternal plasma levels of pregnancy-associated murine protein-2 and alpha-fetoprotein, *Acta Pathol. Microbiol. Immunol., Scand. Sect. B,* 94, 339, 1986.

12. Poulsen, O.M., Hau, J., and Kollerup, J., Effect of homogenization and pasteurization on the allergenicity of bovine milk analysed by a murine anaphylactic shock model, *Clin. Allerg.,* 17, 449, 1987.

13. Hau, J., Cervinkova, Z., O'Brien, D., Stodulski G., and Simek J., Serum levels of selected liver proteins following partial hepatectomy in the female rat, *Lab. Anim.,* 29, 185, 1995.

14. King, N.W., Simian models of acquired immunodeficiency syndrome (AIDS): a review, *Vet. Pathol.,* 23, 345, 1986.

15. Farah, I.O., Kariuki, T.M., King, C.L., and Hau, J., An overview of animal models in experimental schistosomiasis and refinements in the use of non-human primates, *Lab. Anim.,* 35, 205, 2001.

16. Pantelouris, E.M., Absence of thymus in a mouse mutant, *Nature,* 217, 370, 1968.

17. Hau, J., Poulsen, O.M., and Dagnæs-Hansen, N.F., Induction of pregnancy-associated murine protein-1 (PAMP-1) in dwarf (dw) mice by growth hormone, *Lab. Anim.,* 24, 183, 1990.

18. Jensen, H.E., Andersen, L.L.I., and Hau, J., Fetal malformations and maternal alpha-fetoprotein levels in curly tail (ct) mice, *Int. J. Feto-Matern. Med.,* 4, 205, 1991.

19. Migaki, G., *Compendium of Inherited Metabolic Diseases in Animals. Animal Models for Inherited Metabolic Diseases,* Alan R. Liss, New York, 1982, 473.

20. Van der Meer, M., Baumans V., Olivier B., et al., Behavioral and physiological effects of biotechnology procedures used for gene targeting in mice, *Physiol. Behav.,* 73, 719, 2001.

21. Lander, E.S., Array of hope, *Nat. Genet. Suppl.,* 21, 3, 1999.

22. Van Zutphen, L.F.M., Is there a need for animal models of human genetic disorders in the post-genome era?, *Comp. Med.,* 50, 10, 2000.

23. Olson, H. et al., Concordance of the toxicity of pharmaceuticals in humans and in animals, *Regul. Toxicol. Pharmacol.,* 32, 56, 2000.

24. Mann, R.D., *Modern Drug Use. An Enquiry on Historical Principles,* MTP Press, Lancaster, United Kingdom, 1984.

25. Koppanyi, T. and Avery, M.A., Species differences and the clinical trial of new drugs: a review, *Clin. Pharmacol. Ther.,* 7, 250, 1966.

26. Lewis, P., Animal tests for teratogenicity, their relevance to clinical practice, in Hawkins, D.F., Ed., *Drugs and Pregnancy: Human Teratogenesis and Related Problems,* Churchill Livingstone, Edinburgh, 1983, 17.

27. Calabrese, E.J., *Principles of Animal Extrapolation,* Lewis Publishers, Chelsea, Michigan, 1991.

28. Beynen, A.C. and Hau, J., Animal models, in *Principles of Laboratory Animal Science,* Van Zutphen, L.F.M., Baumans, V., and Beynen, A.C., Eds., Elsevier, New York, 2001, chap. 10.

29. Schmidt-Nielsen, K., *How Animals Work,* Cambridge University Press, London, 1972.

30. Schmidt-Nielsen, K., *Animal Physiology, Adaptation and Environment,* Cambridge University Press, London, 1975.

31. Kleiber, M., Body size and metabolism, *Hilgardia,* 6, 315, 1932.

32. Hau, J. and Poulsen, O.M., Doses for laboratory animals based on metabolic rate, *Scand. J. Lab. Anim. Sci.,* 15, 81, 1988.

33. Bartels, H., Metabolic rates of mammals equals the 0.75 power of their body weight, *Expl. Biol. Med.,* 7, 1, 1982.

34. Snider, G.L., Lucey, E.D., and Stone P.J., Animal models of emphysema, *Am. Rev. Respir. Dis.,* 133, 149, 1986.

35. Frenkel, J.K., Choice of animal models for the study of disease processes in man, *Fed. Proc.,* 28, 160, 1969.

36. Hagelin, J., Hau, J., and Carlsson, H.-E., Gradual implementation of the 3 Rs in biomedical research, submitted.

CHAPTER 2

Animal Models in Pharmacology and Toxicology

Otto Meyer and Ove Svendsen

CONTENTS

INTRODUCTION

Current knowledge in the disciplines of pharmacology and toxicology has been achieved largely by using experimental animals. In recent years, new knowledge in pharmacology has accumulated from strong interfaces between molecular pharmacology, receptor pharmacology, and *in vivo* pharmacology, including experimental studies in laboratory animals and humans. A similar strong interface can be seen between *in vitro* and *in vivo* toxicology. Over the years, the animal models in pharmacology and toxicology have become increasingly sophisticated because of continuous changes in endpoints. Many relatively simple animal models that were very important in the past have become redundant and have been replaced by non-animal methodologies with the same or even more specific endpoint.

With the present laboratory technologies, many issues in pharmacology and toxicology can be studied by *in vitro* methods. However, in both disciplines, an understanding of the complex interaction in different physiological or pathophysiological systems requires studies in intact organisms, allowing all relevant events to take place.

The attitude toward animal experimentation in pharmacology and toxicology has changed considerably during recent decades and is under strong public observation. In particular, within the past 10 years, there has been an ever-increasing focus on the 3Rs (reduction, refinement, and replacement) and on humane endpoints in animal experimentation. This is particularly important in the disciplines of pharmacology and toxicology, in which much experimentation in laboratory animals takes place in conscious animals. However, in recent years, focus on humane endpoints and the developments in usage of analgesics and anesthetics have, to a great extent, reduced the burden on the animals.

In contrast to many other disciplines that use laboratory animals, the developments in animal models in pharmacology and toxicology are derived from universities, research institutes, and pharmaceutical and other chemical industries. The development of new pharmaceuticals relies almost exclusively on animal models in those two disciplines. Thus, the regulatory acceptance of any new chemical product, irrespective of its usage, is based on toxicological studies in laboratory animals.

This chapter reviews animal models in pharmacology and toxicology. Animal models in pharmacology are divided into animal models in pharmacodynamics (primary and secondary effects) and pharmacokinetics. Animal models in toxicology mainly include those used for regulatory purposes.

ANIMAL MODELS IN PHARMACOLOGY

Pharmacology is the discipline covering the broad knowledge of how drugs interact with body constituents to produce therapeutic effect, as well as the events of the drug in the body and its ultimate elimination. Pharmacology covers the spectrum from molecular-level effects to the action of the drug on the whole body and relies heavily on knowledge of biochemistry, physiology, pathophysiology, molecular biology, and organic chemistry. The elucidation of molecular mechanisms of drug action, the development of new drugs, and the formulation of clinical guidelines for safe and effective use of drugs in therapy or prevention of disease states and in relief of symptoms are all part of pharmacology. Animal models have for decades been an integral part of this elucidation.

As a consequence of developments in biology and developments in techniques, the majority of animal models in pharmacology today are rather sophisticated in order to describe the endpoints of interest for the scientist. In many models, complicated behaviors have to be learned. In others, combined treatments with other drugs have to take place to describe the endpoint and interpret the results obtained. In addition, different complicated instrumentation of the animals has to take place to apply substances or collect body fluids for analysis. An example is triple microdialysis, with one microdialysis probe in one structure of the brain for determination of monoamine and metabolite levels, another microdialysis probe in the contralateral part of the brain for determination of drug and drug metabolite concentrations in exactly the same structure, and a third microdialysis probe in the jugular vein for determination of drug and drug metabolite concentrations.

Animal models in pharmacology can be divided into two subdisciplines: animal models in pharmacodynamics and animals models in pharmacokinetics. Animal models in pharmacodynamics can further be divided into models for illustration of the primary effect of drugs and models for description of secondary effects (side effects). The latter category also includes animal models in safety pharmacology. From a regulatory point of view, primary and secondary pharmacodynamic and safety pharmacology are defined in CPMP/ICH/539/00, adopted November 2000, available at www.ich.org.

Animal models in pharmacodynamic primary effect are so broad that a complete review would go beyond the scope of this chapter. Animal models have been developed and are available for almost any therapeutic area in human and veterinary medicine. Within recent years, hundreds of new models have been developed using gene technologies, mainly by knockout of specific genes in mice. In addition, new strains of laboratory animals such as the minipig have been introduced as models in diabetes research.[1] This section is limited to models in the following few selected therapeutic areas: infections, mental disorders, neurodegenerative diseases, endocrine diseases, noninfectious inflammation, and pain. A search in MEDLINE via PubMed covering the years 1966 to 2001 with the search words *animal models in pharmacology* resulted in a list of 8400 references. For *animal models in infectious disease*, there were 1597 references; for *mental disorders*, 956 references; and for *diabetes*, 1012 references. This illustrates the enormous amount of literature available on this topic.

In *in vivo* pharmacology, many factors with an impact on biological variation, reproducibility, and predictability have been identified. They can be related to the animal, the environment, and the experimental procedure. It is crucial that scientists using experimental animals for their research have deep insight into these factors. Otherwise, data obtained from animal experimentation may be of no use, and animal lives would be spent unnecessarily. Most of those factors have been described in detail by Claassen[2] and summarized by Svendsen and Hansen.[3]

Animal Models in Pharmacodynamic Primary Effect

Drugs to Treat Infections

This area includes bacterial, mycotic, parasitic, and viral infection models.[4] Bacterial models include the following: peritonitis and sepsis models,[5] syphilis models,[6] tuberculosis,[7] keratitis,[8] urinary tract infections,[9–11] arthritis,[12] and endocarditis.[13] Parasitic models include Leishmaniasis models[14] and Echinococcosis models.[15] Mycotic and viral models include models relevant for human immunodeficiency virus infections.[4]

Drugs to Treat Mental Disorders

For mental disorders, no direct animal models exist. Animal models of mental disorders are mostly indirect models that express only a limited and select part of the pathophysiology of the disease. In many cases, models are based on correlation with aspects of the disease rather than on evidence of pathophysiological mechanisms or on the actual theoretical pathophysiological mechanism.

Animal models for schizophrenia can be divided into *screening models* and *simulation models*. The screening models are based on pharmacological tools (i.e., usage of drugs to produce elements of the disease, such as dopaminergic hyperactivity), whereas simulation models are based on psychological aspects expressed as certain behaviors in animals.[16]

The models that have been used in the discovery of the second generation of antischizophrenic drugs include *mechanistic receptor models* and *symptom models* of antipsychotic activity and extrapyramidal symptoms.[17] The mechanistic receptor models include relative *in vivo* effects on neurotransmitter receptors obtained by administration of specific agonists or antagonists for the receptor in question; and drug discrimination, in which animals are trained to discriminate in two sets of drinking water between a stimulus drug with selectivity for a given neurotransmitter function and substances without this particular activity. The symptom models include (1) inhibition of conditioned avoidance response, in which rats are trained to escape an electric foot shock in a shuttle box; (2) inhibition of dopamine agonist-induced hypermotility or stereotypy and induction of cataleptogenic activity caused by dopamine receptor antagonists; (3) measurement of drug-induced electrophysiological effects on dopamine neurones in ventral tegmental area and substantia nigra, pars compacta; (4) drug-induced dystonia in non-human primates; and (5) cognitive function determined as the effect on spatial learning and memory in the Morris' water maze. These models are detailed below.

Relative *in vivo* effects on neurotransmitter receptors can be described by selecting *in vivo* effects, preferentially those CNS mediated, that are as specific as possible for the receptor in question, most often by using a selective agonist as a tool. In this way, dopamine D_2 antagonism can be measured by inhibition of pergolide-induced circling behavior in 6-hydroxy-dopamine-lesioned rats, and 5-HT_2 antagonism can be measured by inhibition of head twitches induced by a 5-HT_2 agonist or by the 5-HT precursor, 1-5-HTP.[17]

In drug discrimination, two principles have been used: (1) use of a stimulus drug with selectivity for a given neurotransmitter function or (2) use of a stimulus drug with mixed effect on a variety of receptors. D-amphetamine has been used extensively as a stimulus drug selective for dopamine receptors in the limbic dopamine system.

Selective inhibition of conditioned avoidance response vs. unconditioned escape response is an old but still useful test for the characterization of antipsychotic drugs.

Hypermotility, stereotypy, and catalepsy models are often used in the *in vivo* screening of putative antipsychotic drugs. There is strong evidence that hypermotility induced by dopamine agonists is mediated by the limbic dopaminergic system, whereas stereotyped behavior and catalepsy are associated with increased and decreased striatal dopaminergic function, respectively.

The advantage of the electrophysiological model in measuring effects on dopamine neurons in the ventral tegmental area and substantia nigra, pars compacta is that it models the time course of antipsychotic treatment and that the limbic vs. striatal selectivity ratio of the drug can be evaluated in the same group of animals.

Dystonia in non-human primates is considered the most predictive model of the severe extrapyramidal side effects in humans that are induced by some of the older antipsychotic drugs.

Because schizophrenic patients show impairment of cognitive function, improvement of this deficit has become a target in antipsychotic drug development. The effect on spatial learning and memory in Morris' water maze is the preferred model.

Other simulation models for schizophrenia include models for anhedonia, social withdrawal, latent inhibition, and prepulse inhibition. These models have been reviewed by Ellenbroek et al.[18] More detail is beyond the scope of this chapter but may be found in Chapter 7, "Animal Models for Psychological Disorders."

Drugs to Treat Neurodegenerative Diseases

Under this heading, animal models in cerebral ischemia (stroke models) and Parkinson's disease are highlighted. The ischemia models can be divided into *global ischemia* and *focal ischemia* models.[19]

Global ischemia models are differentiated into total-body ischemia, global cerebral ischemia, and forebrain ischemia. Total-body ischemia models include (1) decapitation with studies on the isolated brain; (2) cardiac arrest and resuscitation, excluding possible remaining collateral circulation into the brain; and (3) profound systemic hypotension induced by pharmacological agents.

Global cerebral ischemia models include increased cerebral pressure obtained by cisternal injection of artificial cerebrospinal fluid, asphyxia or cervical compression obtained by simultaneous occlusion of cervical blood vessels by tourniquet and systemic hypotension, and, finally, combination of surgical occlusion of the major arteries. Forebrain ischemia models include four models, all based on artery occlusion: (1) bilateral common carotid occlusion in Mongolian gerbils, (2) four-vessel occlusion in the rat (Pulsinelli's model), (3) bilateral common carotid artery occlusion with hypotension (Smith's model), and (4) bilateral common carotid artery occlusion in spontaneous hypertensive rats.

The most important focal ischemia models in rats include five models: (1) proximal main carotid artery occlusion (Tamura model), (2) intravascular thread (Koizumi model), (3) distal main carotid artery occlusion with bilateral common carotid artery (CCA) occlusion (Chen model), (4) tandem occlusion (Brint model), and (5) photothrombosis (Watson model).

This illustrates the great variety of models within a certain area in which endpoints can be very different. The outcome of these models is highly dependent on temperature, glucose level, blood pressure, and the age and sex of animals.

Parkinson's disease is a manifestation of nigrostriatal dopamine neurone degeneration. The majority of animal models in Parkinson's disease include administration of pharmacological agents or neurotoxins.[20] Reserpine and alpha-methyl-tyrosine cause, by two different mechanisms, depletion of catecholamines in the brain. 6-Hydroxydopamine administered by intracerebral or intraventricular injection causes specific damage to the dopaminergic system via oxidative stress to dopaminergic neurones. Systemic administration of the compound 1-methyl-4-phenyl-1,2,5,6-tetrahydropyridine (MPTP) results in depletion of striatal dopamine and nigrostriatal cell death in a wide variety of animal species, including mice, cats, dogs, sheep, minipigs, and non-human primates. Selective uptake of an MPTP metabolite into dopaminergic neurones via the dopamine transporter leads to its accumulation and accounts for its toxic specificity. Administration of metamphetamine to rats results in long-term depletion of striatal dopamine. The action of this toxin differs from that of MPTP in that dopamine is depleted at the level of dopaminergic terminals, not cell bodies.

Drugs to Treat Endocrine Diseases

The number of animal models in endocrinology is so overwhelming that this section is limited to animal models in diabetes.[21] Diabetes is classified on the basis of clinical symptoms in type 1 diabetes (insulin deficiency) and type 2 diabetes (insulin resistance). Animal models featuring physiological and pathological changes characteristic of each diabetes subtype are available.[22] Specific etiological factors or genetic backgrounds have been selected and combined to produce a particular type of experimental diabetes.

Animal models in type 1 diabetes include genetic, viral, and chemical models. In genetic models (NOD mouse and BB diabetic rat), diabetes occurs spontaneously with a total dependency on exogenous insulin. Chemical agents used in chemical models include agents that specifically damage pancreatic beta cells, cause a temporary reduction in insulin production and secretion, or diminish the metabolic efficacy of insulin in target tissue. Streptozotocin and alloxan are the most widely used substances for destruction of pancreatic beta cells.

Animal models in type 2 diabetes include genetic, chemical, and surgical models. The genetic models are produced through selective breeding, spontaneous mutations, or genetic engineering. Some examples include the db/db mouse, ob/ob mouse, KK mouse, NZO mouse, fa/fa Zucker rat, and fa/fa diabetic Zucker rat. Chemical models are obtained through injection of streptozotocin in low doses, in standard doses together with a protecting agent, or in a single dose to neonatal rats. Recently, minipigs have been included in this type of model.[1]

Drugs to Treat Neurogenic Inflammation (Rheumatoid Arthritis)

The study of joint inflammation and pain has been greatly facilitated by use of various animal models that mimic inflammatory stages in humans.[23–25] The models are generally divided into those that cause acute (e.g., carrageenan, urate crystals, kaolin, latex beads, Freund's complete adjuvant (FCA), interleukin-1) or chronic inflammation (FCA)[26] and others that cause neuropathic pain (e.g., sectioning or partial compression of a nerve trunk) when administered to animals, usually rats.

Rheumatoid arthritis is a chronic immune-mediated disease of unknown etiology and pathogenesis. Nevertheless, it is generally considered a disease of autoimmune origin. Most of the experiments leading to the discovery of neurogenic inflammation and its possible involvement in rheumatoid arthritis have been carried out in rodents with experimentally induced arthritis. One of the most valuable and widely used animal models is adjuvant-induced arthritis in rats.[27]

Drugs to Treat Pain

Over the years, many tests of nociception and pain in animals have been developed. The species most frequently used in pain research are mice and rats. There are two main types of tests. In the first, the response to the stimulation is fixed, and stimulation intensity increases until a defined standard response occurs. Examples include the tail-flick and hot-plate tests. In the second type, the stimulus is standardized, and the strength or duration of the response is measured. Examples include the formalin and writhing tests.

According to Tjølsen and Hole,[28] animal models of nociception and pain can be divided into two classes. The first class includes direct measurement of pain by behavioral responses to (1) acute stimulation of nociceptors, (2) intrathecal injection of nociceptive neurotransmitters, (3) long-term peripheral stimulation, (4) models of neuropathic pain, and (5) models of central pain. The second class is based on physiological correlates of pain and nociception after a noxious stimulus and includes electrophysiological methods and biochemical and histochemical methods.

The acute stimulation of nociceptors can be divided into methods based on reflex response measurements (tail-flick tests, paw-pressure test, tail-pinch test, and shock-titration test) and those based on behavior coordinated at higher levels (hot-plate test, formalin test, chemically induced writhing test, and colonic-distension test for visceral pain).

Long-term peripheral stimulation tests include subcutaneous injection of carrageenan to cause localized inflammation, monoarthritis inflammation, general adjuvant-induced arthritis, and surgical trauma.

Surgical trauma in pigs and rats has been used to create nociceptive models[29,30] with either behavior or neuronal expression of the immediate-early gene c-fos as a marker. Other surgical models have been described by Brennan et al.,[31] Brennan,[32] Lascelles et al.,[33] and Slingsby and Waterman-Pearson.[34]

Animal Models in Pharmacodynamic Secondary Effect

The animal models used for identification of secondary effects are models in intact animals that may be instrumented for the purpose of identifying drug-induced changes of normal physiological parameters such as rate of respiration, respiratory tidal volume, heart rate, electrocardiogram, cardiac output, pulmonary arterial blood pressure and blood flow, renal perfusion, digestive system function, smooth-muscle activity, autonomic and central nervous system activity, and several other critical body functions.

The term "safety pharmacology" has become an integrated activity in the development of new drugs. There is no official definition of the term. However, it is the systematic approach of investigating a new drug for efficacy to potentiate or inhibit activities of physiological or pharmacological responses or interaction with other drugs, whether *in vitro* or *in vivo*.

Safety pharmacological studies are strongly focused and designed to assess the potential adverse effects of a compound on the physiological function of one or more organs or organ systems in either intact or acutely prepared animal models that have proven relevance to humans, whether healthy or sick. Adverse effects of a compound on body function can be a consequence of either primary or secondary pharmacological properties.

Further details can be obtained from "Note for Guidance of Non Clinical Safety Studies for the Conduct of Human Clinical Trials for Pharmaceuticals" (FPMP/ICH/286/1995); "Note for Guidance on the Investigation of Drug Interactions" (CPMP/EWP/560/95, approved Dec. 1997); and "Standard Guidance: ICH Topic S7A CPMP/ICH/539/00."

ANIMAL MODELS IN PHARMACOKINETICS

In pharmacokinetics, healthy animals are used to study absorption, distribution, metabolism, and excretion of drugs. For drugs intended for human use, mice, rats, and dogs are generally used. In certain cases, non-human primates or minipigs are used. For veterinary drugs, pharmacokinetic studies are generally conducted in healthy animals of the actual target species, such as cattle, small ruminants, horses, pigs, dogs, or cats.

In the past, animal models were extensively used for pharmacokinetic studies in drug development. Today, developments in *in vitro* techniques have greatly supplanted such studies. Instead, pharmacokinetics in animal models is strongly integrated in the safety evaluation of new drugs with the aim of describing the actual drug exposure achieved in the safety studies (i.e., toxicokinetics). The most essential pharmacokinetic parameters are studied in the animal species used for toxicity studies: (1) mice or rats for acute toxicity testing; (2) rats, dogs, minipigs, or non-human primates for subchronic toxicity testing; (3) mice, rats, rabbits, minipigs, or non-human primates for teratogenicity testing; and (4) rats for reproduction testing. The main goal is to document the level of drug exposure during the conduct of the toxicity studies to make interpretations from studies in animals to exposure levels in humans.

Pharmacokinetic studies in pharmacodynamic animal models have not been integrated to the same extent because pharmacokinetic studies in animal models are used for safety testing. Even in veterinary medicine, where drugs are given to sick animals, the pharmacokinetic data are generally obtained using healthy animals. However, in recent years, a number of clinically relevant animal models have been developed for different purposes, and some are used to study pharmacokinetic parameters under conditions of actual diseases.[35–38]

ANIMAL MODELS IN TOXICOLOGY

Toxicology is the discipline used to predict undesirable biological or adverse effects in the living organisms as a consequence of exposure to, for instance, chemicals in our environment, both man-made as well as naturally occurring. A practical definition of an adverse change is the following: any treatment-related alteration from baseline that diminishes an organism's ability to survive, reproduce, or adapt to the environment.[39] The discipline forms part of the administration of chemicals in our society, such as medicines, food additives, pesticides, and industrial and household chemicals. In addition, the data from toxicological investigations constitute the essential part of the health evaluation of the use in society of gene-manipulated organisms (GMOs) and products made from GMOs, such as biological pesticides and so on. Thus, the main role of toxicological testing is to identify the hazards in humans as a consequence of exposure to, for instance, chemical substances and, in addition, to establish a dose relationship for the toxic effect to identify the toxic dose.

Toxicological data can come from studies on humans, from *in vitro* studies, or from studies in laboratory animals.

Toxicological data derived from humans will be the most reliable in predicting the potential consequence of human exposure. However, in most cases, reliable human data will not be available for evaluation. First of all, no data on human exposure to a chemical substance exist before the chemical has been introduced in the society, maybe apart from limited data from those persons who were exposed during the synthesis of the chemical.

Real toxicological studies in humans that are conducted to identify the possible adverse effects of chemical substances are only allowed in very few cases for restricted purposes. The prevailing human data come from epidemiological studies. However, such studies are very complicated to perform and resource demanding, and the data are often difficult to interpret, for instance, to identify the cause of an observed or recorded effect. Nevertheless, data from epidemiological studies play an increasing role in the toxicological evaluation of chemical substances as the development of electronic data technology makes it possible to handle huge sets of data from sufficiently large groups of individuals to achieve acceptable sensitivity of the study. Furthermore, the development of sensitivity of analytical methods and the use of biological markers will increase the applicability of human data.

In vitro methods using cells, tissue, or isolated organs, including those employing cells of non-mammalian origin, are used to some extent in toxicological testing of chemicals, such as in testing for genotoxicity. These tests are under constant development. However, such studies are limited by the fact that they cannot reflect the reaction of the intact organism. Many resources are invested in the development of new *in vitro* methods and the refinement of existing methods. Consequently, in the near future, *in vitro* studies will play an increasing although still relatively limited role in the toxicological evaluation of chemicals.

The prevailing amount of toxicological data used in the health assessment of human exposure to, for instance, chemicals will derive from studies in laboratory animals.

EXTRAPOLATION

It has been stated that the ultimate proof that a substance is a human teratogen can come only from information on the consequences of human exposure.[40] This statement is valid regarding toxicological effects in general. The difficulty is then overcome of differences between human and animal species in, for instance, absorption, metabolism, excretion, and sensitivity on the cellular level. However, comparing both data from human exposure and data from dosing experimental animals in the database established over decades has given considerable comfort in addressing, for instance, both cancer and developmental toxicity. Thus, with the exception of a few chemicals, such as the coumarin anticoagulant drugs, those agents well accepted as human teratogens have been shown to be teratogenic in one or more laboratory animal species. Likewise, of the relatively few substances known to cause cancer in humans, several were first demonstrated in laboratory animals, and there are several instances in which a substance that was carcinogenic in animal tests was later related to a particular human cancer found in people exposed to the particular substance. In addition, the biological resemblance or similarity between laboratory animal species and humans (that is, that the cellular structure and biochemistry are remarkably alike across species, starting with the lipoprotein cell membrane, which affects the absorption of xenobiotics into the cell, to metabolic processes like glycolysis, the Krebs cycle, and numerous other aspects of intermediary metabolism) serves as the basis on which data and knowledge can be extrapolated or functions inferred from one species to another. Even though the assumption is valid that one may use data from studies in laboratory animals to predict the outcome in humans, it is always crucial in the evaluation of data to consider the inherent species differences in a pattern of biological reactions to an exposure of substances.

Several biological parameters, including those for absorption and excretion of chemical substances (toxicokinetics), are dependent on the body weight, both in humans and in laboratory animals. Thus, it would be desirable to have data on the toxicokinetics, including data on bioactivation and cytotoxicity in the actual tissue that constitutes the target organ both in the laboratory animal used and in the human. Such data would make it possible to compare the effect in the two species and would constitute the basis for the assessment of the dose–response relationship. However, such data are not available in most cases, and as a consequence of that, the regulatory toxicological evaluation operates with a so-called uncertainty factor to compensate for the lack of knowledge about differential sensitivity among species. Such a factor, called the *no observed adverse effect level* (NOAEL), is applied to the highest dose in studies in laboratory animals that did not result in observed toxicological effect in order to establish a figure for exposure in humans that maintains an acceptable level of safety. A UF size of 100 has traditionally been used. Originally, this factor was empirically based. However, scientific evaluation of the established database over the years has shown that a factor of 100 gives the desired margin of safety for humans.

The dose in studies in laboratory animals are often expressed as milligrams per kilogram of body weight, but other (more recent?) data indicate that the dose expressed in milligrams per square meter of body surface constitutes a better basis for comparing the sensitivity for the exposure to chemicals between animals and humans. Thus, a difference of up to 10 times can be the result when an acceptable figure for exposure to humans is based on the NOAEL for mice, depending on whether the dose is expressed as milligrams per kilogram of body weight or as milligrams per square meter of the body surface; in other words, in some cases, the margin of safety is 10 times lower when establishing an ADI based on the dose, expressed in relation to body surface.

In conclusion, the laboratory animal model is valid to a high degree for prediction of the human situation. However, the evaluation of the data as to consequences in humans should always be done carefully, considering the species differences.

ETHICAL CONSIDERATIONS

The use of laboratory animals for experimental purposes inevitably raises concern for animal welfare. Many, if not all, toxicological tests or test procedures inflict some distress or pain and anxiety on laboratory animals. However, at the same time, laboratory animal experiments give valuable information of vital importance for both humans and, to some extent, animals. Thus, toxicological testing becomes an ethical dilemma, about which societal opinion ranges from extreme anti-laboratory animal experimentation attitudes to beliefs that animals can be used whenever considered relevant. The prevailing opinion is that use of laboratory animals should only take place when necessary to answer particular questions and that the animal's pain and distress must be minimized. This opinion is respected in national and international regulations. For toxicological test methods (test guidelines, TG) implying use of laboratory animals, the following criteria should apply. The results obtained using TGs should provide the scientific information needed for evaluation and sufficient basis for regulatory authorities to make decisions. Finally, the recommended procedure should minimize the suffering of the laboratory animals involved and, where possible and practical, reduce the number of animals used or even replace them. The European Organisation for Economic Co-Operation and Development (OECD) has recently published "Guidance Document on Recognition, Assessment, and Use of Clinical Signs as Humane Endpoints for Experimental

Animals in Safety Evaluation" with the purpose of applying the principles of the "3 Rs" to use of animals in regulatory toxicity tests.

CHOICE OF ANIMAL SPECIES

No ideal animal model exists covering toxicological testing in general. The toxicological databases indicate that the more animal species used, the better the predictive value of the data for the human situation. The choice of suitable laboratory animal species is done on a case-by-case basis, based on the available data and other relevant information.

In principle, all animals can serve as laboratory animals, but only a limited number of species are in use because of practical factors such as size of the animal, required breeding conditions, and economy. In addition, the obtained knowledge of certain animal species traditionally used for years has led to or will determine the choice of animal model.

Laboratory animals are often divided into groups as rodents or non-rodents. In the former group, the mouse and rat are the most used species. Also, guinea pig and hamster are used quite often. In general, rodents have a relatively short lifetime (a few years, with the exception of guinea pigs, which can obtain an age of approximately 8 years), they are easy to breed, have high fecundity, and are easy to house in sufficient quantities of individuals. The dog has traditionally been the most used species within the group of non-rodents. However, the use of pigs has increased in recent years, concurrent with the development of the minipig into a reliable and applicable laboratory animal and because of the fact that the dog is also a very popular pet animal. Monkeys are used only in very limited numbers and only for specific purposes for which a primate species is the only choice. Rabbits are frequently used for specific purposes, including eye irritation and skin irritation. In developmental toxicity studies, the rabbit is used as a representative of the group of non-rodents. However, it is constantly debated whether it is correct from a biological point of view to separate the group to which the rabbit belongs, Lagomorpha, from that of the rodents, Rodentia.

The choice of the most relevant species is dependent on data already obtained and on the available information on the chemical in question. However, a few general examples on specific features of the different species should be mentioned. Dogs and rats are the most efficient species concerning bile excretion. The common types of experimental animals, like mice and rats, used in studies for developmental toxicity have, unlike humans, a yolk sac placenta, which plays a significant role during the organogenesis. Many commonly used animal models such as the rat are obligate nose breathers, whereas many humans breathe via the mouth, thus bypassing the nasopharyngeal area. Concerning dermal absorption, human skin is less permeable than that of most laboratory animals. Finally, concerning metabolism, the cat has a low capacity for glucoronic acid conjugation, the dog has a similar reduced capacity for acetylation of chemical substances, and the pig exhibits a reduced ability for sulfate conjugation.

Within species exist a number of strains and stocks with specific characteristics that determine their applicability to the different toxicological test methods. The individual strains and stocks represent different genetic backgrounds. In addition, the introduction of gene technology has resulted in the development of several new strains, the transgenic animals.

The laboratory animals are often characterized as either inbred or outbred, the latter bred for the purpose of obtaining genetic heterogenicity. Concerning the latter, a large breeding colony is necessary to avoid some degree of inbreeding that leads to a shift in the genetic constitution of the stock. In addition to a drift toward inbreeding, the different stocks can undergo changes as a consequence of individual selection of animals for breeding to obtain a more profitable production. It has been speculated that this practice is the foundation for the increase in litter size in some Wistar-derived rats over the past 20 years and that, together with dietary changes, it has resulted in more heavy animals with a higher spontaneous incidence of diseases and consequently shorter life span (e.g., some Sprague Dawley and Wistar rats).

Inbreeding results in a high level of homozygosity, which results in more homogeneity and consequently less variance within some relevant parameters. However, such breeding practice also has drawbacks in leading to an inbreeding depression that results, for instance, in a decrease in fecundity and litter size.

Both inbred and outbred animals are used in toxicology testing. The choice of one or the other has been debated and, among others, has led to a proposal to use a normal group size, albeit one composed of two or three strains, in safety testing of chemicals. The general principles for choice of animals in regulatory toxicology testing do not answer whether one is more relevant than another. The choice is most often based on tradition and experience within the laboratory. Thus, the inbred rat strain F344 has been used in National Toxicology Program studies in the United States, whereas outbred stocks like Wistar and Sprague Dawley rats are frequently used in many laboratories in Europe.

PHYSIOLOGY AND EXPERIMENTAL CONDITIONS, INCLUDING MICROBIOLOGICAL STATUS AND DIET AND FEEDING CONDITIONS

Many factors are known to influence the outcome of toxicity tests in laboratory animals, some of which are species and strain and stock of animals (already mentioned); body weight; health; stress; husbandry (temperature, light, relative humidity, etc.); diet; dose; vehicle; volume; time and duration of dosing; and so on. Apart from a short comment on the choice of diet, a review of these factors is not a subject for this chapter, and more detailed information may be found in Volume I of this Handbook. The type of diet and its feeding is an important factor in toxicity testing that sometimes has more influence on the parameters measured in the laboratory animals than that of the exposure itself.

The diet of laboratory animals in toxicological tests should fulfill the nutritional requirements for the specific species and be free from contaminants of chemical as well as microbial origin. The dietary composition is, in addition to the nutritional conditions and impact on health of contamination, of importance for the physiological status of the animal. For instance, a high content of dietary fiber in rat diets shortens the food's transit time in the gut, and the dietary composition can influence bile secretion and the intestinal flora as well.

Three main types of diets are used in toxicological tests in rodents. First, there is the so-called chow diet, composed of natural ingredients like cereals and skimmed milk powder with vitamins and minerals added. Second, there is the semisynthetic or semipurified diet, containing defined constituents like casein, soybean oil, and carbohydrates including starches, minerals, vitamins, and sometimes cellulose. The main advantages of the chow diet are good nutritional value and low price. However, the chow diet can vary in quality because the nutritional value of mainly the cereal part of the diet changes depending on harvest condition and control of contaminants. In contrast to the case of the chow diet, the semisynthetic diet is expensive to produce and consequently often has a price on the order of approximately 10 times that of the chow diet. However, the obvious advantage of using the semisynthetic diet is more quality control because of its composition of well-defined constituents and the fact that single ingredients can be interchanged without changing the nutritional value of the diet. This is of importance when testing substances with a nutritional component such as a protein, a carbohydrate, or fat in that a possible toxic effect can be distinguished from the effect of nutrition or malnutrition.

The third type of diet is the synthetic diet. In contrast to the case of the semisynthetic diet, all the ingredients in this diet are composed of chemically well-defined components. Thus, the protein, such as casein, in the semisynthetic diet is replaced by the corresponding amino acids. This type of diet is only used in very few cases, for specific purposes.

The high energy content of the diet, resulting in heavy rats with higher incidence of diseases and decreased survival, has been a problem for long-term toxicity studies in recent years. If the caloric value of the diet is lowered, for instance, by replacing the content of highly digestible carbohydrates in semisynthetic diets with the less digestible starches and in addition increasing the amount of the almost nondigestible cellulose and reducing the fat as well, the rat will simply compensate by eating more. This ability to compensate for the caloric value of the diet is also seen when using a diet with a very high digestible energy content; in other words, the rat consequently will eat less. For long-term toxicity studies, especially of carcinogenicity, it has been proposed that the feeding regimen be changed by introducing dietary restriction (DR), in which the animals are only offered a measured amount of diet, resulting in less intake than under the condition of an *ad libitum* feeding regimen. This feeding practice has been used successfully in some studies in which the incidence of diseases in rats, including cancer, was decreased or, more correctly, delayed in occurrence and the longevity of the animals was simultaneously improved. However, it will probably take years to introduce DR into national and international test guidelines for toxicity testing because of concern that the delayed occurrence of, for example, cancer reflects a decrease in the sensitivity of the test in detecting the carcinogenic potential of a tested chemical and because the considerable database on historical control data is based on data from *ad libitum* feeding studies.

TOXICITY TESTS

The three main tasks of toxicity testing are to elucidate the following: (1) spectrum of toxicity, that is, detection of adverse effects of chemicals in selected laboratory species and description of dose–effect relationships over a broad range of doses; (2) extrapolation, that is, prediction of adverse effects in other species, particularly humans; and (3) safety, the prediction of safe levels of exposure in other species, particularly humans.

The toxicity testing includes in general the following tests:

Acute toxicity
Acute eye irritation or corrosion
Acute dermal irritation or corrosion
Skin sensitization
Repeated-dose toxicity
Carcinogenicity
Reproductive toxicity
Neurotoxicity
Genetic toxicity

In addition, specific studies to elucidate the absorption, distribution, metabolism, and excretion (toxicokinetics), characteristics and studies to demonstrate a possible mode of action and mechanism (toxicodynamics) are important elements in testing for the health assessment of chemicals.

A short review of the *in vivo* toxicity tests will be given, including a description of general conditions such as design of the tests; dose selection; and, when relevant, choice of common species.

The most important guidelines and regulatory requirements are available on the Internet at the following addresses: http://www.emea.eu.int, http://www.oecd.org, and http://www.fda.gov/cber/guidelines.htm.

Tests for Acute Toxicity

Acute toxicity comprises any adverse effect occurring within a short period of time, most often within 14 d, after exposure to a single dose of a chemical, or sometimes after several doses within 24 h. The administration of the test substance can be oral, dermal, or via inhalation. For many years, acute toxicity data have been used to satisfy hazard classification and labeling requirements. Thus, the provision of either a point estimate of the median lethal dose, the dose LD_{50}, which is the lethal dose for 50% of the test animals; or a range estimate of the LD_{50} generally meets the acute toxicity data requirements for classification for regulatory authorities in the areas of industrial chemicals, consumer products, pesticides, etc.

For acute toxicity by inhalation, the LC_{50} is used, expressing the median lethal concentration parallel to that of the LD_{50}. The LC_{50} is normally expressed as milligrams per liter of the ambient air under standard conditions.

LD_{50} or LC_{50} is only one of several parameters used to express acute toxicity. The calculated LD_{50} or LC_{50} parameter does not constitute an absolute figure, as there are great variations among tests for a single chemical, both within the same laboratory and between different laboratories, because of factors such as species or strain and stock of the laboratory animals and their age or test conditions in general.

In recent years, there has been an increasing awareness that the use of death as an endpoint in toxicological testing inflicts unacceptable suffering on laboratory animals. Furthermore, the use of LD_{50} or LC_{50} in general is based more on practical reasons, for deriving a figure for regulatory use, than on science as such, and this has resulted in development of new, alternative tests in which more ethically acceptable procedures for acute toxicity are used. Thus, three new OECD test guidelines for oral acute toxicity have recently been introduced: the Fixed-Dose Procedure (OECD TG 420), the Acute Toxic Class Method (OECD TG 423), and the Up-and-Down Method (OECD TG 425). Over time, the existence of these should lead to a deletion of the traditional acute oral toxicity test (OECD TG 401). All the guidelines involve the administration of a single bolus of test substance to fasted healthy adult rodents by oral gavage, observation up to 14 d after dosing, and recording of body weight and necropsy of all animals. However, the three new, alternative tests provide significant improvements in the number of animals used as compared with that for the traditional test. In addition, they all contain requirements that the OECD Guidance Document on Humane Endpoints should be followed, which should reduce the overall suffering of the animals used. Furthermore, the Fixed-Dose Procedure has an endpoint of toxicity rather than mortality and uses a sighting study to minimize the number of animals required; and the Up-and-Down Method has a stopping rule, which limits the number of animals in the test.

The data from acute toxicity tests are used for regulatory purposes, that is, to establish rules for handling chemical substances in society. In addition, the data from these tests can be used in planning further toxicological testing, including the choice of dose levels. For pharmaceuticals, among others, the data from acute toxicity testing can form the basis for the evaluation of the interval between a therapeutic dose and a toxic one.

In the acute toxicity test, most often, groups of animals of each sex are exposed to several doses of the test substance, either at the same time or one at a time, sequentially, awaiting a possible effect or no effect of the first administered dose. Rats and mice are most commonly chosen for acute toxicity studies. For some chemicals for which high acute toxicity is not expected, the guideline for the traditional acute toxicity test is open to the possibility of a limit test that includes only one fixed dose.

In a sighting study (preliminary or dose range finding) performed to get information on the dose–toxicity relationship, including an estimate of the minimum lethal dose, females will normally be the preferred sex unless information indicates that males are more sensitive.

In the acute toxicity test, a clinical examination and mortality check are made shortly after dosing at frequent intervals and at least once daily thereafter. Cage-side observations include those of any changes in the skin, fur, eyes, mucous membranes, circulatory system, autonomic and central nervous systems, somatomotor activities, behavior, etc. Any pharmacotoxic signs such as tremor, convulsions, salivation, diarrhea, lethargy, sleepiness, morbidity, fasciculation, mydriasis, miosis, droppings, discharges, or hypotonia are recorded. Necropsies are performed on animals that are moribund, those found dead, and those killed at the conclusion of the study. All changes in the size, color, or consistency of any organ are recorded.

Microscopic examination of a lesion may be essential. Therefore, tissues from such lesions must be preserved in an appropriate fixative.

Eye Irritation

This test was developed in 1944 by Draize et al.[41] to study eye irritation in rabbits and is used to identify human eye irritants. The test is easy to conduct and requires no special instruments. Simplicity is probably the main reason for the popularity of the test. However, it is also the limitation of the test. The Draize test can identify most moderate-to-severe human eye irritants, but the test may fail to detect mild or subtle ocular irritation. The result from the Draize test is a criterion for classifying and labeling chemicals.

In the original test, 0.1 ml or 0.1 g test substance is applied to the eye conjunctival sac of albino rabbits. The degree or extent of opacity of the cornea, the redness of the iris, and the chemosis and discharge of the conjunctiva are scored subjectively according to an arbitrary scale at preselected intervals after exposure. Scoring is based on the degree of effects caused by the testing substance. More emphasis is placed on the opacity of the cornea, whereas emphasis is considerably less on other effects, such as conjunctival changes and iritis.

The eye irritation test will inevitably lead to often-severe suffering of laboratory animals, and consequently, to address this concern, the testing procedure has been modified over the years. Thus, the number of animals in the test has been reduced; and if the test chemical is suspected to cause eye irritation, the test allows the initial use of one animal and cessation of further testing if eye irritation clearly is observed. In addition, the introduction to the OECD Test Guideline for eye irritation presents some initial considerations before testing. Thus, it is stated that it is not necessary to test chemicals with an acidity of pH < 2 or chemicals that are strong bases, with a pH > 11. Furthermore, the data from skin irritation tests and from well-validated and accepted *in vitro* tests should be evaluated before the initiation of testing.

Humane concern about using animals in eye irritation tests has prompted many investigators to turn to alternative methods. The development of alternatives is still in its infancy. Recent research has focused on validation of methods, most of which are *in vitro*. However, it is generally agreed that *in vitro* techniques will replace animal testing in the near future only to some extent, so the immediate concern is to further reduce the number of animals used and minimize the pain inflicted on animals during the study. It is the experience of one of the authors that less than 5% of the animals used for this test show any reaction to the treatment.

Skin Irritation

The albino rabbit is the preferred animal species when testing for skin irritation because of its high skin sensitivity and light skin, on which even slight skin irritant effects of a substance usually can be detected.

In general, substances or products are tested for skin irritation using a test design first proposed by Draize et al. in 1944.[41] The substance to be tested is applied in a single dose on a small area (approximately 6 cm^2) of the skin of three rabbits and covered with a gauze patch, which is held in place with nonirritating tape. At the end of the exposure period, normally 4 h, any residual test substance is removed. Each animal serves as its own control. The possible skin reactions of erythema and edema are described and graded according to a classification system on each of the following days. The duration of the study should be sufficient for a full evaluation of the reversibility of the possible effects observed.

Dermal irritation is the production of reversible changes, whereas dermal corrosion is the production of irreversible changes (scar formation) in the skin. If it is suspected that the test substance might produce severe irritancy or corrosion, the OECD test guideline prescribes that a single animal test should be employed. As in the case of the eye irritation test, alternative *in vitro* tests are under development. Thus, a recent OECD draft proposal for *in vitro* skin corrosion tests (the Rat Skin Transcutaneous Electrical Resistance assay and the Human Skin Model Assay) has been introduced.

Skin Sensitization

Allergic contact dermatitis (type IV sensitization) is an immunologically mediated reaction. This is in contrast to the case of irritant contact dermatitis, which is a skin reaction caused by a primary and direct effect of the substance on the skin. In humans, the responses to both types of dermatitis are very similar, characterized by pruritis, erythema, edema, papules, vesicles, bullae, or combinations of these. In animals, the reactions may differ, and only erythema and edema may be seen. Allergic contact dermatitis is a T-cell-mediated cutaneous reaction to a substance, characterized by a delayed response (24–96 h) to a patch test with a nonirritating concentration of the substance.

The guinea pig has been the animal of choice for predictive sensitization tests for several decades. Two types of tests have been developed: (1) adjuvant tests, in which sensitization is potentiated by the injection of Freund's complete adjuvant, and (2) nonadjuvant tests. The test animals are initially exposed to nontoxic doses of the test substance by either or both intradermal injection or epidermal application (induction exposure). After a rest period of 10 to 14 d (induction period), during which an immune response may develop, the animals are exposed to a challenge dose. The extent and degree of skin reaction to the challenge exposure in the test animals are compared with that demonstrated by control animals that undergo sham treatment during induction and receive the challenge exposure. In the OECD Test Guideline, the minimal required number of animals for the adjuvant test, the Guinea Pig Maximization Test, is 10 test animals and five control animals, whereas the minimum for the nonadjuvant test, the Bueler Test, is 20 test animals and 10 control animals. Male or female (nulliparous and nonpregnant) young adult animals can be used.

Mouse models for assessing sensitization potential, such as the Mouse Ear Swelling Test and the Local Lymph Node Assay, have been developed and offer the advantages of an endpoint that is measured objectively, a short duration, and minimal animal treatment. Recently, the OECD has introduced a draft guideline for the Local Lymph Node Assay.

Repeated-Dose Toxicity: 28 Days, 90 Days (Subchronic), and 1 Year (Chronic)

These toxicity studies are designed to examine the adverse effects resulting from repeated exposure over a limited period of time, up to a certain part of the average life span of experimental animals. The dosing can be oral, dermal, or via inhalation. The data from these studies provide valuable information on the cumulative exposure on target organs and on general health hazards likely to occur as a consequence of repeated low-dose exposure to a chemical. As these studies are aimed at detecting any systemic toxic effect, a wide variety of parameters are monitored, such as clinical appearance including ophthalmological examination, body weight, body weight gain, and food consumption; and sometimes water intake, hematology, clinical biochemistry, and pathology including histopathology.

The 90-d exposure was originally chosen because this period generally covers 10% of the life span of the laboratory rat, whereas the 1-year exposure is supposed to cover a major part of the life of laboratory animals. The more recent guideline for the 28-d repeated toxicity study is designed as a first-tier test or screening test to detect the entire spectrum of systemic adverse effects of repeated exposure to the test chemical, including possible neurotoxic effects, immunotoxicity, or effects on the sexual organs. On the basis of the data from the latter study, the dose regimen can be selected for follow-up studies, including more prolonged exposure for the test chemical to further study the observed toxic effect.

All laboratory animals can be used in repeated dose toxicity studies, including rodents (most often rats and mice) and non-rodents, of which the minipig and the dog are the preferred species. The 28-d, 90-d, and 1-year repeated dose toxicity studies are very similar to each other and differ only in the number of animals required (the minimum required numbers are 5, 10, and 20 of each sex for the respective studies, for rodents, and 4 of each sex, for non-rodents, in all the studies) and in the extent of the parameters included. All routes of exposure, that is, oral, dermal, intravenous, or inhalation, can be employed. The oral administration of a test substance can be carried out by gavage, in capsules, or in the diet or drinking water. Dietary administration is a very common route of dosing.

The animals are divided into four groups. One group serves as a control group. The other three groups are given the chemical in increasing doses. The dose levels can be based on data from previous studies, including studies on toxicokinetics, among others. In general, the highest dose should result in toxic effects but not produce an incidence of fatalities, which would prevent a meaningful evaluation. The lowest dose level should not produce any evidence of toxicity. Where there is usable estimation of human exposure, the lowest level should not exceed this. Ideally, the intermediate dose levels should produce minimal observable toxic effects. If more than one intermediate dose is used, those dose levels should be spaced to produce a gradation of toxic effects. Twofold to fourfold intervals are frequently optimal for setting the descending dose levels.

The control group shall be an untreated group or a vehicle-control group, in cases using a vehicle to administer the test substance.

The OECD guidelines for the repeated dose toxicity are as follows: 28-d and 90-d studies include a limit test procedure for chemicals. If a test at one dose level, equivalent to at least 1000 mg/kg body weight per day, produces no observed adverse effects and if toxicity would not be expected based on data from structurally related compounds, then a full study using three dose levels may not be considered necessary. The limit test applies except when human exposure indicates the need for a higher dose level to be used.

Basically, the toxic effects of the test substance can be defined by physical examination, daily observations, ophthalmological examination, determination of diet and water consumption, body and organ weights, hematology, clinical chemistry, urinalysis, and pathology studies. In dogs and minipigs, electrocardiography may be included. When possible, these parameters are evaluated before initiation of the study to obtain baseline information on the animals. Detailed observations of each animal are made at least once and preferably twice daily for the duration of the study. If recovery groups are included in the study, these animals are observed for a period of weeks after withdrawal of treatment.

Daily observations include close scrutiny for changes in the fur, skin, eyes, mucous membranes, and orifices; the respiratory, circulatory, autonomic, and central nervous systems; somatomotor activities; and behavior. Special attention is given to any palpable mass that may be related to tumor incidence. All signs are recorded. If deaths occur during the study, the animals are necropsied within a short period of time and the tissues placed in fixative. Severely moribund animals are killed and necropsied to prevent loss of valuable tissues to autolysis. At the end of a test period, all animals except those in the recovery groups are killed. The recovery groups are observed during the recovery period, bled for hematology and clinical chemistry, and then killed for pathological studies.

Hematological analysis includes hematocrit, hemoglobin concentration, red blood cell count, white blood cell count (total and differential count), morphology of the red blood cells, and a measure of clotting ability such as prothrombin and thromboplastin time or platelet count.

Biochemical measurements comprise electrolyte balance, carbohydrate and protein metabolism, and organ function tests. This information can be important in the establishment of target organ toxicity. The analyses include most if not all of the following parameters: calcium, phosphate, sodium, potassium, chloride, fasting glucose, serum aspartate aminotransferase (AST, SGOT) and alanine aminotransferase (ALT, SGPT), alkaline phosphatase, ornithine carbamyltransferase, gamma-glutamyl transpeptidase, blood urea nitrogen, total protein, albumin, globulin, total bilirubin, blood creatinine, cholesterol, acid–base balance, lipids, cholinesterase (plasma, red blood cell, or brain), and any other biochemical parameters that may facilitate the definition of adverse effects. The number of biochemical parameters examined is based on the class of chemicals and the expected toxicity. For example, cholinesterase activities should be considered if the test substance is an organophosphate or a carbamate, which are expected to be inhibitors of the enzyme.

Urinalysis is generally conducted at the same time as hematology and clinical chemistry. The following parameters are usually determined: specific gravity, osmolarity, or both; acidity; protein; glucose; ketones; bilirubin; epithelial cells; urobilinogen and stones; etc.

All animals are subjected to a gross pathology examination. All tissues from the high-dose group and control animals and any tissues with lesions in other groups are further examined microscopically. These examinations should be extended to animals of all other dosage groups if treatment-related changes are observed in the high-dose group. The different test guidelines include lists of the minimal number of tissues recommended for histopathological examination. However, the clinical and other findings may suggest the need to examine additional tissues. Also, any organs considered likely to be target organs based on the known properties of the test substance should be preserved for histopathological examination.

Carcinogenicity Studies

The objective of long-term carcinogenicity studies is to observe test animals for a major portion of their life span for the development of neoplastic lesions during or after exposure to various doses of a test substance by an appropriate route of administration. Such an assay requires careful planning and documentation of the experimental design, a high standard of pathology, and unbiased statistical analysis. These requirements are well known and have not undergone any significant changes during the past several years. However, in recent years, some development of a testing strategy has taken place in which information about chemical structure and data from short-term *in vitro* and *in vivo* studies for, say, genotoxic effects have been considered for regulatory purposes to decide whether a long-term, resource-demanding carcinogenicity study should be required at all.

The preferred animal species for long-term carcinogenicity studies are rats, mice, and to some extent, hamsters, mainly because these species have a relatively short life span and can be housed in sufficient numbers in the laboratory. In addition, most of the data from other toxicology studies comes from rodents as well. It is very important to know the normal life span of the strain or stock used in these studies because of the long exposure period employed. Furthermore, data on the background tumor incidence are crucial. Thus, a Fischer rat, F344, will not be the most appropriate choice of strain when testing a chemical suspected to cause tumors in the testes because this strain is known to have a rather high spontaneous incidence of interstitial (Leydig cell) tumors that could mask a possible effect of the test chemical.

Both rats and mice are commonly used in risk assessment for humans. There is an ongoing discussion in the scientific community about whether the use of both rodent species is necessary. It has been stated, based on a survey of databases covering studies with pharmaceuticals, that, in general, the rat is more sensitive than the mouse. Use of the male rat and the female mouse has been suggested as an alternative to a standard two-species, two-sex bioassay. Carcinogenic risk assessment on the basis of a life-span study in a single rodent species in combination with short-term genotoxicity and mechanistic information tests, including short- or medium-term *in vivo* rodent tests, such as the model of initiation–promotion or the carcinogenesis model using neonatal or transgenic mice, has also been suggested. Until there is international consensus on newer approaches for carcinogenic risk assessment, both sexes of rats and mice are normally used for testing chemicals such as food additives and pesticides, unless specific considerations suggest otherwise.

All routes of exposure can be applied. The chemicals are normally administered orally and to some extent by dermal application or via inhalation for a period of not less than 24 months for rats, or 18 months for mice and hamsters. Groups employed in the test include a minimum of 50 animals of each sex, with one control group and three test groups of rodents that are no more than 6 weeks of age at the start of the dosing period. The required minimal survival rate of the test animals to ensure sufficient time for development of tumors is 50% at 24 months and 18 months, respectively, for rats and for mice and hamsters. Animals that die during the study shall shortly thereafter be subjected to necropsy to fulfill the requirement that not more than 10% of the animals are unsuitable for histopathological analysis because of autolysis, which will occur quite quickly at room temperature and consequently further necessitate that the animals in the study be observed frequently.

The highest dose level should be sufficiently high to elicit signs of minimal toxicity without substantially altering the normal life span because of effects other than tumors. The highest dose level is often referred to the *maximum tolerated dose,* or MTD. The criteria for setting that dose have been heavily discussed among toxicologists. In the OECD guideline for carcinogenicity studies, the criteria used are those signs of toxicity that may be indicated by alterations in certain serum enzyme levels seen in previous studies or by slight depression of body weight gain (<10%).

For diet mixture, the highest concentration should not exceed 5%, with the exception of nutrients, to avoid interference with the dietary requirement.

The lowest dose should in general not be lower than 10% of the high dose and should not interfere with normal growth, development, and longevity of the animals or otherwise cause any indication of toxicity. The intermediate doses should be established mid-range between the high and low doses.

The carcinogenicity studies include biological parameters such as clinical appearance, body weight and body weight gain, food consumption, clinically detectable tumors, and hematology. The main focus is on the pathological examinations that include necropsy and on histopathology of tissues and organs. Tumors found in the different tissues or organs will be classified, for example, as benign or malignant. The number of tumor-bearing animals can be subdivided according to specific tumor sites or types, as well as by time to tumor occurrence. The evaluation of a possible carcinogenic effect of the chemical is based on the comparison of these parameters between the dosed and control animals.

Reproductive Toxicity Tests

The reproductive toxicity tests constitute an important part of the toxicological testing program in the health assessment of chemicals. Tests for reproductive toxicity should ideally be able to identify one or more of the following effects on reproduction:

- Impairment of male (and female) reproductive functions or capacity, such as adverse effects on libido, sexual behavior, any aspect of spermatogenesis (or oogenesis), or any hormonal activity or physiological response that would interfere with the capacity to fertilize, the fertilization itself, or the development of the fertilized ovum up to and including implantation.
- Induction of noninheritable harmful effects on the progeny, that is, in the widest sense, any effect interfering with normal development, both before and after birth up to puberty, should be included. Both morphological malformations and functional disturbances (e.g., hormonal, neurological) should be evaluated.

Many different experimental methods for investigating toxic effects of chemicals on reproduction and development are in use. Several tests are standardized, and guidelines have been issued by various governmental agencies and international organizations; others are still undergoing scientific evaluation. The following sections focus mainly on standardized and regulatory accepted methods, some of which are presented in Table 2.1. Tests other than those included in Table 2.1 can reveal effects that indicate a chemical's potential to interfere with normal reproduction, such

Table 2.1 Overview of *In Vivo* Tests for Reproductive Toxicity Testing

Test	Exposure Period	Endpoints in Offspring	Animal Species Normally Used
One-, two-, or multigeneration studies	Continuously over one, two, or several generations	Growth, development, and viability Histopathology of sex organs, brain, and target organs Fertility Proposal: estrus cyclicity and sperm quality	Rat and mouse
Prenatal developmental toxicity study (teratogenicity study)	Usually during organogenesis Proposal: from implantation to the day before birth	Resorptions Fetal growth Morphological variations and malformations	Rat, mouse, and rabbit
Developmental neurotoxicity study (behavioral teratology studies)	During pregnancy and lactation	Birth and pregnancy length Physical and functional maturation Behavioral changes caused by central and peripheral nervous system effects Brain weights and neuropathology	Rat
Reproductive or developmental toxicity screening test	At least three dose levels from 2 weeks before mating until day 4 postnatally	Fertility Pregnancy length and birth Fetal and pup growth and survival until day 3	Rat

as the dominant lethal test, fertility assessment by continuous breeding, and repeated dose toxicity testing, in which the gonads are subjected to pathological examination. More recently, new test guidelines for detecting hormonal disruption have been under validation, such as the Rodent Uterotrophic Screening Assay and the Rodent Hershberger Screening Assay for the screening of chemicals that may interact *in vivo* with the estrogen receptor or with the androgen receptor, respectively.

In recent years, many *in vitro* test systems have been proposed as alternatives to animal testing for developmental toxicity. These tests may be useful for screening closely related chemicals and for elucidating the mechanisms underlying the effects, but they cannot replace animal testing in the risk assessment of chemicals.

One-, Two-, and Multigeneration Studies

Various international organizations and countries have drafted guidelines for carrying out one-, two-, and multigeneration studies; these organizations include the U.S. Environmental Protection Agency (EPA) and the OECD.

The purpose of generation studies is to examine successive generations to identify possible effects of a substance on fertility of male and female animals; pre-, peri-, and postnatal effects on the ovum, fetus, and progeny, including teratogenic and mutagenic effects; and peri- and postnatal effects on the mother.

These guidelines have a number of common requirements. The preferred species are the rat and the mouse. Other species may be used if relevant (e.g., in case of differences in toxicokinetics between the preferred species and humans, to clarify ambiguous results or further study observed effects). The test substances are administered by the relevant route to groups of animals (the number of animals per group must be sufficient to yield about 20 pregnant animals at or near term). The chemical is administered over at least one spermatogenic cycle and during the last stages of oocyte maturation before the parent generation animals are mated. The exposure of the females is continued throughout the mating period and gestation, up to weaning of the last generation. At least three treatment groups and a control group (that is, untreated or treated with vehicle in the highest dose used) should be used. Ideally, unless limited by the physicochemical nature or biological effects of the test substance, the highest dose level should induce toxicity but not mortality in the parental animals. The low dose should ideally not induce any observable adverse effects on the parents or offspring.

The animals are observed daily for clinical changes. Body weight is recorded weekly for the parent animals and for offspring; offspring weight is normally recorded at birth, on days 4, 7, and 14 after birth, at weaning, and every week thereafter. Pregnancy rate, duration of pregnancy, number of pups per litter, number of live and dead pups, number of pups with anomalies, and, if necessary, histological examinations of dead or killed animals. The numbers of live pups on day 4 and at weaning are recorded, and the following indices are often calculated:

- Mating index: copulation/estrus cycles required
- Fecundity index: pregnancies/copulations
- Male fertility index: males impregnating females/males exposed to fertile nonpregnant females
- Female fertility index: females conceiving/females exposed to fertile males
- Incidence of parturition: parturitions/pregnancies
- Live birth index: viable pups born/pups born
- Survival index for 24 h, 4 d, 12 d, and 21 d

The number of litters per female per generation varies in the different guidelines from one to two.

Birth weight and postnatal growth are recorded but it is important in the evaluation of the data to consider variations due to different litter sizes or different sex distribution in the litters. A change in offspring body weight is a sensitive indicator of developmental toxicity, in part because it is a continuous variable. In some cases, weight reduction in offspring may be the only indicator of developmental toxicity in a generation study. Although there is always a question remaining as to whether weight reduction is a permanent or transitory effect, little is known about the long-term consequences of short-term fetal or neonatal weight changes. Therefore, weight reduction should be used to establish the NOAEL.

In the recently adopted test guideline for a two-generation reproductive toxicity study, the assessment of effects on sperm quality and estrus cyclicity in offspring has been included in the guideline. In addition, the assessment of the offspring has been improved compared with the case in the earlier version. For example, the recent guideline includes the recording of developmental milestones, including some behavioral parameters and the histopathology of sex organs, brain, and identified target organs.

The one-generation study, and especially the two- and multigeneration studies, include exposure of both sexes during all stages of reproduction, and in that sense these studies are unique. The two- and multigeneration studies are, together with the Test for Developmental Neurotoxicity, the only toxicological tests for rodents that cover the early period of the development of the individual, from the time of weaning up to about the age of 5 to 6 weeks, at which time exposure in repeated toxicity tests normally starts. Thus, these tests allow the assessment of all endpoints, provided that the parameters used are sufficiently sensitive. However, these tests are labor intensive, and there are many in the field who claim that the guidelines for these tests demand too many parameters, which could interfere with the validity of the data. Others claim that there should be more parameters. Altogether, the guidelines for these reproductive tests still have to undergo some revision, such as introduction of new parameters and refinement or replacement of some of those already in. End-points such as neonatal death and malformations constitute a specific problem because the commonly used laboratory animals may eat dead or seriously malformed pups immediately after birth. An effect may, therefore, only be indicated indirectly, by a smaller litter size. If only a few pups were malformed or dead, the reduction in litter size will be small compared with the normal variation in litter size and may therefore go undetected or not reach statistical significance. Preimplantation losses and resorptions are indicated in an indirect way in the form of a decreased litter size, and the sensitivity for these effects may be rather low.

Fertility assessment by continuous breeding has been used to study the depletion of oocytes from the ovary in mice exposed to procarbazine. In this study, prenatally treated mice were continuously housed with untreated male mice, and the cumulative number of offspring was measured by removing the female when it was noticeably pregnant and then returning the female to the male's cage immediately after delivery to establish a pattern of forced repetitive breeding.

The teratology study is the *in vivo* method for studying embryo–fetal toxicity as a consequence of exposure during pregnancy (e.g., growth retardation, anatomical variations, teratogenicity, and lethality). Various international organizations and countries have drafted guidelines for these tests. These guidelines have a number of common requirements. The preferred species include rodents (e.g., the rat and mouse) and non-rodents (e.g., the rabbit). Other species may be used if relevant (e.g., in case of differences in toxicokinetics between the preferred species and humans, in order to clarify ambiguous results or further study observed effects).

Young mature virgin females are artificially inseminated or mated with males. The time of mating is established by observation of the mating (e.g., in rabbits), by identification of a plug (mixture of sperm and cellular material from the vagina in rats and mice), by analysis of a vaginal smear (in rats), or by noting the time of insemination (e.g., in pigs and rabbits). Normally, three dose levels and a control group (untreated or vehicle control; the group size is 20 pregnant animals for rats and mice and 12 for the rabbit) are used to establish a dose–effect relationship. The pregnant female rats are exposed at least during the period of organogenesis, that is, between day 6, when implantation occurs, and day 15. (The corresponding periods for mice and rabbits are days 6–15 and days 6–18, respectively). This period has been found to be the most sensitive to the induction of structural, anatomical malformations (the corresponding sensitive period for humans is between the 18th and 60th day of pregnancy). Days 6 through 15 are the indicated dosing period for pregnant rats. However, this may vary, depending on the substance administered or on whether the effect on a specific organ is to be studied.

The animals are observed daily for clinical changes. Body weight is recorded, and food consumption is recorded throughout the gestation. The uterus is removed by cesarian section, and the uterus and the fetuses are examined the day before anticipated birth. (The dam is examined macroscopically for any structural abnormalities or pathological changes that may have influenced the pregnancy). If dosing is initiated before or at the time of implantation, the preimplantation loss (i.e., the number of embryos lost before implantation) is evaluated.

The total number of implantations, including living embryos, dead embryos, and resorption (embryos that die early and are reassimilated, corresponding to early abortions in humans) is noted. The degree of resorption (i.e., the extent to which the embryo has been resorbed) is recorded to establish the time of death of the embryo during the pregnancy.

The fetuses are sexed, weighed, and examined for gross malformations. Retarded growth and effects on visceral and skeletal development are evaluated, including the degree of ossification of the bones.

The teratology test was designed to detect malformations. In the past, there was a tendency to consider only malformations, or malformations and death as relevant endpoints in teratology studies. Today it is assumed that all four manifestations of developmental toxicity (death, structural abnormalities, growth alterations, and functional deficits) are of concern. As a consequence, the name of the test in the recently adopted version has been changed to "Prenatal Developmental Toxicity Study," and the exposure period has been extended to the day before birth.

The sensitivity of the test for detection of rare events such as malformations is limited because of the relatively small number of animals used. With the normal group sizes of 20 pregnant rats, it is not possible to identify any increase in major malformations unless high dose levels are administered or the substance studied is highly toxic to the embryo or fetus.[42] To assess the developmental toxicity of a chemical, it is therefore important to include information on other developmental effects such as minor anomalies, variations, and fetal death and growth. In addition, malformations of organs developing after the period of major organogenesis, such as the sex organs and the brain, may at present not be detected in the teratology study. An example is the suspected endocrine disrupter dibutylphthalate, for which exposure during the period of male sexual differentiation resulted in major disturbances in the morphological and functional development of the male reproductive system.[43] Consequently, in the updated OECD Guideline, the dosing period has been extended to cover at least the period from implantation to 1 d before the day of scheduled kill, which is 1 d before the expected day of delivery. In the paragraph of the Guideline titled "Principle of the Test," it is stated that, if appropriate, the dosing period should cover the entire period of gestation to the day of scheduled kill, to include the examination of effects from the preimplantation period.

Teratology studies are very suitable for the demonstration of intrauterine death after implantation (resorptions). In studies in which dosing starts before implantation, preimplantation loss may also be assessed.

Fetal weight can be assessed rather exactly in a teratology study, but it is important to include variations due to different litter sizes or sex distribution in control vs. exposed groups in the analysis.

Developmental Neurotoxicity Studies

Prenatal exposure to chemicals may lead to a range of functional disturbances in the offspring. A number of chemicals are known to produce developmentally neurotoxic effects in humans and other species. For example, lead and methylmercury affect brain development, but effects on fertility, the immune system, metabolism of foreign substances, and development as a whole have also been observed.

A guideline for developmental neurotoxicity studies was issued by the U.S. EPA in 1991, and a revised U.S. guideline was proposed in 1995.[44] During recent years, a proposal for OECD TG 426 Developmental Neurotoxicity Study has been developed based on the U.S. guideline.[45]

Developmental neurotoxicity studies are designed to develop data on the potential functional and morphological hazards to the nervous system arising in the offspring from exposure of the mother during pregnancy and lactation. These studies identify changes in behavior caused by effects on the central nervous system and the peripheral nervous system. As behavior is affected by the function of other organs such as the liver, kidneys, and endocrine system, toxic effects on these organs in offspring may also be reflected in general changes in behavior. No single test is able to reflect the entire complex and intricate function of behavior. For testing behavior, therefore, a range of parameters, a *test battery*, is used to identify changes in individual functions.

The most-used animal species are the rat and the mouse. The early guidelines generally recommend groups of 20 animals, with dosing from day 15 of gestation to day 21 after gestation; that is, spanning fetogenesis and the entire lactation period. However, the recommended dosing period does not cover all events because the central nervous system is also susceptible to abnormal development during the period of organogenesis. Consequently, dosing is often started earlier, for example on day 1 or day 6 of the pregnancy. In the "Proposal for a New OECD Guideline 426," the dosing period includes the entire gestation and lactation period. After birth, the number of progeny is recorded, and the litters are adjusted so that each contains the same number of pups. To determine whether the chemical substance tested affects the offspring directly (via the mother's milk) or indirectly (either via a change in milk production or as a result of a change in the behavior of the exposed mothers), *cross-fostering* may be employed. Cross-fostering is a method in which litters from exposed mothers are reared by control mothers and vice versa.

Studies that intend to identify abnormal development are conducted on individual animals over short or long periods. In the rat, studies last until weaning, although this period does not cover the entire period of brain development because the brain does not attain an approximate adult stage until the age of 6 weeks, corresponding to 12 to 15 years of age in humans.

The evaluation of offspring consists of observations to detect gross neurological and behavioral abnormalities; assess physical development, reflex ontogeny, motor activity, motor and sensory function, and learning and memory; and evaluate brain weights and neuropathology during postnatal development and adulthood.

The methodology employed in behavioral teratology is described in several reviews. Behavioral teratology tests may generally be grouped into tests of physical development, simple reflexes, motor function, development of the senses, spontaneous activity, learning and memory, and functions of the neurotransmitter systems.

The "Proposal for a New OECD Guideline 426" is designed to be performed as a separate study. However, the observations and measurements can also be incorporated into, for example, a two-generation study.

The limitations mentioned in the section on generation studies concerning endpoints such as neonatal death, malformations, preimplantation loss, and resorptions also apply to developmental neurotoxicity studies.

The behavioral functions assessed cover many important aspects of the nervous system; however, some functions of relevance (e.g., endocrine disruption such as social interaction and mating behavior) are not included in the guidelines at present.

Other potentially relevant postnatal endpoints, such as kidney function, liver function, and immunotoxicity, are not included in these guidelines.

Screening Tests for Reproductive and Developmental Toxicity

Because the capacity for toxicity testing cannot keep up with the number of chemicals in modern society, there is an increasing demand for new toxicological tests of shorter duration, using fewer resources. Especially for "old" chemicals, for which the patent rights no longer exist, or for chemicals introduced into the market years ago, when no or only few toxicity data were required, it is essential to develop tools for obtaining data for safety assessment. In recent years, such new screening tests for reproductive and developmental toxicity have been developed. By definition, a screening test is limited in scope compared with a conventional test. Data from a screening test indicating possible toxic potential of a substance identify the substance as one of high priority for further evaluation.

Recently, the OECD introduced guidelines for screening tests for reproductive toxic effects, that is, the Reproduction/Developmental Toxicity Screening Tests, as part of the Screening Information Data Sets for high-production-volume chemicals: (1) the Reproduction/Developmental Toxicity Screening Test for initial information on the possible effect of a chemical on reproduction or development, and (2) the Combined Repeated Dose Toxicity Study with the Reproduction/Developmental Toxicity Screening Test, which is a combination of a 28-d toxicity study and Reproduction/Developmental Toxicity Screening Test (OECD TG 421 and OECD TG 422, respectively). Both test guidelines are designed for use with rats.

The general purpose of these tests is to generate preliminary information concerning the effects of a test substance on male and female reproductive performance such as gonadal function, mating behavior, conception, development of conceptus, and parturition. They are not suggested as alternatives to or replacements for the existing test guidelines for generation and teratology studies.

The dosing of the animals is initiated at least 2 weeks before mating and continued until the end of the study on postnatal day 4. The number of animals per group recommended is at least 10 of each sex, and this is expected to provide at least eight pregnant females per group. Effects on fertility and birth are registered. Live pups are counted and sexed, and litters are weighed on days 1 and 4 postpartum. The parameters include, among others, a detailed histological examination of the ovaries, testes, and epididymides of at least the highest-dosed and the control animals.

The test does not provide complete information on all aspects of reproduction and development. In particular, it offers only limited means of detecting postnatal manifestations of prenatal exposure or effect induced during postnatal exposure.

The value of a negative study is more limited than that of data from generation and teratology studies because of the lower number of animals per group, the shorter period of exposure, as well as the limited number of endpoints measured.

Another screening test, the *in vivo* Teratology Screening Test, has been proposed in which pregnant mice or rats are exposed to a test substance from day 8 to day 12 of pregnancy and the progeny are examined after birth.[46] This test was introduced as an alternative method to the above-mentioned teratogenicity tests. The hypothesis underlying this test is that most prenatal effects do not just produce specific defects but also are manifested in the postnatal period as a lack of viability and reduced growth.

In the *in vivo* Teratology Screening Test, pregnant mice (rats can also be used) are exposed to a test substance from day 8 to day 12 of the pregnancy. One dose level is employed (the minimum toxic dose for the mother animal), together with a control group. The mother animals are weighed during the period of exposure. After birth, the litter is weighed on days 1 and 3. Stillborn young and young that die after birth are dissected and examined for defects. The test focuses on malformations as the endpoints of concern. Results from a validation study have shown that effects on offspring viability or body weight indicate a potential for teratogenic effects, that is, malformations. A test guideline for this test has not been established.

Neurotoxicity Study

Neurotoxicity studies are very complex in design because the nervous system constitutes the essential basis for several functions in the organism, and chemicals can affect the nervous system in many different ways. Consequently, as no single test can encompass all aspects of neurotoxicity, many individual tests exist, each developed to test for different specific functional deficits. Toxic effects on the nervous system will most often result in behavioral changes that can be detected with behavioral tests in laboratory animals. However, such changes in behavior could also be a consequence of systemic toxicity. Thus, it is crucial that evaluations of studies on neurotoxicity take into consideration the results of other toxicity studies. Furthermore, histopathological and hematological examinations as well as the analysis of biochemistry will add to one's ability to differentiate whether the observed neurotoxicity is caused by a primary, direct effect on the nervous system or is a consequence of an indirect, secondary effect on the nervous system. Within the OECD program on guidelines for testing health effects of chemicals, the Neurotoxicity Study in Rodents has recently been adopted. In addition, as mentioned previously, both the developmental neurotoxicity studies and the repeated dose toxicity studies include parameters on neurotoxicity.

Genetic Toxicology Testing

The objective of genetic toxicology testing is to identify chemicals that induce mutations and conceivably may affect the incidence of heritable disease in humans. A mutation is a change in the information content of the genetic material that is propagated through subsequent generations of cells or individuals. Subsequently, it has been confirmed that many chemicals that produce cancer have mutagenic activity; and consequently, many of the tests are used to investigate chemicals for both mutagenic and possible carcinogenic activity. Genotoxic chemicals are those that exert their adverse effects through interaction with the genetic material of the cells (i.e., deoxyribonucleic acid [DNA]) by altering its structure, function, or both.

Many tests exist, including *in vitro* test systems, using both mammalian cells as well as bacterial and fungal cells. The test systems are subdivided into two major groups according to whether they test for point or gene mutations or chromosomal aberrations (either structural or numerical), either in somatic or germ cells. Within the OECD program on guidelines for testing health effects of chemicals, there exists a third group of tests for DNA effects.

The *in vivo* tests constitute the essential basis for the classification and labeling of chemical substances for genotoxicity. In addition, the *in vivo* tests for genotoxicity are essential in the testing strategy for carcinogenicity because the prevailing number of substances that have an inherent potential to cause mutations *in vivo* also cause cancer in laboratory animals.

Chromosomal aberrations can be studied in bone marrow cells of rodents dosed with the test chemical, either by counting micronuclei in maturing erythrocytes (micronucleus test) or by ana-lyzing chromosomes in metaphase cells from various tissues, that is, bone marrow, gonads, or peripheral lymphocytes.

Chromosomal aberrations can also be studied in the dominant lethal test by measuring changes in offspring from treated males. In the OECD test guideline Rodent Dominant Lethal Test, male animals are exposed to the test substance and mated with untreated virgin females. The various germ cell stages can be tested separately by the use of sequential mating intervals. The induction of dominant lethal effects causing embryonic or fetal death is evaluated. Dominant lethals are generally accepted to be the result of chromosomal aberrations (structural and numerical anomalies), but gene mutations and toxic effects cannot be excluded. The heritable translocation test (i.e., the Mouse Heritable Translocation Assay) is another example of a test for chromosomal aberrations (structural and numerical) in mammalian germ cells as recovered in the first-generation progeny.

Finally, the Mouse Spot Test should be mentioned. This test detects presumed somatic mutations in fetal cells after transplacental absorption of the chemical substance.

Future Trends in the Use of Laboratory Animals in Regulatory Toxicology

The use of laboratory animals in regulatory toxicology constitutes an essential part of the administration of chemical substances in society. Thus, data from these tests are required as a part of the law to identify toxic chemicals; in other words, to obtain information about the hazard as a consequence of exposure and the dose at which the effect occurs. Concerning information on mode of action, the required regulatory toxicity tests in general have some limitations. More information about mechanism of action causing the toxic effect will improve the interpretation of the data and, consequently, the evaluation of the implication of human exposure. Up until now, the testing for toxicity has predominantly focused on identifying an effect and determining a possible NOAEL. However, the recognition of the importance of the information on mode of action in the health assessment of human exposure to chemicals will gradually change the present, rather descriptive toxicological testing methodology toward a test program that includes more test methods on toxicodynamics. This development will imply the need for the development of new, more specific, more sophisticated test methods that use well-defined laboratory animal models. Such development will change the testing strategy and could eventually lead to a reduction in the use of laboratory animals in regulatory toxicology.

REFERENCES

1. Larsen, M.Ø., The Use of the Göttingen Minipig in Diabetes Research. Development and Character-ization of a Novel Non-Rodent Animal Model of Type 2 Diabetes by Means of Beta-Cell Injury and High Fat Feeding, Ph.D. thesis, Royal Veterinary and Agricultural University, Copenhagen, Denmark, 2001.
2. Claassen, V., Neglected factors in pharmacology and neuroscience research. Biopharmaceutics, animal characteristics maintenance, testing conditions, in *Techniques in the Behavioral and Neural Sciences*, Huston, J.P., Ed., Elsevier, Amsterdam, 1994, p. 486.

3. Svendsen, O. and Hansen, A.K., Biological variation, reproducibility and predictability of *in vivo* drug testing, *Scand. J. Lab. Anim. Sci.,* 25, 86, 1998.

4. Zak, O. and Sande, M.A., Eds., *Handbook of Animal Models of Infection. Experimental Models in Antimicrobial Chemotherapy,* Academic Press, London, 1999, p. 1136.

5. Frimodt-Møller, N., Knudsen, J.D., and Espersen, F., The mouse peritonitis/sepsis model, in *Handbook of Animal Models of Infection. Experimental Models in Antimicrobial Chemotherapy,* Academic Press, London, 1999, p. 127.

6. Alder, J.D., Hamster model of syphilis, in *Handbook of Animal Models of Infection. Experimental Models in Antimicrobial Chemotherapy,* Academic Press, London, 1999, p. 285.

7. Orme, I.M., Murine models of tuberculosis, in *Handbook of Animal Models of Infection. Experimental Models in Antimicrobial Chemotherapy,* Academic Press, London, 1999, p. 315.

8. Kernacki, K.A., Hobden, J.A., and Hazlett, L.D., Murine model of bacterial keratitis, in *Handbook of Animal Models of Infection. Experimental Models in Antimicrobial Chemotherapy,* Academic Press, London, 1999, p. 361.

9. Hopkins, W.J., Mouse model of ascending urinary tract infection, in *Handbook of Animal Models of Infection. Experimental Models in Antimicrobial Chemotherapy,* Academic Press, London, 1999, p. 435.

10. Matsumoto, T., Rat bladder infection model, in *Handbook of Animal Models of Infection. Experimental Models in Antimicrobial Chemotherapy,* Academic Press, London, 1999, p. 447.

11. Findon, G., Subclinical pyelonephritis in the rat, in *Handbook of Animal Models of Infection. Experimental Models in Antimicrobial Chemotherapy,* Academic Press, London, 1999, p. 463.

12. Bremell, T., Experimental models of infectious arthritis, in *Handbook of Animal Models of Infection. Experimental Models in Antimicrobial Chemotherapy,* Academic Press, London, 1999, p. 539.

13. Lefort, A. and Fantin, B., Rabbit models of bacterial endocarditis, in *Handbook of Animal Models of Infection. Experimental Models in Antimicrobial Chemotherapy,* Academic Press, London, 1999, p. 611.

14. Croft, S.L. and Yardley, V., Animal models of visceral Leishmaniasis, in *Handbook of Animal Models of Infection. Experimental Models in Antimicrobial Chemotherapy,* Academic Press, London, 1999, p. 783.

15. Romig, T. and Bilger, B., Animal models of Echinococcosis, in *Handbook of Animal Models of Infection. Experimental Models in Antimicrobial Chemotherapy,* Academic Press, London, 1999, p. 873.

16. Ellenbroek, B.A. and Cools, A.R., Animal models for schizophrenia: an introduction, in *Atypical Antipsychotics,* Ellenbroek, B.A. and Cools, A.R., Eds., Birkenhäuser Verlag, Basel, Switzerland, 2000, p. 35.

17. Arnt, J., Screening models for antipsychotic drugs, in *Atypical Antipsychotics,* Ellenbroek, B.A. and Cools, A.R., Eds., Birkenhäuser Verlag, Basel, Switzerland, 2000, p. 99.

18. Ellenbroek, B.A., Sams-Dodd, F., and Cools, A.R., Simulation models for schizophrenia, in *Atypical Antipsychotics,* Ellenbroek, B.A. and Cools, A.R., Eds., Birkenhäuser Verlag, Basel, Switzerland, 2000, p. 121.

19. Tamura, A., Kawai, K., and Takagi, K., Animal models used in cerebral ischemia and stroke research, in *Clinical Pharmacology of Cerebral Ischemia,* Horst, G.J.T and Korf, J., Eds., Humana Press, Totowa, NJ, 1999, p. 265.

20. Tolwani, R.J., Jakowec, M.W., Petzinger, G.M., Green, S., and Waggie, J., Experimental models in Parkinson's disease: insight from many models, *Lab. Anim. Sci.,* 49, 363, 1991.

21. McNeill, J.H., Ed., *Experimental Models of Diabetes,* CRC Press, Boca Raton, FL, 1999.

22. Rodrigues, B., Poucheret, P., Battell, M.L., and McNeill, J.H., Streptozotocin-induced diabetes: induction, mechanism(s), and dose dependency, in *Experimental Models of Diabetes,* McNeill, J.H., Ed., CRC Press, Boca Raton, FL, 1999, p. 3.

23. Donaldson, L.F., Seckl, J.R., and McQueen, D.S., A discrete adjuvant-induced monoarthritis in the rat — effects of adjuvant dose, *J. Neurosci. Methods,* 49, 5, 1993.

24. Mapp, P.I., Walsh, D.A., Garret, N.E., Kidd, B.L., Cruwys, S.C., Polak, J.M., and Blake, D.R, Effect of three animal models of inflammation on nerve fibres in the synovium, *Ann. Rheum. Dis.,* 53, 240, 1994.

25. Schaible, H.-G. and Grubb, B.D., Afferent and spinal mechanisms of joint pain, *Pain,* 55, 5, 1993.

26. McQueen, D.S., Inflammatory pain and the joint, in *Pain and Neurogenic Inflammation,* Brain, S.D. and Moore, P.K., Eds., Birkhäuser Verlag, Berlin, 1999, p. 137.

27. Billingham, M.E.J., Adjuvant arthritis: the first model, in *Mechanisms and Models in Rheumatoid Arthritis,* Henderson, B., Edwards, J.C.W., and Pettipher, E.R., Eds., Academic Press, New York, 1995, p. 389.

28. Tjølsen, A. and Hole, K., Animal models of analgesia, in *The Pharmacology of Pain,* Dickenson, A. and Besson, J.-M., Eds., Springer-Verlag, Berlin, 1997, p. 1.

29. Rønn, A., Nørgaard, K.M., Lykkegaard, K., and Svendsen, O., Effects of pre- or postoperative morphine and of preoperative ketamine in experimental surgery in rats, evaluated by pain scoring and c-fos expression, *Scand. J. Lab. Anim. Sci.,* 27, 223, 2000.

30. Svendsen, O. and Lykkegaard, K., Neuronal c-fos immunoreactivity as a quantitative measure of stress and pain, *Acta Agric. Scand., Sect. A, Animal Sci.,* (Suppl. 30), 131, 2001.

31. Brennan, T.J., Vandermeulen, E.P., and Gebhart, G.F., Characterization of a rat model of incisional pain, *Pain,* 64, 493, 1996.

32. Brennan, T.J., Postoperative models of nociception, *ILAR J.,* 40, 129–136, 1999.

33. Lascelles, B.D.X., Waterman, A.E., Cripps, P.J., Livingston, A., and Henderson, G., Central sensitization as a result of surgical pain: investigation of the pre-emptive value of pethidine for ovariohysterectomy in the rat, *Pain,* 62, 201, 1995.

34. Slingsby, L.S. and Waterman-Pearson, A.E., The post-operative analgesic effects of ketamine after canine ovariohysterectomy — a comparison between pre- and post-operative administration, *Res. Vet. Sci.,* 69, 147, 2000.

35. Agersø, H., Pharmacokinetics and Tissue Penetration of Amoxycillin in *Actinobacillus pleuropneumoniae* and *Salmonella typhimurium* Infected Pigs, Ph.D. thesis, Royal Veterinary and Agricultural University, Copenhagen, Denmark, 1996.

36. Lauritsen, B., Biochemical Markers as Indicators of the Efficacy of Antibacterial Treatment of *Actinobacillus pleuropneumoniae* Infection in Pigs, Ph.D. thesis, Royal Veterinary and Agricultural University, Copenhagen, Denmark, 2001.

37. Lindecrona, R.H., The Pharmacodynamic Effect of Amoxicillin and Danofloxacin Against *Actinobacillus pleuropneumoniae* and *Salmonella Typhimurium* in an *In Vitro* Pharmacodynamic Model, Ph.D. thesis, Royal Veterinary and Agricultural University, Copenhagen, Denmark, 1998.

38. Petersen, M.B., Pharmacodynamic and Pharmacokinetic Parameters of Benzimidalzoles in the Pig Using Oesophagostomum Dentatum as Model Parasite, Ph.D. thesis, Royal Veterinary and Agricultural University, Copenhagen, Denmark, 1998.

39. U.S. Environmental Protection Agency, Principles of neurotoxicity risk assessment (final report), *Fed. Reg.,* 59, 42360, 1994.

40. Brown, N.A. and Fabro, S., The value of animal teratogenicity testing for predicting human risk, *Clin. Obstet. Gynaecol.,* 26, 467, 1983.

41. Draize, J.H., Woodward, G., and Calvery, H.O., Methods for the study of irritation and toxicity of substances applied topically to the skin and mucous membranes, *J. Pharmacol. Exp. Ther.,* 82, 377, 1944.

42. Palmer, A.K., Regulatory requirements for reproductive toxicity: theory and practice, in *Developmental Toxicology,* Kimmel, C.A. and Buelke-Sam, J., Eds., Raven Press, New York, 1981, p. 259.

43. Mylchrest, E., Sar, M., Catley, R.C., and Foster, P.M.D., Disruption of androgen-related reproductive development by di(*n*-butyl)phthalate during late gestation in rats is different from flutamide, *Toxicol. Appl. Pharmacol.,* 156, 81, 1999.

44. U.S. Environmental Protection Agency, Proposed guideline for neurotoxicity risk assessment (final report), *Fed. Reg.,* 60, 52032, 1995.

45. Organisation for Economic Co-Operation and Development [OECD], OECD Test Guidelines for the Testing of Chemicals. Proposal for New Test Guideline 426: Developmental Neurotoxicity Study. Environmental Health and Safety Division, draft document, Paris, October 1999.

46. Chernoff, N. and Kavlock, R.J., An *in vivo* teratology screen utilizing pregnant mice, *J. Toxicol. Environ. Health.,* 10, 541, 1982.

RECOMMENDED READING

Allaban, W.T., Turturro, A., Leakey, J.F.A., Seng, J.E., and Hart, R.W., FDA points-to-consider documents: the need for dietary control for the reduction of experimental variability within animal assays and the use of dietary restriction to achieve dietary control, *Toxicol. Pathol.,* 24, 776, 1996.

Ashby, J., Alternatives to the 2-species bioassay for the identification of potential human carcinogens, *Hum. Exp. Toxicity,* 15, 183, 1996.

Barclay, R.J., Herbert, W.J., and Poole, T.B., The Disturbance Index: A Behavioural Method of Assessing the Severity of Common Laboratory Procedures on Rodents, UFAW Welfare Research Report 2, Universities Federation for Animal Welfare, Hertfordshire, United Kingdom, 1988.

Calabrese, E.J., Ed., *Principles of Animal Extrapolation,* John Wiley & Sons, New York, 1983.

Carere, A., Mohn, G.R., Parry, J.M., Sors, A.I., and Nolan, C.V., Methods and Testing Strategies for Evaluating the Genotoxic Properties of Chemicals, European Commission, Report EUR 15945, ECSC-EC-EAEC, Brussels, 1995.

CEC, Council Directive 86/609/EEC of 24 November 1986 on the approximation of laws, regulations and administrative provisions of the Member States regarding the protection of animals used for experimental and scientific purposes, *Off. J. Eur. Comm.,* 29, 1, 1986.

Claudio, L., Kwa, W.C., Russell, A., and Wallinga, D., Contemporary issues in toxicology: testing methods for developmental neurotoxicity of environmental chemicals, *Toxicol. Appl. Pharmacol.,* 164, 1, 2000.

Close, B., Banister, K., Baumans, V., Bernoth, E.-M., Bromage, N., Bunyan, J., Erhardt, W., Flecknell, P., Gregory, N., Hackbarth, H., Morton, D., and Warwick, C., Recommendations for euthanasia of experimental animals. Part 1, *Lab. Anim.,* 30, 293, 1996.

Close, B., Banister, K., Baumans, V., Bernoth, E.-M., Bromage, N., Bunyan, J., Erhardt, W., Flecknell, P., Gregory, N., Hackbarth, H., Morton, D., and Warwick, C., Recommendations for euthanasia of experimental animals. Part 2, *Lab. Anim.,* 31, 1, 1997.

Cook, J.C., Klinefelter, G.R., Hardisty, J.F., Sharpe, R.M., and Foster, P.M.D., Rodent Leydig cell tumoriginesis: a review of the physiology, pathology, mechanisms, and relevance to humans, *Crit. Rev. Toxicol.,* 29, 169, 1999.

CPMP/465/95, Note for Guidance on Preclinical Pharmacological and Toxicological Testing of Vaccines, 1997.

CPMP/SWP/1042/99, Note for Guidance on Repeat Dose Toxicity, 1999.

CPMP/SWP/112/98, Safety Studies for Gene Therapy Products, draft, 1998.

Directive 75/318/EEC, The Rules Governing Medicinal Products in the European Union, Vol. 3B, 1998.

FDA, U.S. Food and Drug Administration, FDA Toxicological Principles for the Safety Assessment of Direct Food Additives and Color Additives Used in Food, Redbook I, 1982.

Festing, M.F.W., Genetic factors in neurotoxicology and neuropharmacology: a critical evaluation of the use of genetics as a research tool, *Experientia,* 47, 990, 1991.

Festing, M.F.W., The scope for improving the design of laboratory animal experiments, *Lab. Anim.,* 26, 256, 1992.

Festing, M.F.W., Genetic variation in outbred rats and mice and its implications for toxicological screening, *J. Exp. Anim. Sci.,* 35, 210, 1993.

Gad, S.C., Dunn, B.J., Dobbs, D.W., Reilly, C., and Walsh, R.D., Development and validation of an alternative dermal sensitisation test: the mouse ear swelling test (MEST), *Toxicol. Appl. Pharmacol.,* 84, 93, 1986.

Gulezian, D., Jacobson-Kram, D., McCullough, C.B., Olson, H., Recio, L., Robinson, D., Storer, R., Tennant, R., Ward, J.M., and Neuman, D., Use of transgenic animals for carcinogenicity testing: considerations and implications for risk assessment (review article), *Toxicol. Pharmacol.,* 28, 482, 2000.

Hansen, E. and Meyer, O., Animal model in reproductive toxicity, in *Handbook of Laboratory Animal Science, Vol. II, Animal Models,* Svendsen, P., and Hau, J., Eds., CRC Press, Boca Raton, FL, 1994, p. 17.

Hansen, A.K., Sandøe, P., Svendsen, O., Forsman, B., and Thomsen, P., The need to refine the notion on reduction, in *Humane Endpoints in Animal Experiments for Biomedical Research. Proceedings of the International Conference, 22–25 November 1998, Zeist, The Netherlands,* Hendriksen, C.F.M. and Morton, D.B., Eds., The Royal Society of Medicine Press, 1999, p.139.

Hass, U., Hansen, E.V., and Østergaard, G., Experimental studies in laboratory animals, in Has, U., Brandorff, N.P., Brunborg, G., Ekström, T, Hansen, E.V., Jacobsen, B.M., Jelnes, J.E., Meyer, O., Taskinen, H., and Wiger, R., Eds., *Occupational Reproductive Toxicity — Methods and Testing Strategy for Hazard Assessment of Workplace Chemicals,* Nordic Council of Ministers and National Institute of Occupational Health, Denmark, 1994, p. 21.

Hooks, W. and Harling, R.J., The choice of rat strain for tumorigenicity studies, *Dev. Life Sci.,* 3, 9, 2001.

Hubert, M.-F., Laroque, P., Gillet, J.-P., and Keenan, K., The effect of diet, ad libitum feeding, and moderate and severe dietary restriction on body weight, survival, clinical pathology parameters, and cause of death in control Sprague-Dawley rats, *Toxicol. Sci.,* 58, 195, 2000.

ICH, Harmonized Tripartite Guidelines: S5A: Detection of Toxicity to Reproduction for Medicinal Products; S5B: Reproductive Toxicology: Male Fertility Studies.

ICH, Note for Guidance on Carcinogenicity: Testing for Carcinogenicity of Pharmaceuticals (CPMP/ICH/299/95), ICH Topic S1B, Step 4, Concensus Guideline, European Agency for the Evaluation of Medicinal Products, London, 1997.

Infante, P.F., Use of rodent carcinogenicity test results for determining potential cancer risk to humans, *Environ. Health Perspect.,* 101(Suppl. 5), 143, 1993.

Jacobsen, B.M. and Meyer, O., Extrapolation from *in vivo/in vitro* experiments to human beings, in *Embryo-Foetal Damage and Chemical Substances*, Working Party Report, Ministry of Health, The National Food Agency of Denmark, 98–107, 1989.

Lijinsky, W., Importance of animal experiments in carcinogenesis research, *Environ. Mol. Mutagenesis,* 11, 307, 1988.

Mepham, T.B., Combes, R.D., Balls, M., Barbieri, O., Blokhuis, H.J., Costa, P., Crilly, R.E., de Cock Buning, T., Delpire, C., O'Hare, M.J., Houdebine, L.-M., Van Kreijl, C.F., Van Der Meer, M., Reinhardt, C.A., Wolf, E., and Van Zeller, A.-M., The use of transgenic animals in the European Union. The report and recommendations of ECVAM Workshop 28, *ATLA* 26, 21–43, 1998.

Meyer, O., Implications of animal welfare on toxicity testing, *Hum. Exp. Toxicol.,* 12, 516, 1993.

Meyer, O., Jacobsen, B.M., and Hansen, E.V., Identification of embryo-foetal toxicity by means of animal studies, in Andreasen, P.B., Brandt, N.J., Cohr, K.-H., Hansen, E.V., Hass, U., Jacobsen, B.M., Knudswen, I., Lauritsen, J.G., Melchior, J.C., Meldgaard, L, Meyer, O., Olsen, J.H., Palludan, B., and Poulsen, E., Eds., *Embryo-Foetal Damage and Chemical Substances.* Working Party Report, National Food Agency, Ministry of Health, Publication 181, 77–91, 1989, Søborg, Denmark.

National Research Council, *Nutrient Requirement of Laboratory Animals,* 4th revised ed., National Academy Press, Washington, D.C., 1995.

Newberne, P.M. and Sotnikov, A., Diet: the neglected variable in chemical safety evaluations, *Toxicol. Pathol.,* 24, 746, 1996.

Novacek, M.J., Where do rabbits and kin fit in?, *Nature,* 3, 379, 299, 1996.

Organisation for Economic Co-Operation and Development [OECD], Guidance Document for the Development of OECD Guidelines for Testing of Chemicals. OECD Series on the Test Guideline Programme no. 1, Environment Monograph 76, Paris, 1995.

Organisation for Economic Co-Operation and Development [OECD], OECD Test Guidelines for the Testing of Chemicals. Draft Proposal for a New Guideline: *In Vitro* Skin Corrosion Tests. Environmental Health and Safety Division, draft, Paris, November 1999.

Organisation for Economic Co-Operation and Development [OECD], Guidance Document on the Recognition, Assessment, and Use of Clinical Signs as Humane Endpoints for Experimental Animals Used in Safety Evaluation. OECD Environmental Health and Safety Publications, Series on Testing and Assessment no. 19, Paris, 2000.

Organisation for Economic Co-Operation and Development [OECD], Revised Draft Guidance Document for Neurotoxicity Testing. OECD Environmental Health and Safety Publications, Series on Testing and Assessment no. 20, Paris, 2000.

Organisation for Economic Co-Operation and Development [OECD], OECD Test Guidelines for the Testing of Chemicals, OECD, Paris, 2001, section 4.

Organisation for Economic Co-Operation and Development [OECD], Introduction to the OECD Guidelines on Genetic Toxicology Testing and Guidance on the Selection and Application of Assays, in OECD Test Guidelines for the Testing of Chemicals, Paris, 2001, section 4.

Organisation for Economic Co-Operation and Development [OECD], OECD protocol and guidance for the conduct of the Rodent Hershberger Assay. Phase One Status Report. Environment Directorate. Task Force on Endocrine Disrupters Testing and Assessment (EDTA) of the Test Guidelines Programme: ENV/JM/TG/EDTA (2001) 3, 2001.

Organisation for Economic Co-Operation and Development [OECD], Proposal for the development of a test guideline for the rodent uterotrophic assay. Environment Directorate. Task Force on Endocrine Disrupters Testing and Assessment (EDTA) of the Test Guidelines Programme: ENV/JM/TG/EDTA (2001) 5, 27, Apr. 2001.

Organisation for Economic Co-Operation and Development [OECD], OECD Test Guidelines for the Testing of Chemicals. Revised proposal for new test guideline 429: Skin Sensitisation: Local Lymph Node Assay. Environmental Health and Safety Division, ENV/JM/TG(2001)4, 02-May-2001.

Organisation for Economic Co-Operation and Development [OECD], Guidance document on acute oral toxicity testing. Environment Directorate, OECD Environment, Health and Safety Publications, Series on Testing and Assessment no. 24, Paris, June 2001.

O'Grady, J. and Dárcy, P.F., Eds., *The Textbook of Pharmaceutical Medicine,* 3rd ed., The Queens University of Belfast, Belfast, Ireland, 1998.

Recio, L., Transgenic animal models and their application in mechanistically based toxicology research, CIIT Activities, Chemical Industry Institute of Toxicology, 15, 1, 1995.

Reeves, P.G., Nielsen, F.H., and Fahrey, G.C., Jr., AIN-93 purified diets for laboratory rodents: final report of the American Institute of Nutrition ad hoc writing committee on reformulation of AIN-76 rodent diet, *J. Nutr.,* 123, 1939, 1993.

Riley, E.P. and Vorhees, C., *Handbook of Behavioral Teratology,* Plenum Press, New York, 1986.

Schardein, J.L., Principles of teratogenesis applicable to human exposure to drugs and chemicals, in *Chemically Induced Birth Defects,* Schardein, J.L., Ed., Marcel Dekker, New York, 1, 1985.

Schardein, J.L., Schwetz, B.A., and Kenel, M.F., Species sensitivities and prediction of teratogenic potential, *Environ. Health Perspect.,* 61, 55, 1985.

Spindler, P. et al., First dose in man: toxicological considerations, *Pharmacol. Toxicol.,* 86(Suppl. 1), 8, 2000.

Tilson, H.A., The role of developmental neurotoxicology studies in risk assessment, *Toxicol. Pathol.,* 28, 149, 2000.

Toppari, J., Larsen, J.C., Christiansen, P., Giwercman, A., Grandjean, P., Guillette, L.J., Jégou, B., Jensen, T.K., Jouannet, P., Keiding, N., Leffers, H., McLachan, J.A., Meyer, O., Müller, J., Rajpert-De Meyts, E., Scheike, T., Sharpe, R., Sumpter, J., and Skakkebæk, N.E., Male reproductive health and environmental xenoestrogens, *Environ. Health Perspect.,* 104(Suppl. 4), 1996.

U.S. Environmental Protection Agency (EPA), Guideline § 81–8, 82–7, 83–1, Neurotoxicity Screening Battery, Pesticide Assessment Guidelines, Subdivision F, Hazard Evaluation: Human and Domestic Animals, Addendum 10 Neurotoxicity, EPA 540/09–91–123, March 1991, p. 13. (Available from National Technical Information Service, Service, Springfield, VA 22161. NTIS PB 91–154617.)

U.S. Environmental Protection Agency (EPA), Health Effects Test Guidelines, OPPTS 870.3700, Prenatal Developmental Toxicity Study, Prevention, Pesticides and Toxic Substances (7101), EPA 712-C-98–207, August, 1998.

U.S. Environmental Protection Agency (EPA), Health Effects Test Guidelines, OPPTS 870.3800, Reproduction and Fertility Effects, Prevention, Pesticides, and Toxic Substances (7101), EPA 712-C-98–208, August, 1998.

Van Oosterhout, J.P.J., Van Der Laan, J.W., De Waal, E.J., Olejnizak, K., Hilgenfeld, M., Schmidt, V., and Bass, R., The utility of two rodent species in carcinogenic risk assessment of pharmaceuticals in Europe, *Regul. Toxicol. Pharmacol.,* 25, 6, 1997.

CHAPTER 3

Animal Models in Fetal Growth and Development

Anthony M. Carter

CONTENTS

0-8493-1084-9/03/$0.00+$1.50

INTRODUCTION

Current research on fetal growth and development[1] is focused on two lines of enquiry requiring quite different models. The first of these is the genetic control of growth. Research on this topic has been greatly advanced by gene targeting and transgene expression in the mouse, methods that are described elsewhere in this volume. This chapter focuses on two new tools: conditional gene targeting and expression and microarray technology.

The second focus of research is fetal programming of adult disease. It is now recognized that the developmental alterations associated with fetal growth restriction can have long-term consequences. Low weight at birth has been linked to an increased risk for adult-onset diseases, including hypertension, ischemic heart disease, and non-insulin-dependent diabetes.[2] Much of the current work on the mechanisms underlying this process, termed *fetal programming,* is done in sheep. Indeed, since the pioneering work of Barcroft,[3] Dawes,[4] and others, the chronically instrumented, unstressed sheep fetus has been the model of choice in fetal physiology. Therefore, it will be described in some detail. Rodent models of intrauterine growth restiction are also useful in research on fetal programming, although there is a lack of consensus on the most appropriate models to supplement work in the sheep.

GENE EXPRESSION DURING DEVELOPMENT

With the advent of transgenic and gene-targeting methodologies to determine the biological roles of genes during development,[5] the mouse has become an important experimental model.

Gene Targeting and Transgenic Animals

Conventional gene targeting results in knockout of the gene of interest and the resultant absence of the normal gene product. In brief, the procedures followed are as follows: construction of a gene-targeting vector, containing a mutation in the target gene; introduction of the targeting vector into embryonic stem cells; selection of cell clones that have undergone homologous recombination with the targeting vector; and production of embryonic stem cell–mouse chimeras. Finally, a breeding program is established to yield a transgenic line homozygous for the targeted gene.

The opposite and complementary approach is to cause overexpression of a native gene or expression of a foreign gene. Briefly, this requires construction of a transgene with a promoter and a reporter gene. After microinjection of the construct into an oocyte, the two-cell embryo is transferred to the uterus of a pseudopregnant mouse. A breeding and screening program then yields a transgenic line expressing the transgene under the chosen promoter. In general, the choice of promoters for transgenes has not favored studies of prenatal growth. As an example, expression of a human insulin-like growth factor (IGF) binding protein-1 under the mouse metallothionein promoter first occurs late in gestation.[6] Therefore, models are required in which transgenes are expressed during fetal and placental development.

An intriguing finding from work with knockout and transgenic mice is that many genes are required for development, but only a small number control the rate of growth. Efstratiadis[7] identified 20 growth control genes in mice, half of which were important for fetal growth. These included the genes coding for insulin, IGFs, their receptors, and the receptor substrates. The pathways controlling development of organ systems are presently being mapped. Examples are the genes controlling placental development[8] and left–right patterning of the heart.[9]

Uniparental Disomy

As many as 10% of all genes are subjected to parental imprinting, including several that are critical for fetal development. Thus, for the IGF-II gene (*Igf2*), the phenotype of the offspring is determined by the paternal allele, but the receptor phenotype (*Igf2r*) is determined by the maternal allele.[7] Recently, another set of imprinted genes needed for normal development was found on mouse chromosome 12.[10] The techniques required to investigate imprinted genes include the generation of embryos in which both chromosome sets are inherited from one parent,[11] or of chromosomally balanced conceptuses in which specific chromosomes are derived from the same parent.[12]

Conditional Gene Targeting

Global gene knockout frequently leads to severe abnormalities that cause the embryo to die. This curtails the experiment and precludes further study of the gene. A more useful approach is to block expression of the gene in a single tissue. Tissue-specific gene activation and inactivation is now possible using the Cre recombinase-*lox P* (Cre-*loxP*) system.[13]

Cre recombinase is an enzyme of bacteriophage origin that catalyzes recombination between two of its recognition sites, called *loxP*. Insertion of *loxP* sites into a gene can usually, although not inevitably, be achieved without affecting gene expression. Excision of the region flanked by the *loxP* sites (floxed) will occur only upon expression of Cre recombinase, which can be driven by a tissue-specific promoter. This is called *conditional knockout*.

The simplest strategy is to cross a *loxP* provider and a Cre-expressing transgenic line (Figure 3.1). One set of procedures is needed to make the floxed gene and to establish a transgenic line homozygous for the gene. Another series of procedures establishes a Cre recombinase driven by a promoter expressed in the tissue of interest. For studies of fetal development,[1] promoters might include the α-fetoprotein promoter for fetal liver; the *tie-1* promoter for fetal vessel endothelium; or the *4311* promoter for placental spongiotrophoblast. Here, too, a breeding and screening program is needed to establish a transgenic line expressing Cre recombinase under the chosen promoter. Only then is it possible to do the experiment properly, by crossing the floxed-targeted line with the transgenic line expressing Cre recombinase under the desired promotor. The result should be tissue-specific knockout of the gene in question. Each of these procedures demands considerable time and resources. For some applications, it might be possible to use established Cre transgenic lines (listed at http://www.mshri.on.ca/nagy/Cre-pub.html). An excellent survey of the techniques for producing floxed genes, further applications of the Cre-*loxP* system, and details of the complementary Flp recombinase system are given by Nagy.[13]

Conditional Transgene Expression

A complementary technology allows the reversible overexpression of a transgene. As with the Cre-*loxP* system, it requires the generation of two transgenic strains. In one strain, the transgene of interest is under the control of the *tetO*-CMV promoter. The other strain expresses a hybrid molecule, termed the *tetracycline transcriptional activator*, under a promoter that confers tissue specificity. Crossing the two lines generates some progeny with both transgenes. In these, the gene

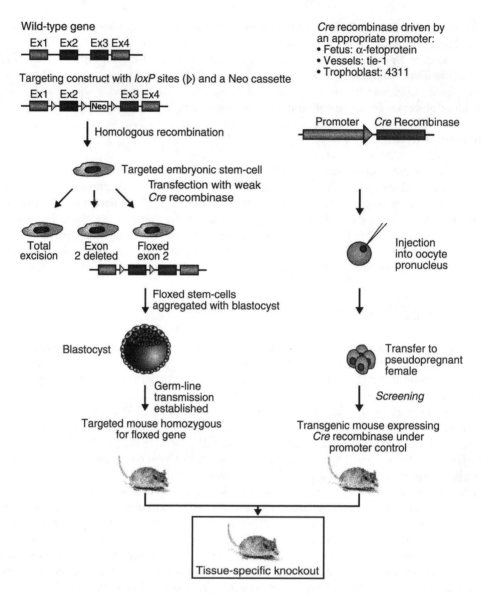

Figure 3.1   Strategy for conditional knockout of a target gene in fetal or placental tissues. Left: An essential exon of the wild-type gene (exon 2) is flanked with *loxP* sites by gene replacement. A neomycin resistance cassette (Neo) equipped with a third *loxP* site is co-introduced. The construct is then inserted into embryonic stem cells by electroporation. Stem cells with homologous recombination are selected and grown. These cells are transfected with a weak *Cre* recombinase, with three possible results: total excision of exon 2 and the Neo cassette; excision of exon 2; and excision of the Neo cassette. The latter cells are aggregated with a blastocyst, which is transferred to the uterus of a pseudopregnant mouse. Finally, a breeding program to establish germ line transmission yields a transgenic line homozygous for the floxed gene. Tissue-specific deletion of exon 2 can then be achieved by crossing with a transgenic line expressing *Cre* recombinase with an appropriate promoter. Right: The *Cre* recombinase gene is linked to a promoter, for example, α-fetoprotein promoter for fetal liver; the *tie-1* promoter for fetal vessel endothelium; or the *4311* promoter for spongiotrophoblast. After microinjection of the construct into an oocyte, the two-cell embryo is transferred to the uterus of a pseudopregnant mouse. A breeding and screening program yields a transgenic line expressing *Cre* recombinase under the chosen promoter. (From Han, V.K.M. and Carter, A.M., *Curr. Opin. Pharmacol.*, 1, 632, 2001. With permission.)

of interest can be turned off and on by administration or withdrawal of tetracycline analogs such as doxycycline.[14]

Microarray Technology

As part of the spin-off from the human genome project, there are now sophisticated tools that allow examination of a large number of genes in a single sample. An example is a study that identified more than 15,000 genes expressed during mouse development.[15] The authors constructed a microarray with cDNA sequences for all 15,000 genes, spotted onto nylon membranes. They then applied the technique to compare differences in expression profiles by the mouse embryo and mouse placenta at embryonic day 12.5. In this way, they were able to identify 289 genes that were more highly expressed in the placenta than in the embryo and 61 genes that were placenta specific. In this one experiment, the number of genes highly expressed in placenta was increased fivefold over those previously known. Potential applications of microarray technology include detecting genes that change expression during embryonic or placental development and identifying downstream target genes in transgenic and targeted mice.

THE SHEEP AS AN EXPERIMENTAL ANIMAL

The sheep is the most widely accepted model in fetal physiology. Much of the pioneering work was done with the ewe anesthetized and the fetus exteriorized.[3,4] However, study of the chronically instrumented sheep fetus is now the norm. It is possible to perform sophisticated experiments in the unstressed fetus, as exemplified by studies of left ventricular function (Figure 3.2).

Breeding

Fetal physiologists are dependent on a steady supply of time-dated pregnant sheep, and most maintain their own flock or make arrangements with a local farm. There are several excellent texts on sheep husbandry[16] and the management of experimental sheep.[17] To ensure a constant supply of pregnant sheep throughout the spring, ewes are introduced to the ram from late September (Northern hemisphere) and for the next 3 to 4 months. A harness containing a colored crayon is strapped to the ram's chest, so that when a ewe is tupped, her fleece is marked. The flock is inspected once a day to note which ewes have been freshly tupped.[4] The estrous cycle is 16 to 17 d in sheep, so most ewes will be tupped during the first 2 weeks after they have been introduced to the ram. Vaginal sponges impregnated with medroxyprogesterone acetate are often used to synchronize estrus. They are kept in for 2 weeks, and mating occurs about 40 h after the sponge has been removed.[17] Some sheep have a second, shorter breeding season that enables work to be resumed in the autumn. To obtain pregnancies out of season, hormone treatment is necessary, possibly in conjunction with artificial alteration of the daylight pattern.[18]

Anesthesia

Animals should be shorn and acclimatized to the laboratory environment for several days before surgery. The ewe must be fasted for 24 h to avoid rumen distention during surgery (bloat), but the animal should not be deprived of water. General anesthesia of the ewe and fetus can be maintained with 1 to 2% halothane in 40% N_2O and 60% O_2 (v/v). A respirator should be coupled to the anesthetic system to assist and control ventilation. To enable insertion of an endotracheal tube, anesthesia can be induced with intravenous sodium thiopental. Some authors favor the use of halothane alone and induce anesthesia with halothane administered by mask.[19] Alternatively, surgery can be performed under epidural anesthesia with 1% (w/v) tetracaine hydrochloride, supplemented

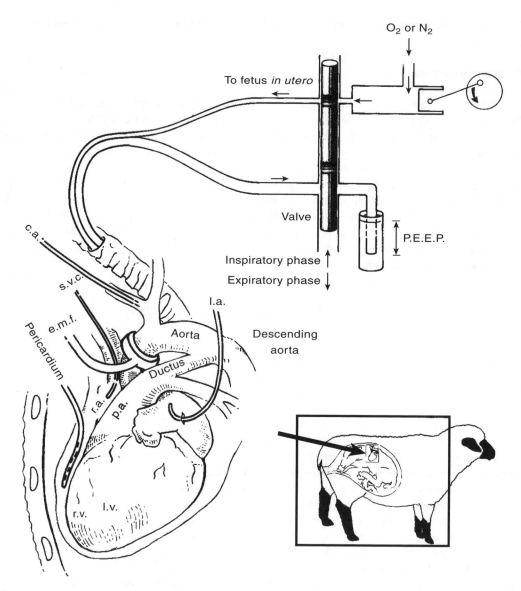

Figure 3.2   Instrumentation of the sheep fetus for studies of left ventricular function. An electromagnetic flow sensor (e.m.f.) was placed on the ascending aorta to measure ventricular output. Catheters were placed in the pericardium, the right atrium (r.a.) via the superior vena cava (s.v.c.), and the left atrium (l.a.). The right ventricle (r.v.), left ventricle (l.v.), and pulmonary artery (p.a.) are indicated. Also shown is a system used to ventilate the fetus *in utero.* (From Morton, M.J., Pinson, C.W., and Thornburg, K.L., *J. Physiol.*, 383, 413, 1987. With permission.)

with intravenous ketamine for sedation and a local anesthetic for fetal skin incisions.[20] Dissociative anesthesia induced and maintained by a continuous intravenous infusion of ketamine is a further possibility.[21]

Surgery

A complete surgical scrub of the animal should be done, and all surgical procedures should be carried out under stringent aseptic conditions.[19] The abdomen is opened by midline incision. A trochar is introduced to make a stab wound through the flank, and catheters and leads are threaded through the trochar sheath. Electrocautery is recommended for incisions in the uterus and fetal skin. The myometrium and endometrium are incised in an area free of cotyledons. The membranes are then cut, and the cut edges are fixed to the uterine wall with Babcock clamps. If the procedure requires delivery of the fetal head or trunk for surgery, an assistant should suspend the uterus by the clamps to minimize loss of amniotic fluid. The Babcock clamps can then be adjusted to attach the uterus and membranes to the fetal skin. Once surgery has been completed, the hysterotomy is closed with a continuous overlay, taking care to pick up the chorionic and amniotic membranes. This is followed by a continuous Lembert suture to appose the serosal tissue and ensure strong healing without adhesion. The abdominal wall is closed with a continuous suture, followed by single sutures to provide additional support. The skin is closed with single sutures or wound clips, and the stab wound with a purse-string suture through the skin. Maternal catheters may be tunneled subcutaneously to exit through this or a separate stab wound.

Postoperative Care

Animals should be housed individually, and we favor using the recovery period to accustom the ewe to the metabolic cage or cart in which the studies will be performed. Four points deserve attention when maintaining the chronically instrumented fetus:[19] (1) the encouragement of proper postoperative feeding and provision of excellent animal care; (2) antibiotic treatment; (3) daily checking and flushing of catheters; and (4) sterile handling of catheters, stopcocks, and flushing solutions.

Postoperative Feeding

To lessen the risk of maternal ketoacidosis, the ewe should be encouraged to stand and eat as soon as possible after surgery. Most animals start to eat before they can stand. A careful record should be kept to ascertain that the ewe continues to eat, drink, urinate, and defecate. Animals that refuse food may be in pain and should be given an analgesic such as flunixin. If feeding is discontinued for more than 24 h, sodium propionate can be given by mouth to counteract the development of ketoacidosis and atonia of the rumen. Failure to defecate may indicate painful postsurgical complications, such as torsion of the small intestine, and immediate euthanasia should be considered in such cases.

Antibiotic Treatment

Antibiotic coverage should be given on the day of surgery and for the next 3 d. We give a combination of streptomycin and penicillin to the ewe as an intramuscular injection and administer an antibiotic to the fetus through the amniotic and venous lines. Many investigators consider it unnecessary to give antibiotics by the intravenous route, as the fetus ingests amniotic fluid and can absorb antibiotics through the gut. If fetuses are lost because of infection, the organisms responsible should be identified to ensure the adequacy of the current antibiotic treatment.

Checking and Handling of Catheters

The exteriorized end of the catheters can be closed with sterile plastic stopcocks and stored in plastic bags or in a cloth pouch stitched to the flank of the ewe. Alternatively, the tip of each catheter can be sealed with a metal pin during storage. Sterile handling of catheters and stopcocks is essential. Catheters should be flushed daily with heparinized saline solution. It is advisable first to withdraw blood from the catheter, thereby removing any clots that it may contain. Blood samples should be taken from maternal and fetal arterial catheters to assess blood gas status and acid–base balance. Values should be corrected to body temperature, normally 39°C for the ewe and 39.5°C for the fetus.

Maternal and fetal blood gases, pH, arterial blood pressure, and heart rate are usually stable within 48 h of surgery.[19] However, other physiological functions take longer to stabilize,[22] and a recovery period of at least 5 d is recommended.

Zoonoses

Animal care personnel should be acquainted with the common symptoms of disease,[17,23] and all personnel should be aware of the risk of zoonotic infection. Several outbreaks of Q fever have been associated with the use of sheep in perinatal research. The birth fluids and placentas of infected sheep contain enormous amounts of *Coxiella burnetii,* and there is massive contamination of the environment at the time of parturition.[24]

Instrumentation

Catheters

The most common catheter materials are polyvinyl and silastic tubing. To avoid kinking, a composite catheter is often used, in which the inner polyvinyl catheter is protected for most of its length by an outer catheter of polyvinyl or polyethylene.[25] Catheters should be color coded to facilitate identification.

Umbilical Blood Vessels

The umbilical vessels send branches across the chorioallantoic sac to supply 40 to 100 discrete cotyledons. To catheterize them, a small incision is made in the uterus, chorion, and amnion and the membranes pulled out until umbilical vessels of about 1 mm diameter are encountered. A fine catheter is inserted into the vessel and advanced into the main umbilical artery or vein.[26] To ensure that the catheter is threaded in the right direction, it is advisable first to search for a sizeable vessel, then to find a tributary and catheterize that.

Lower Body Blood Vessels

The descending aorta and inferior vena cava can be accessed from the corresponding femoral vessels. A useful alternative, requiring less exposure of the fetus, is to insert the catheters through the pedal artery and vein.[27] The vein should be approached from the outside of the foot, where it is quite superficial. The artery lies deeper, close to the bone, and is accompanied by one or two veins. The length of catheter required for the tip to reside in the descending aorta or caudal vena cava equals the length of the foot at all gestational ages.

Upper Body Blood Vessels

Preductal aortic blood can be obtained from a catheter advanced from a radial artery into the brachiocephalic artery or ascending aorta, and a catheter can be advanced from a forelimb vein into the superior vena cava.[28] The carotid artery and jugular vein may be catheterized after exposure of the head and neck. However, they can be accessed through a small uterine incision made directly above the vessels of the fetal neck.[29]

Amniotic Cavity

An amniotic catheter is a useful route for administration of antibiotics. Moreover, registration of amniotic fluid pressure provides an essential reference for fetal arterial blood pressure, especially when measured by an external transducer, because the posture of the ewe is constantly changing. To ensure patency of this catheter, it should be provided with multiple side holes, and the tip should be protected by a length of outer tubing with side holes.

Maternal Blood Vessels

Catheters can be placed in the femoral vessels or in a pedal artery and vein[27] and advanced to the maternal descending aorta and inferior vena cava.

Electrodes

The leads for recording or stimulating electrodes are usually made from Teflon-coated stainless steel wire, which conducts current between points at which the coating has been scraped away. Sets of leads, two for recording and one for reference, can usefully be assembled in a length of polyvinyl tubing. Leads may be sewn to the fetal sternum, nuchal muscle, and uterine wall, respectively, to record fetal electrocardiogram, muscle tone, and uterine electromyogram. To record the fetal electrocorticogram, electrodes are implanted biparietally on the dura through burr holes made with a dental drill. Electro-ocular recordings are obtained from electrodes implanted through the orbital ridge of the zygomatic bone.[30]

Flow Probes

To measure ventricular output, a cuff-type electromagnetic flow transducer can be placed around the main pulmonary trunk, ascending aorta, or both vessels. These procedures require thoracotomy, which is performed in the third intercostal space.[31] Electromagnetic flow transducers may also be applied to the inferior and superior venae cavae and the intra-abdominal portion of the umbilical vein.[32] A transit-time ultrasonic flow probe has been used to measure blood flow in the umbilical artery of the sheep fetus.[33]

MODELS OF FETAL PROGRAMMING FOR ADULT DISEASE

Low weight at birth has been linked to an increased risk for adult-onset diseases, including hypertension, ischemic heart disease, and non-insulin-dependent diabetes mellitus. The pioneering work in this field was epidemiological.[2] It led to the concept of fetal programming for adult disease — the idea that fetal development has important implications for adult health.

The mechanisms whereby fetal adaptations to a poor intrauterine environment predispose to adult hypertension and diabetes are as yet unknown. Therefore, much current research is aimed at understanding the link between fetal responses to hypoxia and poor nutrition and the subsequent development of high blood pressure and impaired glucose tolerance. There are several animal models of fetal growth restriction[34] that may prove useful in exploring these relationships.

Fetal Growth Restriction in Sheep

Ca... Carunclectomy

The sheep placenta is comprised of 40 to 100 discrete cotyledons; the fetal villi develop in apposition to the endometrial caruncles, which are present in the uterus of the nonpregnant ewe. The number of cotyledons formed can be reduced by excising most of the caruncles before tupping. This procedure (carunclectomy) results in the birth of small lambs[35] and has been used recently to study endocrine responses of growth-restricted fetuses.[36]

Hyperthermia

Maintenance of ewes in a hyperthermic environment (40°C for 12 h and 35°C for 12 h) during the period of maximal placental growth caused a reduction in fetal weight at midgestation.[37] This was linked to placental insufficiency, reflected in reduced concentrations of progesterone and ovine placental lactogen in maternal blood. Control ewes were kept in a thermoneutral environment and fed the same amount as that consumed by the hyperthermic animals. It is important to take loss of appetite into account in any experiment that exposes the animal to stress.

Embolization of the Umbilical Circulation

Techniques that restrict fetal growth late in gestation may be more relevant to studies of type 2 human fetal growth restriction. One such model depends on reducing fetal placental blood flow by embolization. It is possible to cause a 33% reduction in fetal placental blood flow by repeated injection of large numbers of microspheres into the umbilical circulation. Over a period of 9 d, this can cause a 20% reduction in fetal weight.[38] An attractive feature of this model is the increase in placental resistance and resultant alteration in the umbilical artery flow velocity profile, which is an early feature of human fetal growth restriction.[39] This model has been used to explore the cardiovascular[40] and endocrine[41] responses of the growth-restricted fetus.

Dietary Restriction

Maternal undernutrition during pregnancy commonly leads to low birth weight, whether the restriction is of calories or protein, or both.[42] However, some organs are more susceptible to dietary restriction early in gestation, and others, at later stages. To explore the interaction of undernutrition and gestational age, at least four groups of animals are needed. Using this approach, it was shown that periconceptual undernutrition could reprogram the fetal IGF axis, with the result that the responses of IGF-1 and the IGF-binding proteins to undernutrition in late gestation were markedly altered.[43]

A recent study[44] using an adolescent sheep model demonstrated that nutrient partitioning between mother and fetus can be dramatically altered in young growing females. Thus, overnourishment of the adolescent dams promoted rapid maternal growth throughout pregnancy but resulted in a major restriction in placental mass and led to a significant decrease in birth weight relative to moderately fed adolescents of equivalent age.

It is worth noting that a moderate reduction (15%) in maternal nutritional intake over the first 70 d of gestation was sufficient to alter fetal cardiovascular development, lowering the blood pressure of the fetus and resetting its baroreflex control mechanisms.[45] Fetal size was not affected. The inference is that fetal programming can occur without a change in growth rate.

Glucocorticoid Exposure

Many physiologists believe that glucocorticoids play a pivotal role in fetal programming. In sheep, fetal exposure to dexamethasone for 2 d, very early in gestation, was sufficient to trigger hypertension in the lambs. They continued to have high blood pressure after they had grown into adults, up to at least 5 years of age. These animals did not develop insulin resistance, suggesting different timing for the programming of hypertension and altered sensitivity to insulin.[46]

Some of the programming effects of prenatal glucocorticoid exposure may be independent of a reduction in fetal growth. In another carefully controlled study,[47] fetal growth restriction occurred when betamethasone was given to the mother but not when betamethasone was given directly to the fetus. However, glucose homeostasis in the lambs was affected by betamethasone administration both to the mother and to the fetus.

To fully understand the link between low birth weight and adult-onset diseases, account must be taken of both the factors that control fetal growth and those that impact on organ systems critical to blood pressure control and glucose homeostasis. Thus, even if glucocorticoids do play a central role in fetal programming, there must necessarily be interaction with the IGF system. Indeed, the IGF system and the hypothalamic-pituitary-adrenal (HPA) axis likely are equally important in this context.[1]

Fetal Growth Restriction in Rodents

Dietary Restriction

There are several rodent models of fetal growth restriction based on dietary restriction during pregnancy. As an example, when pregnant rats were fed a diet containing only 6% protein, compared with 20% in the controls, the newborn pups had a low birth weight. They did show catch-up growth postnatally. However, the number of glomeruli in the kidney was reduced in male and female rats examined at 8 weeks of age. These rats became hypertensive by 8 weeks of age, and their blood pressure continued to rise in the succeeding months.[48] It seemed as if this reflected hemodynamic adaptations to maintain renal function despite reduced nephrogenesis.

A dietary restriction model has been validated for the guinea pig in which females are fed 70% of the ad libitum intake of a control group from 4 weeks before conception until day 34 of gestation, then 90% until day 60 (term is 67 d).[49]

Uterine Artery Ligation

In rodents, the placentae of each uterine horn are supplied from an arterial arcade formed by the uterine and ovarian arteries. If the uterine artery is ligated during gestation, the ovarian artery is able to maintain a viable pregnancy. However, placental blood flow is reduced, resulting in fetal growth restriction. This was first demonstrated for the rat[50] and later applied to the guinea pig.[51] Fetal body weight is reduced by about 40% in guinea pigs, but with brain sparing and an increase in the ratio of brain weight to liver weight. This model has been well characterized in terms of fetal endocrine and cardiovascular responses.[52]

Hypoxic Hypoxia

Approximately 140 million people live at high altitude (>2500 m), most of them in developing countries. These populations have an increased incidence of fetal growth restriction and preeclampsia, resulting in a high maternal and infant mortality that poses a major public health problem.[53] Therefore, the link between hypoxic hypoxia and poor fetal growth at high altitude needs to be explored. High-altitude hypoxia can be simulated in guinea pigs by keeping them in a hypobaric chamber from day 6 of gestation onwards.[54]

PERSPECTIVES

We are on the verge of understanding the sequence of genes and gene products that direct fetal development in the mouse. This knowledge will provide a basis for interpreting human data and may be especially useful in human stem cell research. With time, it may prove possible to integrate information on temporal and spatial patterns of expression at the mRNA and protein level from molecular studies. Currently, such studies often implicate a protein or group of proteins in a developmental process without furthering our understanding of their precise role.

The mouse is an unsatisfactory model for functional, physiological studies and will remain so even if advances in nanotechnology make it possible to study the mouse fetus *in utero*. This is because many events in human fetal development take place postnatally in rats and mice. In this respect, the sheep remains a better model. To bridge the gap between mouse, sheep, and human, however, it is worth considering the hystricomorph rodents as alternative models for fetal research. These animals, which include the guinea pig, give birth to precocial young with open eyes, a coat of fur, and full dentition. Some of the lesser-known South American species have large fetuses that should be easy to catheterize. Among these, the paca (*Agouti paca*), which weighs 5 to 10 kg and carries a single fetus with a birth weight of 640 to 900 g,[55] deserves particular attention as a potential model of fetal growth and development.

REFERENCES

1. Han, V.K.M. and Carter, A.M., Control of growth and development of the feto-placental unit, *Curr. Opin. Pharmacol.,* 1, 632, 2001.
2. Barker, D.J.P., *Fetal and Infant Origins of Adult Disease,* British Medical Journal, London, 1992.
3. Barcroft, J., *Researches on Prenatal Life,* Blackwell Scientific Publications, Oxford, United Kingdom, 1946.
4. Dawes, G.S., *Foetal and Neonatal Physiology,* Year Book Medical Publishers, Chicago, 1968.
5. Bronson, S.K. and Smithies, O., Altering mice by homologous recombination using embryonic stem cells, *J. Biol. Chem.,* 269, 27155, 1994.
6. Dai, Z., Xing, Y., Boney, C.M., Clemmons, D.R., and D'Ercole, A.J., Human insulin-like growth factor-binding protein-1 (hIGFBP-1) in transgenic mice: characterization and insights into the regulation of IGFBP-1 expression, *Endocrinology,* 135, 1316, 1994.
7. Efstratiadis, A., Genetics of mouse growth, *Int. J. Dev. Biol.,* 42, 955, 1998.
8. Rossant, J. and Cross, J.C., Placental development: lessons from mouse mutants, *Nat. Rev. Genet.,* 2, 538, 2001.
9. Chang H., Zwijsen, A., Vogel, H., Huylebroeck, D., and Matzuk, M.M., *Smad5* is essential for left-right asymmetry in mice, *Dev. Biol.,* 219, 71, 2000.
10. Georgiades, P., Watkins, M., Burton, G.J., and Ferguson-Smith, A.C., Roles for genomic imprinting and the zygotic genome in placental development, *Proc. Natl. Acad. Sci. U.S.A.,* 98, 4522, 2001.
11. Fundele, R., Surani, M.A., and Allen, N.D., Consequences of genomic imprinting for fetal development, in *Genomic Imprinting,* Reik, R. and Azim Surani, A., Eds., IRL Press, Oxford, United Kingdom, 1997, chap. 6.
12. Catanach, B.M. and Beechey, C.V., Genomic imprinting in the mouse: possible final analysis, in *Genomic Imprinting,* Reik, R. and Azim Surani, A., Eds., IRL Press, Oxford, United Kingdom, 1997, chap. 7.
13. Nagy, A., Cre recombinase: the universal reagent for genome tailoring, *Genesis,* 26, 99, 2000.
14. Ryding, A.D., Sharp, M.G., and Mullins, J. J., Conditional transgenic technologies, *J. Endocrinol.,* 171, 1, 2001.
15. Tanaka, T.S., Jaradat, S.A., Lim, M.K., Kargul, G.J., Wang, X., Grahovac, M.J., Pantano, S., Sano, Y., Piao, Y., Nagaraja, R., Doi, H., Wood, W.H., Becker, K.G., and Ko, M.S., Genome-wide expression profiling of mid-gestation placenta and embryo using a 15,000 mouse developmental DNA microarray, *Proc. Natl. Acad. Sci. U.S.A.,* 97, 9127, 2000.
16. Goodwin, D.H., *Sheep Management and Production,* Hutchinson, London, 1979.
17. Hecker, J.F., *The Sheep as an Experimental Animal,* Academic Press, New York, 1983.
18. Mears, G.J., van Petten, G.R., Harris, W.H., Bell, J.U., and Lorscheider, F.L., Induction of oestrus and fertility in the anoestrous ewe with hormones and controlled lighting and temperature, *J. Reprod. Fertil.,* 57, 461, 1979.
19. van Petten, G.R., Mathison, H.J., Harris, W.H., and Mears, G.J., Chronic preparation of the pregnant ewe and fetus for pharmacological research: the placental transfer and fetal effects of bunitrolol, *J. Pharmacol. Meth.,* 1, 45, 1978.

20. Rudolph, C.D., Roman, C., and Rudolph, A.M., Effect of acute umbilical cord compression on hepatic carbohydrate metabolism in the fetal lamb, *Pediatr. Res.,* 25, 228, 1989.

21. Noakes, D.E. and Young, M., Measurement of fetal tissue protein synthetic rate in the lamb *in utero*, *Res. Vet. Sci.,* 31, 336, 1981.

22. Mellor, D.J. and Slater, J.S., The use of chronic catheterization techniques in foetal sheep, *Br. Vet. J.,* 129, 260, 1973.

23. Radostits, O.M., Gay, C.C., Blood, D.C., and Hinchcliff, K.W., *Veterinary Medicine: A Textbook of the Diseases of Cattle, Sheep, Pigs, Goats and Horses,* 9th ed., Saunders, London, 2000.

24. Fiset, P. and Woodward, T.E., Q fever, in *Bacterial Infections of Humans. Epidemiology and Control,* 3rd ed., Evans, A.S. and Brachman, P.S., Eds., Plenum Medical Book Company, New York, 1998, chap. 29.

25. Rankin, J.H.G. and Schneider, J.M., Effect of surgical stress on the distribution of placental blood flows, *Respir. Physiol.,* 24, 373, 1975.

26. Rudolph, A.M. and Heymann, M.A., Validation of the antipyrine method for measuring fetal umbilical blood flow, *Circ. Res.,* 21, 185, 1967.

27. Bristow, J., Rudolph, A.M., and Itskovitz, J., A preparation for studying liver blood flow, oxygen consumption, and metabolism in the fetal lamb *in utero*, *J. Dev. Physiol.,* 3, 255, 1981.

28. Ashwal, S., Majcher, J.S., Vain.N., and Longo, L.D., Patterns of fetal lamb regional cerebral blood flow during and after prolonged hypoxia, *Ped. Res.,* 14, 1104, 1980.

29. Itskovitz, J., LaGamma, E.F., and Rudolph, A.M., The effect of reducing umbilical blood flow on fetal oxygenation, *Am. J. Obstet. Gynecol.,* 145, 813, 1983.

30. Richardson, B.S., Patrick, J.E., Bousquet, J., Homan, J., and Brien, J.F., Cerebral metabolism in fetal lamb after maternal infusion of ethanol, *Am. J. Physiol.,* 249, R505, 1985.

31. Morton, M.J., Pinson, C.W., and Thornburg, K.L., *In utero* ventilation with oxygen augments left ventricular stroke volume in lambs, *J. Physiol.,* 383, 413, 1987.

32. Reuss, M.L., Rudolph, A.M., and Dae, M.W., Phasic blood flow patterns in the superior and inferior venae cavae and umbilical vein of fetal sheep, *Am. J. Obstet. Gynecol.,* 145, 70, 1983.

33. Maulik, D., Yarlagadda, P., Nathanielsz, P.W., and Figueroa, J.P., Hemodynamic validation of Doppler assessment of fetoplacental circulation in a sheep model system, *J. Ultrasound Med.,* 8, 171, 1989.

34. Carter, A.M., Placental blood flow and fetal oxygen supply in animal models of intra-uterine growth retardation, in *Placenta: Basic Research for Clinical Application,* Soma, H., Ed., Karger, Basel, Switzerland, 1991, p. 23.

35. Alexander, G., Studies on the placenta of the sheep (*Ovis aries* L.): effect of surgical reduction in the number of caruncles, *J. Reprod. Fertil.,* 7, 307, 1964.

36. Ross, J.T., Phillips, I.D., Simonetta, G., Owens, J.A., Robinson, J.S., and McMillen, I.C., Differential effects of placental restriction on IGF-II, ACTH receptor and steroidogenic enzyme mRNA levels in the foetal sheep adrenal, *J. Neuroendocrinol.,* 12, 79, 2000.

37. Regnault, T.R.H., Orbus, R.J., Battaglia, F.C., Wilkening, R.B., and Anthony, R.V., Altered arterial concentrations of placental hormones during maximal placental growth in a model of placental insufficiency, *J. Endocrinol.,* 162, 433, 1999.

38. Block, B.S., Schlafer, D.H., Wentworth, R.A., Kreitzer, L.A., and Nathanielsz, P.W., Regional blood flow distribution in fetal sheep with intrauterine growth retardation produced by decreased umbilical placental perfusion, *J. Dev. Physiol.,* 13, 81, 1990.

39. Trudinger, B.J., Stevens, D., Connelly, A., Hales, J.R.S., Alexander, G., Bradley, L., Fawcett, A., and Thompson, R.S., Umbilical artery flow velocity waveforms and placental resistance: the effects of embolization of the umbilical circulation, *Am. J. Obstet. Gynecol.,* 157, 1443, 1987.

40. Carter, A.M., Challis, J.R.G., and Svendsen, P., Regional adrenal blood flow responses to adrenocorticotropic hormone after chronic embolization of the fetal placental circulation in sheep, *J. Endocrinol.,*148, 517, 1996.

41. Gagnon, R., Murotsuki, J., Challis, J.R.G., Fraher, L., and Richardson, B.S., Fetal sheep endocrine responses to sustained hypoxemic stress after chronic fetal placental embolization, *Am. J. Physiol.,* 272, E817, 1997.

42. Harding J.E. and Johnston, B.M., Nutrition and fetal growth, *Reprod. Fertil. Dev.,* 7, 539, 1995.

43. Gallaher, B.W., Breier, B.H., Keven, C.L., Harding, J.E., and Gluckman, P.D., Fetal programming of insulin-like growth factor (IGF)-I and IGF-binding protein-3: evidence for an altered response to undernutrition in late gestation following exposure to periconceptual undernutrition in the sheep, *J. Endocrinol.*, 159, 501, 1998.

44. Wallace, J.M., Nutrient partitioning during pregnancy: adverse gestational outcome in overnourished adolescent dams, *Proc. Nutr. Soc.*, 59, 107, 2000.

45. Hawkins, P., Steyn, C., Ozaki, T., Saito, T., Noakes, D.E., and Hanson, M.A., Effect of maternal undernutrition in early gestation on ovine fetal blood pressure and cardiovascular reflexes, *Am. J. Physiol. Regul. Integr. Comp. Physiol.*, 279, R340, 2000.

46. Gatford, K.L., Wintour, E.M., De Blasio, M.J., Owens, J.A., and Dodic, M., Differential timing for programming of glucose homoeostasis, sensitivity to insulin and blood pressure by *in utero* exposure to dexamethasone in sheep, *Clin. Sci. (Lond.)*, 98, 553, 2000.

47. Moss, T.J., Sloboda, D.M., Gurrin, L.C., Harding, R., Challis, J.R.G., and Newnham, J.P., Programming effects in sheep of prenatal growth restriction and glucocorticoid exposure, *Am. J. Physiol. Regul. Integr. Comp. Physiol.*, 281, R960, 2001.

48. Vehaskari, V.M., Aviles, D.H., and Manning, J., Prenatal programming of adult hypertension in the rat, *Kidney Int.*, 59, 238, 2001.

49. Roberts, C.T., Sohlstrom, A., Kind, K.L., Grant, P.A., Earl, R.A., Robinson, J.S., Khong, T.Y., Owens, P.C., and Owens, J.A., Altered placental structure induced by maternal food restriction in guinea pigs: a role for circulating IGF-II and IGFBP-2 in the mother?, *Placenta*, 22(Suppl. A), S77, 2001.

50. Wigglesworth, J.S., Experimental growth retardation in the foetal rat, *J. Pathol. Bacteriol.*, 88, 1, 1964.

51. Detmer, A. and Carter, A.M., Factors influencing the outcome of ligating the uterine artery and vein in a guinea pig model of intrauterine growth retardation, *Scand. J. Lab. Anim. Sci.*, 19, 9, 1992.

52. Carter, A.M., Current topic: restriction of placental and fetal growth in the guinea pig, *Placenta*, 14, 125, 1993.

53. Moore, L.G., Niermeyer, S., and Zamudio, S., Human adaptation to high altitude: regional and life-cycle perspectives, *Am. J. Phys. Anthropol. Suppl.*, 27, 25, 1998.

54. Rockwell, L.C., Keyes, L.E., and Moore, L.G., Chronic hypoxia diminishes pregnancy-associated DNA synthesis in guinea pig uteroplacental arteries, *Placenta*, 21, 313, 2000.

55. Miglino, M.A., Carter, A.M., dos Santos Ferraz, R.H., and Fernandes Machado, M.R. Placentation in the capybara (*Hydrochaerus hydrochaeris*), agouti (*Dasyprocta aguti*) and paca (*Agouti paca*), *Placenta*, 23, 416–428, 2002.

CHAPTER 4

Animal Models of Nephrological Disorders

Cynthia E. Glover

CONTENTS

INTRODUCTION

A model, by definition, is a simplified representation of a complex system.[1] Renal pathology and physiology are very complex systems, with complex interactions between major organ systems including the hematopoetic system, the skeletal system, and the cardiovascular system. Animal studies of kidney diseases provide simplified models of a large number of diseases and development, permitting examination of particular variables to better understand the pathogenesis of the disease in question and to evaluate potential treatment options. Animal models permit studies to be conducted *in vivo* under controlled conditions so that specific aspects of disease mechanisms and responses to treatment can be evaluated.[2]

The animal model can only be devised and applied to the level of understanding of the disease in question.[3] As understanding of the system increases, new problems and potential mechanisms of action are recognized. Researchers need to explore and understand these actions to further refine their impressions of the pathogenesis and potential therapies. Therefore, models need to be refined and new applications created for extant models as the comprehension of mechanisms and treatment options grows. No model exactly replicates the human disease for which it is intended to mimic, and renal models are no different in this regard. The advantages and disadvantages of the model need to be considered when interpreting results.

Select models for several major renal diseases are discussed in this survey. Because of the complexity of this system, many models have been omitted; several other disease states have not even been considered. However, this chapter gives the reader an overview of potential modeling systems currently in use and briefly reviews some classic models.

MODELS OF GLOMERULONEPHRITIS

Chronic glomerulonephritis is one of the major causes of chronic renal failure in humans. Glomerular disease can be divided into primary and secondary glomerulonephritis. In primary glomerulonephritis, such as immunoglobin A (IgA) nephropathy, the kidney is the primary organ involved. In secondary glomerulonephritis, systemic disease such as diabetes mellitus or systemic lupus erythematosus involves the kidney as well as other organs.

A major mechanism of glomerular injury involves the deposition of antigen–antibody complexes, either *in situ* against the glomerular basement membrane or due to trapping of circulating immune complexes. These mechanisms are frequently exploited in studies using animal models to investigate glomerulonephritis.

Models of Primary Glomerulonephritis: IgA Nephropathy

IgA nephropathy (also known as Berger's disease)[4] is the most common form of glomerulonephritis in human patients. Patients have a wide spectrum of lesions, from minimal immune complex deposition in the mesangial matrix to terminal renal failure in up to 25% within 10 years.[5] Chronic mesangial glomerulonephritis lesions are characterized by granular, electrodense deposits of IgA, along with C3, in the glomerular mesangium. Similar glomerular changes are seen in secondary glomerulonephropathies in Henoch–Schönlein purpura, cirrhotic liver diseases, and chronic inflammatory diseases of the lungs. Fifty to sixty percent of patients also have either or both IgG or IgM deposition, or both. Clinically, patients experience recurrent episodes of hematuria, particularly in association with infections of the upper or lower respiratory tract or other mucosa. In about half of patients, there is a microscopic hematuria that progresses to proteinuria.

IgA nephropathy is related to an abnormality of IgA production that is induced by antigenic stimulation of the mucosal immune system. Repeated or persistent antigenic stimulation then leads to overproduction of IgA; nephropathy results when there is extensive overproduction of IgA antibodies or there is a defect of clearance of IgA immune complexes by the mononuclear phagocytic system. Circulating immune complexes are trapped and deposited by the mesangial matrix or are formed *in situ*.

Because mild IgA deposits are found in the glomeruli of both humans and rodents without causing dysfunction,[6,7] it is reasoned that the deposits in glomerulonephritis cases have some nephritogenic properties. The deposition of complement C3 in these lesions may activate the membrane attack complex, resulting in glomerular disease.[4,8] Other research[9] implicates secretory, or polymeric, IgA, as opposed to monomeric IgA, as being critical in the pathogenesis.

Rifai developed the first experimental animal model of IgA nephropathy in 1979.[5,9,10] BALB/c mice were preimmunized with anti-dinitrophenol (DNP) IgA, then dosed with DNP-conjugated bovine serum albumin (DNP-BSA). Treated mice developed mesangial deposits of IgA, C3, and DNP-BSA, with focal areas of mesangial thickening. This model demonstrated the development of mesangial deposits from circulating immune complexes. The model mimics the condition seen in human patients, in whom there is an increase in the serum IgA and mesangial IgA deposits in a granular pattern, as well as IgA deposits in blood vessels of the muscles and skin.

A second model, developed by Isaacs et al. and Isaacs and Miller,[5,10–12] used active immunization of CD1 and Swiss-Webster mice with bacterial-derived dextran to induce IgA immune complex formation. These mice developed mesangial granular IgA deposits, with C3 deposition in about half. In a related experiment, Lewis rats on a prolonged intravenous bacterial polysaccharide immunization protocol developed dose-dependent proteinuria and hematuria, without glomerular IgA deposition.[13] These rats consistently recovered within 40 d after ceasing the polysaccharide administration.

Emancipator et al.[10,14] demonstrated the role of mucosal IgA production in IgA nephropathy. BALB/c mice were orally immunized with ovalbumin, bovine gamma globulin, or horse spleen ferritin in drinking water over a 14-week period. An 8- to 16-fold increase in specific IgA antibody was detected in immunized mice, along with specific IgA antibody and antigen deposition in the glomerular mesangium. In other chronic oral immunization studies, rats were immunized over an 8-week period with bovine gamma globulin in the drinking water.[6,10] In Wistar and Lewis rats, an IgA response is seen along with IgG (whereas in Sprague-Dawley and Fischer rats, the effect is in IgG only). Glomerular IgA and IgG deposits are proportional to the levels seen in the serum. Lewis rats display IgA/IgG along with C3, similar to the case of human patients with IgA nephropathy, as well as to the case of mice treated with a similar protocol. The treated Lewis rats have microhematuria but negligible azotemia or proteinuria. The glomeruli have more thromboxane and less prostaglandin E_2 than is the case in controls, with a proportional decrease in glomerular filtration rate and renal plasma flow. Angiotensin antagonist treatment, an antagonist of glomerular contraction, increases the glomerular filtration rate. The clinical correlation between diminished glomerular filtration rate and the progression to glomerulosclerosis suggests that glomerular contraction plays an important role in the development of chronic renal failure in IgA nephropathy.

Alimentary antigens in the form of diet may play a role in influencing circulating IgA immune complement in IgA nephropathy patients. Gliadin is a component of gluten, and anti-gliadin IgA has been found in human patients. Patients on a gluten-free diet[5,15] decreased circulating IgA immune complex but experienced further progression of renal failure. BALB/c mice fed gluten-containing diets,[16] including standard chows, developed detectable levels of serum and glomerular anti-gliaden IgA. Mice given oral immunization with ovalbumin or gliadin developed a more intense IgA deposition. The role of environmental microbial contamination in susceptible patients was demonstrated by orally administering vomitoxin (a mycotoxin found in cereal grains contaminated with the fungus *Fusarium graminearum*) in food for 12 weeks to BALB/c[17] and B6C3F$_1$ mice.[17,18] Vomitoxin in mice induces high serum IgA, IgA immune complex formation, and glomerular IgA deposition. Analogous to male predisposition to IgA nephropathy in humans, male B6C3F$_1$ mice were more sensitive to the development of vomitoxin-induced nephropathy, demonstrating higher serum IgA, hematuria, and mesangial IgA and C3 deposition than female mice at similar doses. Mice injected with IgA antibodies induced by vomitoxin exposure also developed nephropathy.[17] The implication is that alimentary antigens do play a role in the development of IgA nephropathy, although other factors likely influence its progression.

A spontaneous model of IgA nephropathy is the Japanese ddY mouse.[10,19] Mesangial proliferative glomerulonephritis, with deposition of IgA and C3, develops by 40 weeks of age. Increased levels of interleukin (IL)-6, either exogenous or overexpressed as a transgene, results in increased IgA synthesis and mesangial proliferative glomerulonephritis late in life. The antigen has an affinity for binding to mesangial structures, promoting immune complex deposition. There is a correlation between the degree of polymeric IgA and the severity of the lesions, as seen on histology. Selective breeding of ddY mice for high serum IgA has led to a strain (designated HIGA) with earlier onset of glomerular IgA deposition, by about 25 weeks of age.[20,21] The RF/J strain, first reported in 1960 by Gude and Lupton,[22] similarly develops glomerulonephritis at 8 to 12 months of age and likewise shows a correlation between the serum polymeric IgA and the development of glomerulosclerosis, as well as up-regulation of TGF-β in mesangial lesions.[23]

A model described by Stad et al.[6,24] allows insight into antigen-mediated targeting of the immune deposits to the mesangium in rats. Mesangial cells express Thy-1; a hapten-conjugated anti-Thy 1 monoclonal antibody thus binds to the mesangium. Injection of a hapten-specific polymeric IgA (p-IgA) in male Wistar rats results in glomerulonephritis with IgA and C3 deposition, as well as proteinuria. The proteinuria correlates with the amount of C3 expressed, implying a nephritogenic role for C3.

Models of Primary Glomerulonephritis: Miscellaneous Models

Preimmunization schemes, as well as administration of nephrotoxic agents, have been used to evaluate the role of oxidative stress in induced glomerular disease. Rodents preimmunized with bovine gamma globulin develop an immune complex glomerulonephritis,[6,10,14,25] as described above. Rats injected with sheep anti-rat glomerular basement membrane (GBM) IgG likewise developed an anti-GBM nephritis;[8,25] proteinuria was decreased when the rats were pretreated with catalase. Ito et al.[26] produced a crescentic glomerulonephritis resembling rapidly progressing glomerulonephritis in humans using rabbit anti-rat GBM serum and rabbit gamma globulin in Freund's Complete Adjuvant.

Puromycin aminonucleoside (PA) has been used for several years for production of experimental glomerulonephritis, due in part to its role in the production of oxygen free radicals. A single intravenous injection into Wistar and Sprague-Dawley rats produces proteinuria in 3 to 5 d.[27-29] Histologic examination shows visible hyaline droplets in the glomeruli and proximal tubules, loss of the interdigitating foot processes, and focal and segmental glomerulosclerosis. Diamond et al.[30] demonstrated the role of oxidative injury in this model by inducing nephrosis and administering oxygen free-radical scavengers to observe their protective effects.

A progressive glomerular injury model produces chronic aminonucleoside nephrosis analogous to minimal-change nephrotic syndrome.[25] Sprague-Dawley rats are given intravenous injections of PA. Rats have a nephrotic syndrome for 2 to 3 weeks, then a period of remission. By 8 weeks after injection, the treated rats have a recurrent proteinuria, with glomerulosclerosis development by 18 weeks after injection. In a second model,[25] weaning rats are placed for 4 weeks on a diet deficient in selenium and vitamin E. This produces a decrease in glutathione peroxidase activity, resulting in increased ammonia production and hypertrophy of the glomeruli and tubules.

Sheep have been shown to develop spontaneous glomerulonephritis. In the 1960s, 90% of sheep at an abattoir displayed an age-related proliferative glomerular nephritis with generalized or focal mesangial thickening, scarring of the glomerulus, and IgG and complement deposition on the glomerular capillary wall.[31-33] Similar to the case of many human patients, these sheep were asymptomatic; many human cases are detected when proteinuria is found on urinalysis that is run for other reasons. In a flock of Finnish Landrace sheep, lambs born in successive lambings developed a rapidly progressive glomerulonephritis as well as central nervous system disease resembling human mesangiocapillary glomerulonephritis.[32,34,35] Macroscopically, the kidneys were pale and enlarged. On microscopy, kidneys from affected lambs had membranoproliferative glomerulonephritis with crescent formation, with diffusely thickened capillary basement membranes and proliferation of mesangial cells. These lambs were found to be deficient in the C'3 component of complement. Renal failure occurred by 6 to 8 weeks of age.

Models of Secondary Glomerulonephritis: Systemic Lupus Erythematosus

Systemic lupus erythematosus (SLE) is an autoimmune disease that induces B- and T-cell autoreactivity and dysfunction in multiple organ systems. Clinical complications of glomerulonephritis develop in 50 to 80% of SLE patients; 10 to 20% of patients suffer end-stage renal failure as a result of this disease. The spectrum of renal involvement runs the gamut from no lesions at all to proliferative and crescentic glomerulonephritis. Most patients develop proteinuria, Ig and complement in glomeruli, and immune aggregates in the mesangium, subendothelium, and glomerular capillary walls. Immune complex deposition may result from trapping of circulating immunoglobulins, binding of autoantibodies with antigens in the glomerulus, or direct binding of autoantibodies to intrinsic glomerular antigens.[2,36] Animal models of SLE are used to study abnormalities in immunoregulation and to carry out prospective studies of glomerular changes. For instance, an increased glomerular procoagulant activator, or factor X activator, has been observed in mouse strains used as models of lupus nephritis (BXSB, MLR/lpr, and NZBxWF$_1$) but not in control mice (BALB/c) without disease.[37] The factor X activator is localized to the glomerular mesangium and capillary walls, and is theorized to play a role in the pathogenesis of lupus nephritis. Because the factor X activator is only found in areas with glomerular disease, a hypothesis is that inflammatory cells within the lesions release cytokines that induce glomerular X factor expression.

New Zealand Black (NZB) and New Zealand Black × New Zealand White (NZB/NZW) F1 mice develop a spontaneous disease resembling human autoimmune hemolytic anemia and SLE with glomerulonephritis.[31,36] Anti-erythrocyte autoantibodies are produced early in life; later, a membranous or proliferative glomerulonephritis, without renal function impairment, develops. (NZB/NZW) F1 mice tend to develop a pronounced, chronic glomerular disease with progressive renal failure, with mesangial proliferation, glomerulosclerosis, tubular atrophy, and interstitial inflammation. Signs of illness in female mice begin at approximately 6 months of age, and such mice typically die of end-stage renal failure. Fifty percent mortality is seen at 8.5 months of age, and 90% mortality at just over 1 year.[38] In males, illness begins at just over 1 year of age, with 50% mortality at 15 months. As in human SLE, glomerular lesions form because of the deposition of immune complexes and complement. Because of its resemblance to the human disease, this model is frequently used to evaluate potential therapeutic regimens.

Another classic spontaneous model of SLE is the MRL lpr/lpr mouse.[4,39–41] Mice that are homozygous for the lymphoproliferative (lpr) trait, because of a defect in the *fas* gene, produce lymphadenopathy, splenomegaly, and hypergammaglobulinemia. By 6 months of age, they have developed severe immune complex glomerulonephritis, with mesangial and endothelial cell proliferation, crescent formation, and tubulointerstitial nephritis and vasculitis. IgG and C3 deposition is present in the glomeruli. Mice die of end-stage renal failure by 9 months of age. The mouse model, however, does not exactly mirror SLE in that neither the Fas antigen mutation nor lymphoproliferation is part of the human disease.[39]

Additional spontaneous models include MRL/1 mice, BXSB mice, and SCJ/Kj mice. MRL/1 and BXSB mice develop an inherited, spontaneous autoimmunity that resembles SLE, with circulating immune complexes, glomerulonephritis with C3, IgG, and immune complex deposition, and decreased IL-2 production.[42]

The MRL/1 mouse was derived mainly from LG/J mice, with AKR/J, C57BL/6, and C3H contributions.[43] MRL/1 mice develop lupus-like signs at 3 to 4 months of age, with 50% mortality at just over 5 months, and 90% mortality by 7 months in females and by 9 months in males. The glomerulonephritis in these mice is of a subacute, proliferative form with IgG and C3 deposition.[38]

BXSB mice were derived from a C57BL/6 and SB/Le (satin-beige) F1 cross, which was bred for coat color and then found to have lupus-like characteristics.[40,41,43] Males are affected earlier and to a greater extent than females, possibly because of the effect of the *yaa* gene on the male chromosome.[44] Fifty percent of males die at 5 months, and 90% by 8 months; females become ill at about 1 year of age, with 50% mortality at 15 months and 90% at 2 years. Death is due to an acute, proliferative glomerulonephritis with deposition of immune complexes.[38,42]

The spontaneous crescentic glomerulonephritis-forming mouse/Kinjoh strain (SCG/Kj) is an inbred strain derived from a (BXSB × MRL-lpr/lpr) F1 hybrid, selectively bred from parents with a high frequency of crescentic glomerulonephritis.[4,39,45] The SCG/Kj mice develop an early onset of rapidly progressing crescentic glomerulonephritis and a necrotizing vasculitis of the small arteries and arterioles that affects multiple organs including the spleen, heart, uterus, and ovaries. These mice succumb to renal failure by 120 to 135 d of age. Renal lesions include hypertrophy of the glomerular epithelium, extraglomerular hemorrhage, and crescentic proliferation in Bowman's space. Fine granular deposits of IgG, IgM, and C3 are found within the glomeruli, with deposition of IgG along the GBM.

Induced models of SLE can be created by using chemical, metal ion, or pharmacological agents to induce a systemic autoimmune response, including the induction of membranous glomerulonephropathy. As in humans, administration of agents such as procainamid, hydralazine, gold salts, or D-penicillamine to Brown Norway rats can induce a systemic lupus-like syndrome, including glomerulonephritis in some cases.[2] Pristane (2,6,10,14-tetramethylpentadecane) intraperitoneal injection has been shown to induce a lupus-like disease in SJL and BALB/c mice,[46,47] as well as in many other inbred mouse strains. Treated mice develop lipogranulomas, with macrophages producing IL-6 and IL-10. Signs of lupus-like disease in these mice include the presence of characteristic autoantibodies (anti-Su, anti-U1NRP, and anti-Sm)[48] within 6 months of injection. Arthritis, severe diffuse or segmental glomerulonephritis with immune complex deposition, and proteinuria, analogous to SLE-associated glomerulonephritis, are also seen.

A model of pauci-immune, anti-neutrophil cytoplasmic antibody (ANCA)-associated crescentic glomerulonephritis can be induced in Brown Norway rats.[39,49] ANCA in human glomerulonephritis is directed toward myeloperoxidase (MPO), as well as proteinase 3, in the GBM.[50,51] Rats are immunized with human MPO in Complete Freund's Adjuvant.[52] Subsequent unilateral perfusion of one kidney with a lysosomal extract containing MPO, along with proteinase 3 and elastase with hydrogen peroxide, results in proteinuria within 24 h and in a proliferative, necrotizing glomerulonephritis in the perfused kidney within 10 d; the unperfused kidney serves as a control. IgG and C3 could be detected in lesions 24 h after perfusion but waned by 10 d after perfusion. Lack of IgG in the glomerular lesions resembled those of pauci-immune ANCA-associated crescentic glomerulonephritis in humans. Ischemia/reperfusion injury during the perfusion process also contributed to the glomerular lesions.[53] Kobayashi et al.[54] obtained similar results using rabbit anti-rat MPO serum followed by nephrotoxic serum injection in Wistar rats. This model demonstrates the pathogenic role of MPO-ANCA in vasculitis and subsequent renal pathology. A similar experiment in spontaneous hypertensive rats by Yang et al.[55] suggests the contribution of hypertension in aggravating the lesion, although the pathogenesis of the glomerulonephritis was attributed to immune deposition rather than ANCA.

Chronic graft versus host disease is a common induced model, produced by injecting parental donor (DBA/2) lymphocytes into (C57BL/10 × DBA/2) F1 mice.[36,56] The incompatibility between donor and recipient produces a lupus-like disease resembling SLE, with autoantibodies directed against laminin-1 binding along the GBM.[57,58] Upregulation of CD54 (intercellular adhesion molecule-1) parallels that seen in human biopsy specimens. CD54 upregulation is followed by CD11a (lymphocyte function antigen-1)-positive leukocytes. Within 6 to 8 weeks after injection, IgG deposition is present in the glomeruli. Mice develop typical signs of glomerulonephritis, including mesangial proliferation, GBM thickening with spike formation, and glomerulosclerosis. At approximately 3 months after injection, the mice die of renal failure with proteinuria, ascites, and hyperlipidemia.

Murine monoclonal autoantibodies administered to recipient mice induce dense subendothelial deposits ("wire loop lesions") similar to the lesions of human SLE-associated nephritis. These mice also display leukocyte infiltrate of the kidney, intraluminal thrombi, mesangial deposition of PAS-positive material, and glomerular and extraglomerular vascular wall deposition of fine granular material.[2]

Models of Secondary Glomerulonephritis: Diabetes Mellitus

Diabetic nephropathy is a common sequel of type 2 diabetes. Approximately 30% of patients with type 2 diabetes mellitus for 10 years or more develop renal complications.[59] One hypothesis for this tendency toward developing renal disease is that glucose sensitizes the kidney to have an increased response to a secondary insult.[60] Several models involving inherited diabetes mellitus are extant. Inheritance patterns and chromosomal intervals contributing to type 2 diabetes have been mapped in animal models. These models do develop kidney disease analogous to their human counterparts.

Goto Kakizaki (GK) rats, a non-obese strain, are genetically susceptible to type 2 diabetes and secondary glomerulonephritis.[59,60] This strain is useful for the study of the effects of non-insulin-dependent diabetes without confounding factors such as hyperlipidemia or hypertension.[61] The Goto Kakizaki strain was produced by selective breeding of a colony of nondiabetic Wistar rats with glucose intolerance.[62] Hyperglycemia results in thickening of the GBM, glomerular hypertrophy, and early podocyte damage, but without renal hypertrophy, proteinuria, glomerulosclerosis, or interstitial fibrosis.

Spontaneous hypertensive rats develop hypertension, obesity, insulin resistance, and increased triglyceride levels.[59] Renal disease begins at an early age, with proteinuria, progressive glomerulopathy, and tubular damage leading to uremia. On histology, the mesangium is widened and hypercellular; there is focal necrosis, hyalinization and collagen deposition, and arteriolar nephrosclerosis. Vascular glomerular lesions progress to glomerulosclerosis, fibrosis of the interstitium, and tubular atrophy.

In KK mice, a polygenic inbred strain, glucose intolerance begins as early as 2 to 5 months of age, with a blood glucose level approximately twice that of normal.[31, 63] These mice display increased urine production and proteinuria, which increases with the duration of the disease. Histological examination of the kidney reveals an increase in the mesangial matrix as well as hypercellularity, with nodules or accumulations beginning at the hilus and expanding segmentally. There is mesangial deposition of IgG and C3. Later in the disease, splitting of the basement membrane of capillary walls and spike formation is seen, similar to membranous glomerulopathy in humans.

Db/db (homozygous diabetic) mice develop severe diabetes due to a mutational inactivation of the leptin receptor gene (*lpr*).[64,65] The phenotype includes obesity, insulin resistance, and diabetes, with secondary derangement of renal function and morphological changes. Proteinuria begins early, before evidence of renal lesions, which include extracellular matrix expansion. The pathogenesis of renal lesions may include a renal sensitivity to insulin in the face of a hyperinsulinemic state.

To show that glomerular changes are due to the internal environment, a variety of experiments have been performed. Alloxan was given to an inbred strain of rats over a 6-month period to induce a diabetic state. Kidneys were then cross-transplanted with those from nontreated rats. Glomerular changes increased when untreated kidneys were placed in a diabetic rat but were reduced when diabetic kidneys were placed in an untreated rat.[31]

Streptozotocin can be given in a single intravenous injection to induce diabetes in rats.[66] Rats become diabetic in 2 weeks. The distal tubules of the kidney show an accumulation of glycogen by 2 weeks after injection, becoming more marked with time. Glomerular lesions are seen after 4 to 6 weeks. Tubular degeneration and marked glomerulosclerosis develop beginning at 4 months. IgG and albumin are deposited in the GBM. Rats do not develop papillary necrosis or papillitis as do human diabetic patients. Renal neoplasms also form in a portion of streptozotocin-treated rats.

Models of Secondary Glomerulonephritis: Miscellaneous Models

Secondary glomerulonephritis may be seen spontaneously as a sequel of viral infection, as a result of deposition of antiviral antibody complex in the glomerulus. More than 75% of horses experimentally infected with equine infectious anemia, a persistent viral infection, showed cellular proliferation, increased mesangial matrix, neutrophil and mononuclear cell infiltration, basement membrane thickening, and granular deposits of gamma globulin and C3 in the GBM.[31,32,67] With swine fever (chronic hog cholera), most animals die acutely, but survivors demonstrate glomerulonephritis with a lymphocytic/plasmacytic and neutrophilic infiltrate, mesangial cell proliferation and mesangial matrix increase, basement membrane thickening, and anti-host gamma-globulin deposition.[31,32,68] The severity of the glomerular lesions has been shown experimentally to increase with the length of survival. Severe glomerular lesions are associated with tubular degeneration and lymphoid infiltration in the interstitium. The renal damage is apparently caused by a combination of direct viral damage to the glomerular and tubular epithelium, failure of the mesangium to adequately process macromolecular substances such as antigen–antibody complexes or fibrin, and the attraction of lymphocytes and neutrophils to the injured kidney.

An association between upper respiratory infections and clinical relapsing glomerulonephritis has been explored by orally immunizing BALB/c mice for 14 weeks with protein antigens of various sizes (using ovalbumin, bovine gamma globulins, and ferritin).[10] Mice displayed a significant increase in specific IgA-producing plasma cells in the lamina propria of the bronchial and intestinal mucosae, along with circulating specific IgAs. Mice also demonstrated diffuse mesangial IgA deposition in the glomeruli, without C3 deposition. Immunogens were also found in the glomerular deposits, showing the pathogenicity of IgA immune complexes. Mice did not develop the proteinuria or hematuria seen in human patients.

Human IgA nephropathy patients experience hematuria with febrile influenza-type infections or pharyngitis. The transient viremia results in an acute IgA deposition in the kidneys. A model of viral infection with resultant IgA nephropathy is found in mink with Aleutian mink disease.[10,31,69,70] This is a persistent parvoviral infection resulting in diffuse arteritis, chronic hepatitis, and glomerular and interstitial nephritis. The glomerulonephritis is characterized by mesangial cell proliferation, increased matrix, and gamma-globulin and C3 deposition in the capillaries and mesangium. Interstitial nephritis, with tubulorhexis and infiltration by monocytes, is also seen, although IgA deposition in the renal tubules is not demonstrated. An experimental reproduction of viral infection and renal sequelae was created in 129/J mice exposed to Sendai virus.[5,10,71,72] In one experiment, naive mice were infected intranasally or by exposure to infected mice. Mesangial IgA in the mouse kidneys was seen, similar to the pattern in human IgA nephropathy. This demonstrated the validity of the model. In a later experiment in the same group, 129/J mice were immunized intranasally for Sendai virus, then challenged intravenously with live virus or viral envelope protein or challenged naturally by exposure to infected mice. Mesangial IgA was predominant, and viral antigens were also found in small amounts in some glomerular deposits. Hematuria developed in those mice exposed to intact virions but not in those exposed to viral envelope proteins only, inferring that the viral particle promotes some changes in glomerular function that are not fully understood.

Human patients with cirrhosis are often hypergammaglobulinemic and demonstrate concurrent mesangial IgA deposits.[73] These patients also have a higher incidence of endotoxemia, with increases in serum IgA antibodies against bacterial antigens such as those from *Escherichia coli, Pseudomonas aeruginosa,* and *Klebsiella pneumoniae.*[4] IgA eluates taken from the kidneys at autopsy contain IgA preferentially binding to these types of Gram-negative bacterial cell walls. Rats with liver cirrhosis induced by carbon tetrachloride intoxication also had increased serum IgA and glomerular IgA and C3 deposition.[4,74,75] The glomeruli show thickened GBMs and increased mesangial matrix.

Alcoholic rats (Tsukamoto-French rat model) provide another model of this disease.[4,73,76] The Tsukamoto-French model was developed to investigate ethanol-induced liver disease, but it also adeptly illustrates IgA nephropathy secondary to chronic alcohol intoxication. Wistar rats are implanted with an intragastric cannula, through which liquid diets and alcohol can be infused for a 6-week period. Alcohol has the effect of increasing natural killer (NK) cell activity, hence increasing IgA synthesis by B lymphocytes. The result is an increase in IgA deposition in the kidney. Wistar rats receiving intragastric ethanol infusion for 42 d doubled the NK cell activity.[77] Mesangial IgA deposition was seen in the treated rats but not in the controls. The liver is preferentially involved in IgA clearance, so a dysfunction in clearance, as in patients with alcoholic liver cirrhosis, may result in glomerular IgA deposition.[74,78] Amore[29] showed that Lewis rats receiving intragastric whiskey three times weekly demonstrated IgA localization in the mesangium and impairment of IgA clearance by the liver, even with minimal hepatic lesion formation.

ANIMAL MODELS OF ACUTE RENAL FAILURE

Acute renal failure is most commonly caused by acute tubular necrosis (ATN), which in turn may be caused by ischemia or nephrotoxicosis.[79] Sepsis, burns, or circulatory collapse can produce ischemia sufficient for ATN. Lesions in humans are mild compared with most animal models of acute renal failure,[80] and include patchy tubular necrosis in the proximal tubules and ascending limbs of Henle. Nephrotoxic ATN can show variable necrosis in the proximal tubules. A variety of pharmacological agents, ethylene glycol, mercury, lead, or other agents may be involved. Rhabdomyolysis resulting in massive myoglobulinuria may also incite ATN. Mortality can vary, depending on the underlying cause, and may be as high as 50%.[3,81]

In the rat, as well as the mouse, a reversible model of ischemic tubular damage is produced by occlusion of the renal artery, a model using warm ischemia-reflow to produce injury.[3,82] Body temperature has been shown to be a determinant in the severity of renal injury in this model, which illustrates the need for temperature control in experiments to obtain consistent results.[82] Hyperthermia exacerbates renal injury, whereas hypothermia is protective. Renal injury is most apparent after reflow, possibly because of an imbalance between the demand for oxygen in the reperfusion period and the supply available to tissues.[83] The transient hypotension produced by the occlusion results in severe renal hypoperfusion, compromising renal oxygen delivery and depleting adenosine triphosphate (ATP) in the tubular cells. This energy depletion sets off a complex injury cascade, culminating in the lesions of ATN, including extensive necrosis of the proximal tubules, which varies with the duration of occlusion. The distal tubules are less affected. This model does mimic the decrease in glomerular filtration rate as seen in human cases of ATN. Both the rat model and human cases develop casts in the collecting ducts, which may cause obstruction leading to further renal injury and tubular leakage.[3,84,85]

Cold ischemia-reflow models produce small, discrete lesions in the proximal tubules. Medullary and deep cortical blood flow is reduced, with continued glomerular filtration. This model resembles the changes observed in renal transplant cases. Rat kidneys, after 2, 4, and 16 h of cold ischemia, showed small areas of reversible injury in the proximal and distal tubules; 24 h after transplantation, there were small areas of necrosis in the proximal tubules and more widespread necrosis in the loops of Henle and collecting ducts.[78,86,87] The functional and morphological impairment of the transplanted kidney may be due to tissue edema blocking blood flow through the vasa recta and altering blood flow to the medulla.

Nephrotoxic models of ATN are more difficult to produce. Administration of aminoglycosides, radiocontrast agents, and endotoxins do not reliably produce acute renal failure in the rat. Combinations of insults are required to produce consistent results. A distal nephron model in an isolated perfused rat kidney uses a combination of nitric oxide, prostaglandin inhibition, and radiocontrast administration to produce decreased medullary oxygen availability with retained glomerular filtration sufficient to produce renal failure with corresponding medullary ascending limb damage.[79]

Another consistent model involves intramuscular glycerol injection, producing rhabdomyolysis and subsequent renal failure with extensive tubular necrosis and the production of tubular casts.[3,80,88]

ANIMAL MODELS OF PERITONEAL DIALYSIS

Peritoneal dialysis, including continuous ambulatory peritoneal dialysis, is a frequently used method of fluid replacement therapy for patients in chronic renal failure. However, long-term peritoneal dialysis carries with it its own host of dysfunctions, including fibrosis of the peritoneal membrane, loss of ultrafiltration, and infection.[89–91] A study of chronic peritoneal dialysis that was performed in nonuremic rats twice daily for 4 weeks found a decrease in the permeability of the peritoneum to glucose and total protein, damage to the peritoneal membrane due to exposure to dialysis solutions, and thickening of the peritoneum.[90]

Rats and rabbits are the most common species used *in vivo* studies.[89,90,92] Rats are easy to maintain, and there are good descriptions of rat models of renal failure. However, they have a large peritoneal surface area relative to their size, which makes recovery and analysis of infused dialysate difficult. Rabbits can tolerate peritoneal catheters for extended periods and are relatively resistant to peritonitis. Uremic models can be created using subtotal nephrectomy (5/6 nephrectomy).[93] Rats can also be made uremic by 5/6 nephrectomy, either by unilateral nephrectomy and infarction, surgical ablation of the upper and lower thirds of the contralateral kidney,[94] or electrocautery.[95] A study of chronic peritoneal dialysis in uremic rats[90] was accomplished by inserting a silicone catheter into the abdominal cavity of partially nephrectomized Wistar rats. Mortality over the first 4 weeks was similar between dialyzed and nondialyzed rats, but survival over the next 4 weeks was improved in the rats receiving dialysis. Other techniques involve performing an omentectomy before catheter placement to ensure catheter patency without omental occlusion.[91] A further model of continuous ambulatory dialysis was produced in uremic rats by surgical insertion of a permanent silicon indwelling cannula with placement of a sterile catheter via the cannula for dialysis.[96] The cannula remained patent, and intermittent dialysis was successfully accomplished over a 21-d evaluation period.

Peritoneal transport studies have been accomplished in nonuremic rats. In a model used in Stockholm, Sweden,[90] anesthetized, normal Sprague-Dawley rats were infused for 4-h periods, with frequent sampling of blood and dialysate. Studies using various osmotic agents and additives in the dialysis solution were carried out. The study suggested that a higher net ultrafiltration was obtained using a 4% oligopeptide solution, similar to a 3.86% glucose solution but more effective than a 2.27% glucose solution. Additives to reduce peritoneal fluid absorption and hence improve the efficiency of peritoneal dialysis were examined. The addition of 0.01% hyaluronan improved efficiency significantly, as did atrial natriuretic peptide. Addition of amphotericin B to dialysate solution had been reported to increase ultrafiltration in rabbits[97] but did not have the desired effect in rats. A biocompatibility study using dialysis fluid with 3.86% glucose in rats found a decrease in fluid removal and decreased small-solute clearance, suggesting functional peritoneal changes induced by exposure to the dialysis solution.

Implant-associated infections, including those associated with continuous peritoneal dialysis, are often associated with biofilm formation on the implant.[98] These infections tend to be persistent and resistant to antibiotic treatment. A model of biofilm infection on a catheter was developed in New Zealand white rabbits.[99] Tenckhoff catheters were surgically implanted in the peritoneal cavity of the rabbits. Biofilm production and spread was observed over a 3-week period. Peritoneal dialysis was also performed in one group over a 2-week period, and again bacterial growth could be evaluated. The colonization by skin bacteria, *Staphylococcus epidermidis,* produced peritoneal infection in dialyzed rabbits. Gagnon and Richards[98] developed a model of biofilm infection in C57BL/6J mice. The mice were surgically implanted with a section of silastic peritoneal catheter completely within the peritoneal cavity; the implant was infected with *S. epidermidis.* This model was used in the evaluation of treatment regimens as a demonstration of the usefulness of this relatively inexpensive model of implant-associated infections. A further complication in the problem of peritonitis stems from the immunosuppression that results in renal failure. Mice with induced renal failure showed delayed clearance and a decreased inflammatory response to intraperitoneal inoculations of *S. epidermidis*.[100]

ANIMAL MODELS OF RENAL CELL CARCINOMA

Renal cell carcinoma accounts for about 85% of renal tumors in humans, predominantly in males in their fifties and sixties. Thirty thousand new cases are diagnosed annually in the United States. Clear cell carcinomas, with clear or granular-appearing cytoplasm, make up 70 to 80% of renal cell carcinomas. Papillary carcinoma makes up 10 to 15%, and the remaining 5% are chromophobe renal carcinomas arising from the intercalated cells of the collecting ducts.[81] Renal cell carcinomas tend to metastasize widely.

The ideal model, that most like the human disease, is a spontaneous neoplasm with histological characteristics of an adenocarcinoma, with predictable growth and metastasis rates. Animal models of neoplastic disease ideally have the following characteristics:[1] (1) the lesions should be histologically similar to the human counterpart, (2) the lesion should occur in the same organ or tissue, and (3) the model should display similar growth and metastatic characteristics as the human neoplastic counterpart. Models used for preclinical studies should be slow growing, so that there is time to initiate treatment and evaluate its effects.[101]

Spontaneous renal neoplasia is rare in rodents; most models involve disease induced by chemicals, radiation, viruses, or hormones, although some rat and mouse strains that are susceptible to spontaneous tumorogenesis have been developed.

Chemically Induced Tumor Models

Chemical induction acts directly or by metabolic changes to produce mutagenic products, which cause altered DNA formation in the kidney.[1] Most oncogenic agents produce similar types of tumors, and clear-cell tumors are common. Short-chain alkyl or alkenyl halides most frequently induce tubular adenomas or carcinomas. Amine compounds are more likely to be associated with either medullary or papillary lesions or with urinary bladder tumors. Nitrosamines, polycyclic hydrocarbons, mycotoxins, and heavy metals have also been used for tumorogenesis in animal models.[102]

Dimethylnitrosamine (DMN) treatment given to adult Swiss mice has successfully produced renal adenomas.[102] Nephroblastomas were formed in rats dosed with DMN in the drinking water.[102] In another model, young Wistar/Porton albino/Fischer 344/Nb rats were given a protein-deprived diet (glucose and sucrose diet). After injection with dimethylnitrosamines, 90 to 100% developed renal mesenchymal tumors, analogous to the human congenital mesoblastic nephroma of infancy.[1,103] Porton rats given high doses of DMN in the feed for short periods developed both well-differentiated, expansile tumors of the renal epithelium and anaplastic kidney tumors, which metastasized to the lung in one case.[104]

Lead enhances other oncogens and impairs NK cell activity. Added to *N*-(4'-fluoro-4-biphenyl)acetamide, 1% lead acetate produces renal adenocarcinomas in 100% of treated rats.[1,102] Rats induced with chronic lead intoxication[1,102] develop solid and tubular tumors of the renal cortical tubules; tubular-type tumors regularly metastasize to the lungs, whereas solid forms metastasize via the lymphatics to the adrenal glands, liver, spleen, and contralateral kidney.

Streptozotocin (*N*-nitroso-methylamide) is derived from *Streptomyces achromogenes*. It is widely used in animal models for its diabetogenic properties, but it also has tumorogenic properties.[102] Streptozotocin injected intravenously in CBA/H/T6J mice produces cortical epithelial tumors with a solid (carcinoma) or papillary (adenoma) histological pattern.[1,102] These tumors have a low incidence of metastasis, usually to the lung. Females are more susceptible to tumorogenesis; 100% develop neoplasia, compared with 73% of males. This model is used to study tumor pathogenesis and for determining biochemical and molecular mechanisms in carcinogenesis. An orthotopic, transplantable preclinical model was developed by injecting streptozotocin in BALB/c mice.[101] A histologically confirmed renal cell carcinoma that resulted from this treatment was successfully adapted to serial orthotopic transplantation. This isolate, designated SIRCC-1, had the desirable slow growth *in vivo,* as well as high vascularity and metastasis to the lung.

Hormone-Induced Tumor Models

Male Syrian golden hamsters, or gonadectomized males or females, are susceptible to developing estrogen-dependent renal neoplasia when given stilbestrol.[1,103] These tumors originate in the cortical tubular epithelium. Tumors can be transplanted after pretreating the recipient with diethylstilbestrol. Recipients develop bilateral, multiple cortical tumors that rupture and locally metastasize; implant metastases are found on the viscera and abdominal wall. Distant metastases by hematogenous route are not found. With continued passage, these tumors lose their dependence on exogenous estrogen and depend more on endogenous estrogen produced in the adrenal cortex and testis.

Spontaneous Tumor Models

A hereditary, spontaneous tumor of the proximal convoluted tubules was described in a line of Wistar rats by Eker in 1954.[1,105,106] The autosomal dominant trait was mapped to chromosome 10. This gene is lethal in homozygotes. Heterozygous rats develop renal tumors between 4 and 10 months of age.[107] These tumors are described as solid, cystadenomas, and incipient tumors. Metastases are identical to the primary tumor, with the addition of areas of microcalcification. Exposing Eker rats to nitrosamines or streptozotocin can induce chromophobic renal cell tumors. Increased incidence of renal cell carcinomas in Eker rats exposed to *N*-nitrosodimethylamine and ionizing radiation points to a loss of heterozygosity in heterozygotes.[106] The two events (one inherited, one somatic) result in tumor formation. The Eker rat is considered a good model of human renal neoplasia because of its histological similarity. Like human renal cell carcinomas, the tumors in Eker rats overexpress transforming growth factor-α (TGF-α).[106]

The White tumor model[1,108] is a spontaneous adenocarcinoma in the renal cortical tubules of male Wistar-Lewis rats. The tumor does not metastasize, but three types of metastasis models have been developed. In the first model, tumor fragments are placed in the peritoneal cavity of a splenectomized rat; tumor development is 100% in about 9 weeks. Tumors display peritoneal seeding and invasion into the diaphragm, bowel, and muscle wall. In the second model, a single-cell suspension is injected in the tail vein. Tumor development is in 8 to 12 weeks, with a rate of about 30%. Alternatively, single-cell suspensions may be injected under the renal capsule. Response rate is about 80%, with a median development time of 63 d. The White model has been used to evaluate potential chemotherapeutic combinations for cancer treatment.

Claude described two types of spontaneous adenocarcinomas in the renal cortex of BALB/cf/Cd mice.[1,109] These tumors are designated C+ and C–. The C+ tumor invades both kidneys with multiple tumors in each, with a concurrent inhibition in body and organ growth. The C– tumor is a fast-growing, solitary tumor of one kidney, with no inhibition of body or organ growth. Claude's models gave rise to two additional models: the MKT-CD1, or Soloway's model,[1] and the RAG model.[1] The MKT-CD1 model is a spontaneous renal cortical adenocarcinoma in BALB/cf/Cd × BALB/c An N female mice. This tumor resembles human renal cell carcinoma both grossly and histologically and has similar slow-growth characteristics. Because of the inbred strain of these mice, tumors may be transplanted without tumor inhibition by histocompatibility antigens. The RAG model is in

BALB/cf/Cd × BALB/c Crgl mice. This is a heteroploid mouse cell line tumor of 68 to 75 chromosomes.

The RENCA model is a granular cell adenocarcinoma of the renal tubular cells in BALB/c Cr mice.[1] This tumor is characterized by rapid growth and presence of giant and multinucleated cells. On electron microscopy, particles suggestive of virus have been noted, but no tumor could be induced with cell-free extracts. Metastases are found in the lymph nodes and thence to the lungs, liver, spleen, mediastinum, urinary bladder, and serosal surfaces of the gastrointestinal system.

Virally Induced Tumor Models

In 1952, Lucke[39] described a herpesvirus-related, temperature-related adenocarcinoma of the renal tubular cortex in *Rana pipiens*. "Winter" tumors show cytopathological characteristics indicating the presence of the virus, whereas "summer" tumors lack viral characteristics. Metastases via vascular channels are found in the lungs and liver. Tumor implants and dissociated tumor cells were placed in frog embryos by Tweedell[110] but were frequently rejected and failed to produce tumors. However, cell fractions of winter tumors, containing intranuclear inclusion bodies, did produce rapidly growing adenocarcinomas that were histologically identical to Lucke's tumors in mature frogs.

ANIMAL MODELS OF POLYCYSTIC KIDNEY DISEASE

Renal epithelial cysts are the most common abnormality seen in the kidneys.[111] Acquired cysts develop in about 50% of patients on dialysis, and cysts may also be the primary cause of renal failure in inherited cystic disease. Autosomal dominant polycystic kidney disease (ADPKD) is the most common type of inherited cystic disease, affecting 1 in 500 to 1000 individuals.[81,111,112] The inheritance pattern is autosomal dominant and is due to mutations in the PKD-1 gene in 85% and to mutations in the PKD-2 gene in 10%. Most patients are asymptomatic until adulthood. Extrarenal abnormalities in ADPKD patients include hypertension, hepatic cysts, intracranial berry aneurysms, and mitral valve prolapse. In the kidneys, cysts develop in the tubule segments and in Bowman's capsule.[111] Early in development, most cysts are connected to an afferent and efferent tubule segment, although once the cyst reaches 2 mm in diameter, it detaches from either end and secretes fluid via the epithelial lining. Microscopically, alterations in the basement membrane, including thickening, multilamination, and infiltration by inflammatory cells, and fibroblasts, are commonly observed.

Naturally Occurring Models of Polycystic Kidney Disease

Animal models of renal cystic disease include several strains with heritable, spontaneous disease that bear some resemblance to the human counterpart and may help to understand its pathogenesis. Transgenic mice and new strains are being developed to mimic the human disease more closely.

The disease in Han:SPRD cy rats is due to an incomplete autosomal-dominant trait.[111,113] These rats develop cystic disease with focal interstitial infiltration with macrophages, fibroblasts, and leukocytes. Extrarenal pathologies include hyperparathyroidism, osteodystrophic fibrosis, and metastatic calcification affecting the lungs, stomach, blood vessels, heart, and kidneys.[112] Heterozygous males die of uremia by 6 months to 1 year of age, but heterozygous females develop milder cystic enlargement and do not develop severe uremia. Homozygotes, both male and female, are severely ill and die by 3 weeks of age.

The *cpk* mutation was the first model described.[112,114,115] This autosomal-recessive mutation arose spontaneously in a colony of C57BL/6J mice at Jackson Laboratory and later was transferred to a line of congenic DBA/2J mice. Both male and female cpk:cpk mice develop a rapidly progressing cystic enlargement of the kidneys.[111] Death due to renal failure usually occurs by 4 weeks of age. Epidermal growth factor (EGF) is decreased in the distal convoluted tubules, preventing maturation and differentiation of the collecting duct cells,[116] yet EGF is increased in cystic fluid, which may affect cystic enlargement.[112] The saccules thus formed proliferate and distort the collecting ducts and parenchyma, leading to compromised renal function.

The *pcy* mutation arose in the diabetic KK strain and was later transferred to DBA/2J mice.[112,114,117] Inheritance is autosomal recessive. Pcy:pcy mice develop a slowly progressive polycystic kidney disease resembling human ADPKD.[111,112] These mice occasionally also develop cerebral aneurysms. Kidney enlargement is apparent by 8 weeks of age. Macroscopically, cystic formation gives the kidneys a cobblestone-like appearance. Cysts, associated with alterations in the tubular basement membranes, enlarge until renal failure develops at around 8 months of age in males and 6.5 months in females. Thickening of the basement membranes and sporadic enlargement of Bowman's capsule is observed; renal interstitial infiltration by inflammatory cells and fibroblasts is also seen.

A colony of CFW mice spontaneously developed a dominant mutation leading to polycystic kidney disease with adult onset.[112,114,118] Extrarenal lesions reminiscent of ADPKD in humans, including arterial aneurysms and hepatic cysts, occur in up to 20% of affected CFW_{wd} mice. Most mice die by 18 months of age. Environmental factors have been shown to promote disease; in a germ-free environment, only 4% of mice developed renal cysts, but when transferred to conventional housing, 99% developed the disease. Extrarenal lesions were observed only in those mice that were reared in conventional housing or that were moved to conventional housing from a germ-free environment.

The KAT and KAT2J mouse models each have autosomally recessive mutation that confers progressive cystic kidney disease closely resembling ADPKD.[119] KAT2J mice are runts at birth and grow slowly, remaining small throughout life. One third of those that survive weaning die before 100 d of age, and nearly all mice die by 1 year of age. Kidneys in older mice are pale, with cysts replacing much of the parenchyma. KAT mice are also slow to grow, but 22% do survive beyond 1 year of age. Renal cystic lesions are similar to KAT2J mice but are not as severe or extensive.

Induced Models of Polycystic Kidney Disease

Experimental models of PKD can also be induced in transgenic lines of mice or by chemical administration.[112,114] Transgenic mice with a phenotype including polycystic kidneys have been developed using constructs involving the SV40 large T antigen and *c-myc*. Steroid injection and oral administration of 2-amino-4,5-diphenylthiazole HCl (DPT) and nordihydroguaiaretic acid (NDGA) have also been used to create experimental polycystic kidney disease.

A transgenic mouse line used to study choroid plexus tumors was found also to develop cystic lesions in the kidneys.[112,120] A DNA construct using SV40 large T antigen was used to create this line. The mice developed choroid plexus tumors at 3 to 4 months of age. Renal lesions were also noted in a majority of the mice, consisting of tubular epithelial cell proliferation and dilation with cyst formation and of focal glomerular sclerosis.

C-myc overexpression in the kidney in transgenic mice gave rise to polycystic kidneys in 18 transgenic lines.[112,114,121] A *c-myc* transgene was used to create transgenic mice with the intent of evaluating erythroid cell differentiation. The *c-myc* construct, using an SV40 enhancer, led to the development of polycystic kidney disease in a consistent manner. Death due to renal failure occurred between 6 weeks and 3 months of age. The kidneys were markedly enlarged and cystic, although extrarenal lesions such as cerebral aneurysms or hepatic cysts were not found.

TgN737Rpw mice, created by an insertional gene mutation as part of a large-scale program at Oak Ridge National Laboratory, developed scruffy fur, growth retardation, polydactyly, and renal cysts.[112,114,122] The syndrome in mice resembled that of autosomal-recessive polycystic kidney disease (ARPKD), which affects approximately 1 in 10,000 live births and results in infant death and hepatic fibrosis.[81,122] Macroscopically, the kidneys of homozygous mice were pale and slightly enlarged, with cysts that destroyed the surrounding parenchyma. The livers of these mice were slightly pale, with an evident reticular pattern. Histologically, the collecting tubules of the kidneys were dilated with cystic formation, and the livers showed biliary dysplasia and portal hepatic fibrosis. These findings are analogous to those of human ARPKD.

Because mutations in *PKD1* and *PKD2* are associated with ADPKD in humans, there is tremendous interest in developing rodent models with analogous mutations. *PKD1* encodes for polycystin 1, which is expressed in the epithelium and vascular smooth muscle. A mutation in *PKD1* was introduced on C57BL/6 and BALB/c backgrounds.[123] Although heterozygote mice showed no discernable phenotype, homozygotes displayed an embryonic lethality associated with cyst development in the kidneys and pancreatic ducts and pulmonary hypoplasia, implying a role for polycystin in the maturation of renal tubules. A separate mutation in *PKD1* was associated with embryonic mortality in homozygotes caused by vascular leakage;[124] these mice also had renal and pancreatic cyst formation. *PKD2* encodes for polycystin-2. Mice with mutations of *PKD2* have been developed.[125] Heterozygous mice developed renal cysts, the severity of which correlated with the level of polycystin-2 expression in the kidneys. Hepatic cysts were also commonly observed. Homozygotes displayed embryonic lethality with renal cyst formation and, in some, hepatic cyst formation or bile duct proliferation. These results suggest that polycystin-2 also has a role in the maturation of renal tubular structures.

DPT administered to Sprague-Dawley rats in diet or by gavage for 5 weeks created renal cysts in the collecting ducts in 1 to 8 weeks; basement membrane changes resembled those in human ADPKD and in spontaneous heritable polycystic kidney diseases in mice.[112,126] The DPT administration resulted in a marked and progressive, segmental cystic dilation of the collecting and distal tubules, although evidence of tubular obstruction was absent. The kidneys retained normal glomerular and tubular function. It is speculated that the cystic dilation was due to a chemically induced defect affecting the elastic properties of the tubular basement membrane.

NDGA also induces renal cysts in rats that are given the compound in the diet.[112,127,128] Cysts develop as soon as 5 to 7 weeks in the proximal tubules, with thickened, convoluted basement membranes and epithelial cell necrosis, which may contribute to tubular blockage. Inflammatory cell infiltrates were also seen in the interstitium. Cysts developed more rapidly in rats that were raised in a germ-free environment and then transferred to conventional housing than they did in rats that were raised in conventional facilities, implying an immunological component to the disease.

Steroids injected into neonatal rodents in the first week of life can induce polycystic kidney disease.[112,114,129] The mechanism is somewhat controversial; it is uncertain whether the glucocorticoids directly induce the pathology or whether the mineralocorticoid activity indirectly causes renal cysts to form. Some forms of glucocorticoids, such as *tertiary*-butyl-prednisolone, more efficiently produce renal cystic disease. Variations in susceptibility by strain have also been shown in an experiment using 18 different inbred mouse strains.[129] This experiment illustrates the multifactorial pathogenesis of polycystic kidney disease, combining both genetic and environmental factors to induce clinical signs.

Animal Models of Renal Physiology: Hypertension

Hypertensive nephrosclerosis is a leading cause of end-stage renal failure, and the renal injury may add to further hypertension, leading to a cycle of hypertension and renal injury.[130] Not all models of hypertension are designed to study the role of the kidney, but renal pathology does affect the blood pressure via the renin–angiotensin system, and vice versa. Angiotensin II acts as a vasoconstrictor, which can be important in maintaining renal blood flow and glomerular filtration.[131] In fact, in human patients with bilateral renal artery stenosis, or renovascular hypertension, the use of angiotensin-converting enzyme inhibitors to maintain normal blood pressure can result in renal failure due to diminished filtration pressure.

The Goldblatt renal hypertensive model was developed in dogs in the 1930s.[132] The Goldblatt model was adapted to rats, in a two-kidney, one-clip (2K1C) and in a one-kidney, one-clip (1K1C) model, by Mikshe in 1970.[132] The 2K1C model has been used to evaluate the changes in the kidney during hypertension-induced renal failure.[130] Four weeks after the clipping procedure in Sprague-Dawley rats, Mai et al.[130] found progressive increases in size, moderate glomerular mesangial expansion, and widespread tubular atrophy and dilatation in the contralateral (unclipped) kidneys.

A two-kidney, two-clip rat model was developed by Helmchen in 1982 and used again by Satter et al.[131] to evaluate pharmacological therapies for control of hypertension with respect to their effects on renal injury.[131] In this model, 0.25-mm-diameter silver clips were surgically placed around both renal arteries to induce hypertension. The animals were then placed on a low-sodium diet, treated with potential antihypertensive therapies, and evaluated for response to medication and development of renal disease.

Mice make excellent models in which to study the regulation of the renin–angiotensin system. Renin is secreted in response to signals from the macula densa, a collection of specialized epithelial cells in the distal tubule, as part of the tubuloglomerular feedback loop.[133] In most species, including humans, a single gene, *ren-1*, encodes renin; but in wild mice and in several laboratory mouse strains, a second gene, *ren-2*, joins *ren-1* to encode for renin.[132,134] Transgenics can be created to enhance, alter, or delete the expression of either gene. Inactivation of *ren-2* had no phenotypic effects,[135] but inactivation of *ren-1* resulted in hypotension in female mice and in hypercellularity and altered cell morphology in the macula densa.[133] The kidney morphology was otherwise unaffected.

The 2K1C and 1K1C models have been adapted to simulate hypertension in mice.[132] This model was developed on C57BL/6 mice, which carry only *ren-1*, and entailed placing a 0.12-mm-diameter clip on a single renal artery, with or without contralateral nephrectomy. The 2K1C model was shown to have increased plasma renin, although the 1K1C model did not. Both models developed cardiac hypertrophy. These mouse models may be used for evaluation of potential transgenic mouse models to study the hypertension problem in more detail.

The functions of the renin–angiotensin system, including angiotensin II effects, are mediated by AT_1 receptors. Humans have AT_1 receptors only, but rodents have two isoforms, AT_{1A} and AT_{1B}.[136] Angiotensin II functions in the regulation of sodium and water homeostasis. AT_{1A}/AT_{1B} double-knockout mice, as well as other lines that do not produce angiotensin II, develop hydronephrosis that worsens with age.[134] There is atrophy of the renal papillae and inner medulla, along with concurrent impairment of urine-concentrating ability.[136,137] AT_{1A} receptor-deficient mice, such as the *agtr1a (–/–)*, also demonstrate sodium sensitivity, a sodium-dependent change in blood pressure. Aldosterone is increased in response to a decrease in sodium.

Animal Models of Renal Physiology: Development

Congenital anomalies of the kidneys and urinary tract affect approximately 0.5% of pregnancies and are responsible for the major causes of kidney failure in infants.[138] Theories to explain the development of such anomalies include urinary outflow obstruction and defects in the interaction between the metanephric mesoderm and ureteral bud.[139,140] Mackie and Stephens,[141] studying congenital renal malformations in human infants, proposed that ureteral budding from the wolffian duct, if occurring at an abnormal site, would result in urinary outflow obstruction or vesicoureteral reflux, resulting in congenital defects including megaureter and renal hypoplasia.[139,142]

Obstruction of the urinary tract during fetal development produces fibrosis and alterations in the growth of the developing kidney. The renin–angiotensin system interacts with TGF-β to produce these congenital changes.[143] Models of congenital urinary tract obstruction include rabbits, opossum, and sheep, as well as transgenic (knockout) mice.

Surgical models of fetal urinary obstruction have been carried out in large animals for several years. Beck,[144] in the 1970s, carried out experiments in which surgical ureteral ligation in fetal sheep was shown to produce hydronephrosis, with renal contraction. Dilation and thickening of the ureter was also observed when obstruction occurred early in development. In another group, persistent urinary obstruction created in fetal sheep by ureteral and urethral ligation led to the development of hydronephrotic, cystic, or dysgenetic kidneys.[145] Hydronephrotic kidneys were enlarged, with partial effacement of the medulla and dilation of tubules. Cystic kidneys had distorted renal architecture between the cysts, with almost total elimination of the medulla. Dysgenetic kidneys were small, with distortion of the cortex, dilated tubules, and fetal medullary structures.

Vesicoureteral reflux due to bladder outlet obstruction has also been modeled in fetal sheep,[146] demonstrating resultant hydronephrosis with thinning of the cortex and loss of medullary tissue and thickened, tortuous ureters. Furthermore, partial bladder outlet obstruction was associated with increased mRNA levels for renin and AT_2.[147] AT_2 activates TGF-β1, which may be a mechanism for renal fibrosis. Persistence of the AT_2 and AT_1 expression pattern that is usually seen in early development also suggests attempts at compensatory adaptation by the developing kidney.

Experimental obstructive hydronephrosis has also been evaluated in newborn rats and adult rabbits. Newborn Sprague-Dawley rats underwent partial ureteric obstruction, and the kidneys were examined 9 weeks later.[148] Hydronephrosis, with flattening of the renal papilla and thinning of the cortices, was a consistent finding. In experimentally obstructed New Zealand white rabbits, decreases in urine-concentrating ability were thought to be related to observed changes in all segments of the nephron.[149] Chronic obstruction produced papillary necrosis and fibrosis.[150]

The fetal or newborn opossum provides an attractive model for the study of fetal urinary obstruction.[151] Because the young are born shortly after conception and complete their development while attached to the teat, these marsupials are readily accessible to surgical manipulation. This model has been used to identify the roles of insulin-like growth factor and platelet-derived growth factor on obstructed developing kidneys.[143,152] Histologic evaluation of kidneys with early obstruction as compared with those with late obstruction showed ductal hyperplasia and medullary and cortical aplasia; obstruction late in development produced less severe medullary dysplasia.[153] These studies may suggest potential therapeutic interventions or markers for early detection of obstruction.

Angiotensin has been shown to affect development of kidney structure in rodents.[136,137,154,155] Renin expression is highest in the kidneys of fetal and neonatal rats, and angiotensin I (AT_1) and angiotensin II (AT_2) levels are also higher in the kidneys of newborn rats than in adults. The distribution of AT_1 and AT_2 during development suggests specific roles for each: AT_2 receptor expression is highest in undifferentiated mesenchyma and declines with maturation, suggesting a role for AT_2 in morphogenesis regulation; whereas AT_1 receptor expression is higher in more differentiated structures, suggesting that AT_1 is involved in regulating late stages of renal vascular development and in regulating the hemodynamic and reabsorption functions of the renal angiotensin system.[155] As noted earlier, AT_1 nullizygote mice develop shortened papillae and subsequent hyposthenuria.[137] *Agtr2*-null mutant mice develop hydronephrotic kidneys with stenosis at the uteropelvic junction, renal hypoplasia, multicystic kidneys, and renal aplasia.[138]

The *atg–/–* mouse demonstrates the role of the renin–angiotensin system in fetal development.[134] *Atg–/–* mice, which fail to produce angiotensinogen, develop delays in glomerular maturity that are most apparent postnatally.[154] Knockout mice are produced in normal numbers, but few survive to weaning. Those that do survive are hypotensive and display several structural abnormalities in the kidney, including hypertrophy of the renal arteries, atrophy of the papillae, and focal areas of tubular atrophy. No such phenotype is seen when either *ren-1* or *ren-2* are disrupted, but complete renin knockouts show similar renal pathology, suggesting a compensatory role by the residual gene. Angiotensin-converting enzyme-deficient mice are noted to have a similar phenotype.

The wolffian duct, before ureteral budding, is surrounded by undifferentiated mesenchymal cells that express AT_2 receptors. AT_2, as part of its role in morphogenesis, promotes apoptosis. It has been proposed that as a result of failure of this apoptosis, the necessary signaling between the wolffian duct and the metanephric blastema to induce ureteral budding would be interrupted, resulting in ectopic ureteral budding.[139,142] This ectopic budding has been observed in *Agtr2*-null mutant embryos, lending support to this hypothesis.

A naturally occurring model of obstructive hydronephrosis is seen in the *cph* mouse.[156] This autosomal mutation arose in a colony of C57BL/6J mice at the Jackson Laboratory. Homozygous mice are phenotypically distinguishable by 2 weeks of age, having smaller size, distended abdomens, and colorless urine. Most affected mice die of renal failure by 1 to 2 months of age, although some do survive to adulthood. The obstruction arises from a stenosis at the ureteropelvic junction. Kidneys show erosion of the papilla and thinning of cortical tissue.

Fish models give another perspective on development and repair mechanisms.[157] The pattern of mammalian regeneration has been studied in rats given nephrotoxic doses of mercuric chloride, resulting in sloughing of the epithelium and leaving a denuded basement membrane of the proximal tubule. In 3 to 4 d, basophilic, flattened squamous cells were observed in the injured sites; by 5 to 7 d, these had become short, cuboidal basophilic cells. Normal morphology returned by 3 to 4 weeks after injury. Creatinine clearance began improving 7 to 10 d after injury. Fish have shown similar repair processes. Renal function parameters such as creatinine clearance are difficult to assess in fish, but clinical signs such as exophthalmia, ascites, decreased packed cell volume, and hypoproteinemia correlate with the mammalian observations.

CONCLUSIONS

Most modeling of renal pathophysiology is done in rodents. These models can be refined with the use of transgenic (knockout) models for specific aspects of the problem in question. Naturally occurring models may also provide some new avenues into understanding these diseases. From fish to mink, there are a wide variety of conditions that may mimic some aspect of human renal disease.

In several cases, treatment that shows good potential in the model has a lesser response in clinical practice. In other cases, differences between the animal model and the human condition overshadow any understanding derived from the model system. Further improvement in developing animal models that more closely mimic human diseases is an ongoing process. As our understanding of the pathogenic mechanisms involved in renal disease grows, we can expect to develop more sophisticated models that will further enhance our understanding of these important human conditions.

REFERENCES

1. Rangel, M.C. and Pontes, J.E., Animal models of renal cell carcinoma, *Seminars in Urology*, 7, 237–246, 1989.
2. Foster, M.H., Relevance of systemic lupus erythematosus nephritis animal models to human disease, *Seminars in Nephrology*, 19, 12–24, 1999.
3. Lieberthal, W. and Nigam, S.K., Acute renal failure. II. Experimental models of acute renal failure: imperfect but indispensable, *American Journal of Physiology, Renal Physiology*, 278, F1–F12, 2000.
4. Endo, Y., IgA nephropathy — human disease and animal model, *Renal Failure*, 19, 347–371, 1997.
5. Montinero, V., Gesualdo, L., and Schena, F.P., The relevance of experimental models in the pathogenetic investigation of primary IgA nephropathy, *Annales de Medicine Interne*, 150, 99–107, 1999.
6. Scivittaro, V., Amore, A., and Emancipator, S.N., Animal models as a means to study IgA nephropathy, *Contributions to Nephrology*, 104, 65–78, 1993.
7. Sinniah, R., Occurrence of mesangial IgA and IgM deposits in a control necropsy population, *Journal of Clinical Pathology*, 36, 276–279, 1983.
8. Rehan, A., Johnson, K.J., Wiggins, R.C., Kunkel, R.G., and Ward, P.A., Evidence for the role of oxygen radicals in acute nephrotoxic nephritis, *Laboratory Investigation*, 51, 396–403, 1984.

9. Rifai, A., Small, P.A., Jr., Teague, P.O., and Ayoub, E.M., Experimental IgA nephropathy, *Journal of Experimental Medicine*, 150, 1161–1173, 1979.

10. Fornasieri, A. and D'Amico, G., Experimental IgA mesangial nephropathy: the role of antigen and antibody, *Contributions to Nephrology*, 111, 149–154, 1995.

11. Isaacs, K., Miller, F., and Lane, B., Experimental model for IgA nephropathy, *Clinical Immunology and Immunopathology*, 20, 419–426, 1981.

12. Isaacs, K. and Miller, F., Dextran-induced IgA nephropathy, *Contributions to Nephrology*, 40, 45–50, 1984.

13. Pasi, A., Dendorfer, U., Holthöfer, H., Nelson, P.J., Tazzari, S., Armelloni, S., Fornasieri, A., D'Amico, G., and Schlöndorff, D., Characterization of nephropathy induced by immunization with high molecular weight dextran, *Nephrology, Dialysis, Transplantation*, 12, 1849–1855, 1997.

14. Emancipator, S.N., Gallo, G.P., and Lamm, M.E., Experimental IgA nephropathy induced by oral immunization, *Journal of Experimental Medicine*, 157, 572–582, 1983.

15. Coppo, R., Roccatello, D., Amore, A., Quattrocchio, G., Molino, A., Gianoglio, B., Amoroso, A., Bajardi, P., and Piccoli, G., Effects of a gluten-free diet in primary IgA nephropathy, *Clinical Nephrology*, 33, 72–86, 1990.

16. Coppo, R., Mazzucco, G., Martina, G., Roccatello, D., Amore, A., Novara, R., Bargoni, A., Piccoli, G., and Sena, L.M., Gluten-induced experimental IgA glomerulopathy, *Laboratory Investigation*, 4, 499–506, 1989.

17. Yan, D., Rumbeiha, W.K., and Pestka, J.J., Experimental murine IgA nephropathy following passive administration of vomitoxin-induced IgA monoclonal antibodies, *Food and Chemical Toxicology*, 36, 1095–1106, 1998.

18. Greene, D.M., Azcona-Olivera, J.I., and Pestka, J.J., Vomitoxin (deoxynivalenol)-induced IgA nephropathy in the B6C3F$_1$ mouse: dose response and male predilection, *Toxicology*, 92, 245–260, 1994.

19. Imai, H., Nakamoto, Y., Asakura, K., Miki, K., Yasuda, T., and Miura, A.B., Spontaneous glomerular IgA deposition in ddY mice: an animal model of IgA nephritis, *Kidney International*, 27, 756–761, 1985.

20. Muso, E., Yoshida, H., Takeuchi, E., Yashiro, M., Matsushima, H., Oyama, A., Suyama, K., Kawamura, T., Kamata, T., Miyawaki, S., Izui, S., and Sasayama, S., Enhanced production of glomerular extracellular matrix in a new mouse strain of high serum IgA ddY mice, *Kidney International*, 50, 1946–1957, 1996.

21. Miyawaki, S., Muso, E., Takeuchi, E., Matsushima, H., Shibata, Y., Sasayama, S., and Yoshida, H., Selective breeding for high serum IgA levels from noninbred ddY mice: isolation of a strain with an early onset of glomerular IgA deposition, *Nephron*, 76, 201–207, 1997.

22. Gude, W.G. and Lupton, A.C., Spontaneous glomerulosclerosis in aging RF mice, *Journal of Gerontology*, 15, 373–376, 1960.

23. Kamata, T., Muso, E., Yashiro, M., Kawamura, T., Oyama, A., Matsushima, H., Takeuchi, E., Yoshida, H, and Sasayama, S., Up-regulation of glomerular extracellular matrix and transforming growth factor-β expression in RF/J mice, *Kidney International*, 55, 864–876, 1999.

24. Stad, R.K., Bruijn, J.A., van Gijlswijk-Janssen, D.J., van Es, L.A., and Daha, M.R., An acute model for IgA-mediated glomerular inflammation in rats induced by monoclonal polymeric rat IgA antibodies, *Clinical and Experimental Immunology*, 92, 514–521, 1993.

25. Diamond, J.R., The role of reactive oxygen species in animal models of glomerular disease, *The Journal of Laboratory and Clinical Medicine*, 124, 468–469, 1994.

26. Ito, M., Yamada, H., Okamoto, K., and Suzuki, Y., Crescentic type nephritis induced by anti-glomerular basement membrane (GBM) serum in rats, *Japanese Journal of Pharmacology*, 33, 1145–1154, 1983.

27. Lannigan, R., Kark, R., and Pollak, V.E., The effect of a single intravenous injection of aminonucleoside of puromycin on the rat kidney: a light- and electron-microscope study, *Journal of Pathology and Bacteriology*, 83, 357–362, 1962.

28. Diamond, J.R. and Karnovsky, M.J., Focal and segmental glomerulosclerosis following a single intravenous dose of puromycin aminonucleoside, *American Journal of Pathology*, 122, 481–487, 1986.

29. Ryan, G.B. and Karnovsky, M.J., An ultrastructural study of the mechanisms of proteinuria in aminonucleoside nephrosis, *Kidney International*, 8, 219–232, 1975.

30. Diamond, J.R., Bonventre, J.V., and Karnovsky, M.J., A role for oxygen free radicals in aminonucleoside nephrosis, *Kidney International*, 29, 478–483, 1986.

31. Robinson, R.R. and Dennis, V.W., Spontaneously occurring animal models of human kidney diseases and altered renal function, *Advances in Nephrology from the Necker Hospital*, 9, 315–366, 1980.

32. Slauson, D.O. and Lewis, R.M., Comparative pathology of glomerulonephritis in animals, *Veterinary Pathology*, 16, 135–164, 1979.

33. Lerner, R.A. and Dixon, F.J., Spontaneous glomerulonephritis in sheep, *Laboratory Investigation*, 15, 1279–1289, 1966.

34. Angus, K.W., Sykes, A.R., Gardiner, A.C., and Morgan, K.T., Mesangiocapillary glomerulonephritis in lambs. I. Clinical and biochemical findings in a Finnish Landrace flock, *Journal of Comparative Pathology*, 84, 309–317, 1974.

35. Angus, K.W., Gardiner, A.C., Morgan, K.T., and Gray, E.W., Mesangiocapillary glomerulonephritis in lambs. II. Pathological findings and electron microscopy of the renal lesions, *Journal of Comparative Pathology*, 84, 319–330, 1974.

36. Peutz-Kootstra, C.J., de Heer, E., Hoedemaeker, P.J., Abrass, C.K., and Bruijn, J.A., Lupus nephritis: lessons from experimental animal models, *The Journal of Laboratory and Clinical Medicine*, 137, 244–260, 2001.

37. Perampalam, S., Wang, L., Myers-Mason, N., Yeow, J.N., Stanietsky, N., Phillips, J., Weitz, J.I., Ackerley, C., Levy, G.A., and Cole, E.H., Identification of a unique glomerular factor X activator in murine lupus nephritis, *Journal of the American Society of Nephrology*, 10, 2332–2341, 1999.

38. Andrews, B.S., Eisenberg, R.A., Theofilopoulos, A.N., Izui, S., Wilson, C.B., McConahey, P.J., Murphy, E.D., Roths, J.B., and Dixon, F.J., Spontaneous murine lupus-like syndromes. Clinical and immmunopathological manifestations in several strains, *Journal of Experimental Medicine*, 148, 1198–1215, 1978.

39. Specks, U., Are animal models of vasculitis suitable tools?, *Current Opinion in Rheumatology*, 12, 11–19, 2000.

40. Murphy, E.D. and Roths, J.B., New inbred strains, *Mouse News Letter*, 58, 51–52, 1978.

41. Theofilopoulos, A.N. and Dixon, F.J., Murine models of systemic lupus erythematosus, *Advances in Immunology*, 37, 269–390, 1985.

42. Makino, M., Fujiwara, M., and Watanabe, H., Studies on the mechanisms of the development of lupus nephritis in BXSB mice. I. Analysis of immunological abnormalities at the onset period, *Journal of Clinical and Laboratory Immunology*, 122, 127–131, 1987.

43. Dixon, F.J., Andrews, B.S., Eisenberg, R.A., McConahey, P.J., Theofilopoulos, A.N., and Wilson, C.B., Etiology and pathogenesis of a spontaneous lupus-like syndrome in mice, *Arthritis and Rheumatism*, 21(Suppl. 5), S64–S67, 1978.

44. Honda, S., Nemoto, K., Mae, T., Kinjoh, K., Kyogoku, M., Kawamura, H., Miyazawa, S., Weerashinghe, A., Watanabe, H., Narita, J., Koya, T., Arakawa, M., and Abo, T., Mice with early onset of death (EOD) due to lupus glomerulonephritis, *Clinical and Experimental Immunology*, 116, 153–163, 1999.

45. Kinjoh, K., Kyogoku, M., and Good, R.A., Genetic selection for crescent formation yields mouse strain with rapidly progressive glomerulonephritis and small vessel vasculitis, *Proceedings of the National Academy of Sciences of the United States of America*, 90, 3413–3417, 1993.

46. Shaheen, V.M., Satoh, M., Richards, H.B., Yoshida, H., Shaw, M., Jennette, J.C., and Reeves, W.H., Immunopathogenesis of environmentally induced lupus in mice, *Environmental Health Perspectives*, 107(Suppl. 5), 723–727, 1999.

47. Satoh, M., Kumar, A., Kanwar, Y.S., and Reeves, W.H., Anti-nuclear antibody production and immune-complex glomerulonephritis in BALB/c mice treated with pristane, *Proceedings of the National Academy of Sciences of the United States of America*, 92, 10934–10938, 1995.

48. Satoh, M. and Reeves, W.H., Induction of lupus-associated autoantibodies in BALB/c mice by intraperitoneal injection of pristane, *Journal of Experimental Medicine*, 180, 2341–2346, 1994.

49. Kettritz, R., Yang, J.J., Kinjoh, K., Jennette, J.C., and Falk, R.J., Animal models in ANCA-vasculitis, *Clinical and Experimental Immunology*, 101(Suppl. 1), 12–15, 1995.

50. Falk, R.J., ANCA-associated renal disease, *Kidney International*, 38, 998–1010, 1990.

51. Tervaert, J.W.C., Goldschmeding, R., Elema, J.D., van der Giessen, M., Huitema, M.G., van der Hem, G.K., The, T.H., von dem Borne, A.E.G.Kr., and Kallenberg, C.G.M., Autoantibodies against myeloid lysosomal enzymes in crescentic glomerulonephritis, *Kidney International*, 37, 799–806, 1990.

52. Brouwer, E., Huitema, M.G., Klok, P.A., deWeerd, H., Tervaert, J.W.C., Weening, J.J., and Kallenberg, C.G.M., Antimyeloperoxidase-associated proliferative glomerulonephritis: an animal model, *Journal of Experimental Medicine*, 177, 905–914, 1993.

53. Brouwer, E., Klok, P.A., Huitema, M.G., Weening, J.J., and Kallenberg, C.G.M., Renal ischemia/reperfusion injury contributes to renal damage in experimental anti-myeloperoxidase-associated proliferative glomerulonephritis, *Kidney International*, 47, 1121–1129, 1995.

54. Kobayashi, K., Shibita, T., and Sugisaki, T., Aggravation of rat nephrotoxic serum nephritis by anti-myeloperoxidase antibodies, *Kidney International*, 47, 454–463, 1995.

55. Yang, J.J., Jennette, J.C., and Falk, R.J., Immune complex glomerulonephritis is induced in rats immunized with heterologous myeloperoxidase, *Clinical and Experimental Immunology*, 97, 466–473, 1994.

56. Bruijn, J.A., van Elven, E.H., Hogendoorn, P.C.W., Corver, W.E., Hoedemaeker, P.J., and Fleuren, G.J., Murine chronic graft-versus-host disease as a model for lupus nephritis, *American Journal of Pathology*, 130, 639–641, 1988.

57. Bruijn, J.A., Kootstra, C.J., Sutmuller, M.J., Van Vliet, A.I., Bergijk, E.C., and de Heer, E., Matrix and adhesion molecules in kidney pathology: recent observations, *Journal of Laboratory and Clinical Medicine*, 130, 357–364, 1997.

58. Kootstra, C.J., Sutmuller, M., Baelde, H.J., de Heer, E., and Bruijn, J.A., Association between leukocyte infiltration and development of glomerulosclerosis in experimental lupus nephritis, *Journal of Pathology*, 184, 219–225, 1998.

59. Shike, T., Funabiki, K., and Tomino, Y., Animal models, *Contributions to Nephrology*, 134, 9–15, 2001.

60. Riley, S.G., Evans, R.A., Davies, M., Floege, J., and Phillips, A.O., Goto-Kakizaki rat is protected from proteinuria after induction of anti-thy1 nephritis, *American Journal of Kidney Diseases*, 39, 985–1000, 2002.

61. Phillips, A.O., Baboolal, K., Riley, S., Gröne, H., Janssen, U., Steadman, R., Williams, J., and Floege, J., Association of prolonged hyperglycemia with glomerular hypertrophy and renal basement membrane thickening in the Goto Kakizaki model of non-insulin-dependent diabetes mellitus, *American Journal of Kidney Diseases*, 37, 400–410, 2001.

62. Goto, Y., Kakizaki, M., and Masaki, N., Production of spontaneous diabetic rats by repetition of selective breeding, *Tohoku Journal of Experimental Medicine*, 119, 85–90, 1976.

63. Reddi, A.S., Oppermann, W., Patel, D.G., Ehrenreich, T., and Camerini-Davalos, R.A., Diabetic microangiopathy in KK mice. III. Effect of prolonged glyburide treatment on glomerulosclerosis, *Experimental and Molecular Pathology*, 29, 92–101, 1978.

64. Feliers, D., Duraisamy, S., Faulkner, J.L., Duch, J., Lee, A.V., Abboud, H., Choudhury, G.G., and Kasinath, B.S., Activation of renal signaling pathways in db/db mice with type 2 diabetes, *Kidney International*, 60, 495–504, 2001.

65. Chen, H., Chalat, O., Tartaglia, L.A., Woolf, E.A., Weng, X., Ellis, S.J., Breitbart, R.E., Duyk, G.M., Tepper, R.I., and Morgenstern, J.P., Evidence that the diabetes gene encodes the leptin receptor: identification of a mutation in the leptin receptor gene in db/db mice, *Cell*, 84, 491–495, 1996.

66. Yong, L.C.J. and Bleasel, A.F., Pathological changes in streptozotocin induced diabetes mellitus in the rat, *Experimental Pathology*, 30, 97–107, 1986.

67. Banks, K.L., Henson, J.B., and McGuire, T.C., Immunologically mediated glomerulitis of horses. I. Pathogenesis in persistent infection by equine infectious anemia virus, *Laboratory Investigation*, 26, 701–707, 1972.

68. Cheville, N.F., Mengeling, W.L., and Zinober, M.R., Ultrastructural and immunofluorescent studies of glomerulonephritis in chronic hog cholera, *Laboratory Investigation*, 22, 458–467, 1970.

69. Portis, J.L. and Coe, J.E., Deposition of IgA in renal glomeruli of mink affected with Aleutian disease, *American Journal of Pathology*, 96, 227–236, 1979.

70. Mori, S., Nose, M., Miyazawa, M., Kyogoku, M., Wolfinbarger, J.B., and Bloom, M.E., Interstitial nephritis in Aleutian mink disease. Possible role of cell-mediated immunity against virus-infected tubular epithelial cells, *American Journal of Pathology*, 144, 1326–1333, 1994.

71. Jessen, R.H., Nedrud, J.G., and Emancipator, S.N., A mouse model of IgA nephropathy induced by Sendai virus, *Advances in Experimental Medicine and Biology*, 216B, 1609–1618, 1987.

72. Jessen, R.H., Emancipator, S.N., Jacobs, G.H., and Nedrud, J.G., Experimental IgA-IgG nephropathy induced by a viral respiratory pathogen. Dependence on antigen form and immune status, *Laboratory Investigation*, 67, 379–386, 1992.

73. Amore, A., Roccatello, D., Picciotto, G., Emancipator, S.N., Ropolo, R., Cacace, G., Suriani, A., Gianoglio, B., Sena, L.M., Cirina, P., Mazzucco, G., Alfieri, V., Piccoli, G., Coppo, R., and De Filippi, P.G., Processing of IgA aggregates in a rat model of chronic liver disease, *Clinical Immunology and Immunopathology*, 84, 107–114, 1997.

74. Gormly, A.A., Smith, P.S., Seymour, A.E., Clarkson, A.R., and Woodroffe, A.J., IgA glomerular deposits in experimental cirrhosis, *American Journal of Pathology*, 104, 50–54, 1981.

75. Ogata, S., Takeda, M., Lee, M.-J., Itagaki, S.-I., and Doi, K., Histopathological sequence of hepatic and renal lesions in rats after cessation of the repeated administration of CCl_4, *Experimental and Toxicologic Pathology*, 47, 493–499, 1995.

76. Smith, S.M., Yu, G.S.M., and Tsukamoto, H., IgA nephropathy in alcohol abuse. An animal model, *Laboratory Investigation*, 62, 179–184, 1990.

77. Razani-Boroujerdi, S., Tokuda, S., and Smith, S.M., Increased natural killer cell activity in a model of immunoglobulin A nephropathy secondary to chronic alcohol consumption, *Alcoholism: Clinical and Experimental Research*, 17, 860–863, 1993.

78. Woodroffe, A.J., IgA, glomerulonephritis, and liver disease, *Australian and New Zealand Journal of Medicine*, 11(Suppl. 1), 109–111, 1981.

79. Rosen, S. and Heyman, S.N., Difficulties in understanding human "acute tubular necrosis": limited data and flawed animal models, *Kidney International*, 60, 1220–1224, 2001.

80. Solez, K., Morel-Maroger, L., and Sraer, J.-D., The morphology of "acute tubular necrosis" in man: analysis of 57 renal biopsies and a comparison with the glycerol model, *Medicine*, 58, 362–376, 1979.

81. Cotran, R.S., Kumar, V., and Collins, T.C, *Robbins Pathologic Basis of Disease,* 6th ed., W.B. Saunders, Philadelphia, 1999.

82. Zaeger, R.A. and Altschuld, R., Body temperature: an important determinant of severity of ischemic renal injury, *American Journal of Physiology*, 25, F87–F93, 1986.

83. Shanley, P.F., Rosen, M.D., Brezis, M., Silva, P., Epstein, F.H., and Rosen, S., Topography of focal proximal tubular necrosis after ischemia with reflow in the rat kidney, *American Journal of Pathology*, 122, 462–468, 1986.

84. Donahoe, J.F., Venkatachalam, M.A., Bernard, D.B., and Levinsky, N.G., Tubular leakage and obstruction after renal ischemia: structural-functional correlations, *Kidney International*, 13, 208–222, 1978.

85. Finn, W.F. and Chevalier, R.L., Recovery from postischemic acute renal failure in the rat, *Kidney International*, 16, 113–123, 1979.

86. Harvig, B., Engberg, A., and Ericsson, J.L.E., Effects of cold ischemia on the preserved and transplanted rat kidney. Structural changes of the proximal tubule, *Virchows Archive B Cell Pathology*, 34, 153–171, 1980.

87. Harvig, B., Engberg, A., and Ericsson, J.L.E., Effects of cold ischemia on the preserved and transplanted rat kidney. Stuctural changes of the loop of Henle, distal tubule and collecting duct, *Virchows Archive B Cell Pathology*, 34, 173–192, 1980.

88. Nath, K.A., Balla, G., Vercellotti, G.M., Balla, J., Jacob, H.S., Levitt, M.D., and Rosenberg, M.E., Induction of heme oxygenase is a rapid, protective response in rhabdomyolysis in the rat, *Journal of Clinical Investigation*, 90, 267–270, 1992.

89. Wieczorowska-Tobis, K., Breborowicz, A., Pawlaczyk, K., Kuzlan-Pawlaczyk, M., Polubinska, A., and Oreopoulos, D.G., Animal models for peritoneal dialysis, *Peritoneal Dialysis International*, 19, S365–S369, 1999.

90. Lamiere, N., Van Biesen, W., Van Landschoot, M., Wang, T., Heimbürger, O., Bergström, J., Lindholm, B., Hekking, L.P.H., Havenith, C.E.G., and Beelen, R.H.J., Experimental models in peritoneal dialysis: a European experience, *Kidney International*, 54, 2194–2206, 1998.

91. Wieczorowska-Tobis, K., Dorybalska, K., Polubinska, A., Radkowski, M., Breborowicz, A., and Oreopoulos, D.G., *In vivo* model to study the biocompatiblility of peritoneal dialysis solutions, *The International Journal of Artificial Organs*, 20, 673–677, 1997.

92. Garosi, G. and DiPaolo, N., The rabbit model in evaluating the biocompatibility in peritoneal dialysis, *Nephrology, Dialysis, and Transplantation*, 12, 664–665, 2001.

93. Gotloib, L., Crassweller, P., Rodella, H., Oreopoulos, D.G., Zellerman, G., Ogilvie, R., Husdan, H., Brandes, L., and Vas, S., Experimental model for studies of continuous peritoneal dialysis in uremic rabbits, *Nephron*, 31, 254–259, 1982.

94. Griffin, K.A., Picken, M.M., Churchill, M., Churchill, P., and Bidani, A.K., Functional structural correlates of glomerulosclerosis after renal mass reduction in the rat, *Journal of the American Society of Nephrology*, 11, 497–506, 2000.

95. Boudet, J., Man, N.K., Pils, P., Sausse, A., and Funck-Brentano, J.-L., Experimental chronic renal failure in the rat by electrocoagulation of the renal cortex, *Kidney International*, 14, 82–86, 1978.

96. Miller, T.E., Findon, G., and Rowe, L., Characterization of an animal model of continuous peritoneal dialysis in chronic renal impairment, *Clinical Nephrology*, 37, 42–47, 1992.

97. Maher, J.F., Przemyslaw, H., Bennett, R.R., and Chakrabarti, E., Amphotericin selectively increases peritoneal ultrafiltration, *American Journal of Kidney Diseases*, 4, 285–288, 1984.

98. Gagnon, R.F. and Richards, G.K., A mouse model of implant-associated infection, *The International Journal of Artificial Organs*, 16, 789–798, 1993.

99. Read, R.R., Eberwein, P., Dasgupta, M.K., Grant, S.K., Lam, K., Nickel, J.C., and Costerton, J.W., Peritonitis in peritoneal dialysis: bacterial colonization by biofilm spread along the catheter surface, *Kidney International*, 35, 614–621, 1989.

100. Gallimore, B., Gagnon, R.F., and Richards, G.K., Response to intraperitoneal *Staphylococcus epidermidis* challenge in renal failure mice, *Kidney International*, 32, 678–683, 1987.

101. Gruys, M.E., Back, T.C., Subleski, J., Wiltrout, T.A., Lee, J.-K., Schmidt, L., Watanabe, M., Stanyon, R., Ward, J.M., Wigginton, J.M., and Wiltrout, R.H., Induction of transplantable mouse renal cell cancers by streptozotocin: *in vivo* growth, metastases, and angiogenic phenotype, *Cancer Research*, 61, 6255–6263, 2001.

102. Hiasa, Y. and Ito, N., Experimental induction of renal tumors, *Critical Reviews in Toxicology*, 17, 279–343, 1987.

103. Nogueira, E., Cardesa, A., and Mohr, U., Experimental models of kidney tumors, *Journal of Cancer Research and Clinical Oncology*, 119, 190–198, 1993.

104. Magee, P.N. and Barnes, J.M., Induction of kidney tumours in the rat with dimethylnitrosamine, (*N*-nitrosodimethylamine), *Journal of Pathology and Bacteriology*, 84, 19–31, 1962.

105. Bannasch, P. and Zerban, H., Pathogenesis of renal cell adenomas and carcinomas in animal models, *Contributions to Nephrology*, 128, 99–125, 1999.

106. Everitt, J.I., Goldsworthy, T.L., Wolf, D.C., and Walker, C.L., Hereditary renal cell carcinoma in the Eker rat: a unique animal model for the study of cancer susceptibility, *Toxicology Letters*, 82/83, 621–625, 1995.

107. Walker, C., Recio, L., Funaki, K., and Everitt, J., Cytogenetic and molecular correlates between rodent and human renal cell carcinoma, *Progress in Clinical and Biological Research*, 376, 289–302, 1992.

108. White, R.V. and Olsson, C.A., Renal adenocarcinoma in the rat. A new tumor model, *Investigative Urology*, 17, 405–412, 1980.

109. Claude, A., A spontaneous, transplantable renal carcinoma of the mouse. Electron microscope study of the cells and of an associated virus-like particle, *Journal of Ultrastructure Research*, 6, 1–18, 1962.

110. Tweedell, K.S., Induced oncogenesis in developing frog kidney cells, *Cancer Research*, 27, 2042–2052, 1967.

111. Grantham, J.J., Pathogenesis of renal cyst expansion: opportunities for therapy, *American Journal of Kidney Diseases,* 23, 210–218, 1994.

112. Aziz, N., Animal models of polycystic kidney disease, *BioEssays*, 17, 703–712, 1995.

113. Cowley, B.D., Jr., Gudapaty, S., Kraybill, A.L., Barash, B.D., Harding, M.A., Calvet, J.P., and Gattone, V.H., II, Autosomal-dominant polycystic kidney disease in the rat, *Kidney International*, 43, 522–534, 1993.

114. Schieren, G., Pey, R., Bach, J., Hafner, M., and Gretz, N., Murine models of polycystic kidney disease, *Nephrology, Dialysis, Transplantation*, 11(Suppl. 6), 38–45, 1996.

115. Fry, J.L., Jr., Koch, W.E., Jennette, J.C., McFarland, E., Fried, F.A., and Mandell, J., A genetically determined murine model of infantile polycystic kidney disease, *The Journal of Urology*, 134, 828–833, 1985.

116. Gattone, V.H., II, Andrews, G.K., Fu-wen, N., Chadwick, L.J., Klein, R.M., and Calvet, J.P., Defective epidermal growth factor gene expression in mice with polycystic kidney disease, *Developmental Biology*, 138, 225–230, 1990.

117. Takahashi, H., Calvet, J.P., Dittemore-Hoover, D., Yoshido, K., Grantham, J J., and Gattone, V.H., II, A hereditary model of slowly progressive polycystic kidney disease in the mouse, *Journal of the American Society of Nephrology*, 1, 980–989, 1991.

118. Werder, A.A., Amos, M.A., Nielsen, A.H., and Wolfe, G.H., Comparative effects of germfree and ambient environments on the development of cystic kidney disease in CFW_{wd} mice, *Journal of Laboratory and Clinical Medicine*, 103, 399–407, 1984.

119. Vogler, C., Homan, S., Pung, A., Thorpe, C., Barker, J., Birkenmeier, E.H., and Upadhya, P., Clinical and pathologic findings in two new allelic murine models of polycystic kidney disease, *Journal of the American Society of Nephrology*, 10, 2534–2539, 1999.

120. MacKay, K., Striker, L.J., Pinkert, C.A., Brinster, R.L., and Striker, G.E., Glomerulosclerosis and renal cysts in mice transgenic for the early region of SV40, *Kidney International*, 32, 827–837, 1987.

121. Trudel, M., D'Agati, V., and Costantini, F., c-myc as an inducer of polycystic kidney disease in transgenic mice, *Kidney International*, 39, 665–671, 1991.

122. Moyer, J.H., Leo-Tischler, M.J., Kwon, H.-Y., Schrick, J.J., Avner, E.D., Sweeney, W.E., Godfrey, V.L., Cacheiro, N.L.A., Wilkinson, J.E., and Woychik, R.P., Candidate gene associated with a mutation causing recessive polycystic kidney disease in mice, *Science*, 264, 1329–1333, 1994.

123. Lu, W., Peissel, B., Babakhanlou, H., Pavlova, A., Geng, L., Fan, X., Larson, C., Brent, G., and Zhou, J., Perinatal lethality with kidney and pancreas defects in mice with a targetted Pkd1 mutation, *Nature Genetics*, 17, 179–181, 1997.

124. Kim, K., Drummond, I., Ibraghimov-Beskrovnaya, O., Klinger, K., and Arnaout, M.A., Polycystin 1 is required for the structural integrity of blood vessels, *Proceedings of the National Academy of Sciences of the United States of America*, 97, 1731–1736, 2000.

125. Wu, G., D'Agati, V., Cai, Y., Markowitz, G., Park, J.H., Reynolds, D.M., Maeda, Y., Le, T.H., Hou, H., Jr., Kucherlapati, R., Edelmann, W., and Somlo, S., Somatic inactivation of Pkd2 results in polycystic kidney disease, *Cell*, 93, 177–188, 1998.

126. Carone, F.A., Rowland, R.G., Perlman, S.G., and Ganote, C.E., The pathogenesis of drug-induced renal cystic disease, *Kidney International*, 5, 411–421, 1974.

127. Goodman, T., Grice, H.C., Becking, G.C., and Salem, F.A., A cystic nephropathy induced by nordihydroguaiaretic acid in the rat. Light and electron microscope investigations, *Laboratory Investigation*, 23, 93–107, 1970.

128. Evan, A.P. and Gardner, K.D., Jr., Nephron obstruction in nordihydroguaiaretic acid-induced renal cystic disease, *Kidney International*, 15, 7–19, 1979.

129. McDonald, A.T.J., Crocker, J.F.S., Digout, S.C., McCarthy, S.C., Blecher, S.R., and Cole, D.E.C., Glucocorticoid-induced polycystic kidney disease — a threshold trait, *Kidney International*, 37, 901–908, 1990.

130. Mai, M., Geiger, H., Hilgers, K.F., Veelken, R., Mann, J.F.E., Dämmrich, J., and Luft, F.C., Early interstitial changes in hypertension-induced renal injury, *Hypertension*, 22, 754–765, 1993.

131. Sattar, M.A., Yusof, A.P.M., Gan, E.K., Sam, T.W., and Johns, E.J., Acute renal failure in 2K2C Goldblatt hypertensive rats during antihypertensive therapy: comparison of an angiotensin AT receptor antagonist and clonidine analogues, *Journal of Autonomic Pharmacology*, 20, 297–304, 2000.

132. Wiesel, P., Mazzolai, L., Nussberger, J., and Pedrazzini, T., Two-kidney, one clip and one-kidney, one clip hypertension in mice, *Hypertension*, 29, 1025–1030, 1997.

133. Clark, A.F., Sharp, M.G.F., Morley, S.D., Fleming, S., Peters, J., and Mullins, J.J., Renin-1 is essential for normal renal juxtaglomerular cell granulation and macula densa morphology, *The Journal of Biological Chemistry*, 272, 18185–18190, 1997.

134. Tharaux, P.L. and Coffman, T.M., Transgenic mice as a tool to study the renin-angiotensin system, *Contributions to Nephrology*, 135, 72–91, 2001.

135. Sharp, M.G.F., Fettes, D., Brooker, G., Clark, A.F., Peters, J., Fleming, S., and Mullins, J.J., Targeted inactivation of the Ren-2 gene in mice, *Hypertension*, 28, 1126–1131, 1996.

136. Oliverio, M.I., Kim, H.-S., Ito, M., Le, T., Andoly, L., Best, C.F., Hiller, S., Kluckman, K., Maeda, N., Smithies, O., and Coffman, T.M., Reduced growth, abnormal kidney structure, and type 2 (AT$_2$) angiotensin receptor-mediated blood pressure regulation in mice lacking both AT$_{1A}$ and AT$_{1B}$ receptors for angiotensin II, *Proceedings of the National Academy of Sciences of the United States of America*, 95, 15496–15501, 1998.

137. Tsuchida, S., Matsusaka, T., Chen, X., Okubo, S., Niimura, F., Nishimura, H., Fogo, A., Utsunomiya, H., Inagami, T., and Ichikawa, I., Murine double nullizygotes of the angiotensin type 1A and 1B receptor genes duplicate severe abnormal phenotypes of angiotensin nullizygotes, *Journal of Clinical Investigation*, 101, 755–760, 1998.

138. Nishimura, H., Yerkes, E., Hohenfellner, K., Miyazaki, Y., Ma, J., Hunley, T.E., Yoshida, H., Ichiki, T., Threadgill, D., Phillips, J.A., III, Hogan, B.M.L., Fogo, A., Brock, J.W., III, Inagami, T., and Ichikawa, I., Role of the angiotensin type 2 receptor gene in congenital anomalies of the kidney and urinary tract, CAKUT, of mice and men, *Molecular Cell*, 3, 1–10, 1999.

139. Pope, J.C., IV, Brock, J.W., III, Adams, M.C., Miyazuki, Y., Stephens, F.D., and Ichikawa, I., Congenital anomalies of the kidney and urinary tract — role of the loss of function mutation in the pluripotent angiotensin type 2 receptor gene, *The Journal of Urology*, 165, 196–202, 2001.

140. Chevalier, R.L., Editorial: congenital anomalies of the kidney and urinary tract, *The Journal of Urology*, 165, 203–204, 2001.

141. Mackie, G.G. and Stephens, F.D., Duplex kidneys: a correlation of renal dysplasia with position of the ureteral orifice, *The Journal of Urology*, 114, 274–280, 1975.

142. Miyazai, Y. and Ichikawa, I., Role of the angiotensin receptor in the development of the mammalian kidney and urinary tract, *Comparative Biochemistry and Physiology Part A*, 128, 89–97, 2001.

143. Peters, C., Animal models of fetal renal disease, *Prenatal Diagnosis*, 21, 917–923, 2001.

144. Beck, A.D., The effect of intra-uterine urinary obstruction upon the development of the fetal kidney, *The Journal of Urology*, 105, 784–789, 1971.

145. Peters, C.A., Carr, M.C., Lais, A., Retik, A.B., and Mendell, J., The response of the fetal kidney to obstruction, *The Journal of Urology*, 148, 503–509, 1992.

146. Gobet, R., Cisek, L.J., Zotti, P., and Peters, C.A., Experimental vesicoureteral reflux in the fetus depends on bladder function and causes renal fibrosis, *The Journal of Urology*, 160, 1058–1062, 1998.

147. Gobet, R., Park, J.M., Nguyen, H.T., Chang, B., Cisek, L.J., and Peters, C.A., Renal renin-angiotensin system dysregulation caused by partial bladder obstruction in fetal sheep, *Kidney International*, 56, 1654–1661, 1999.

148. Josephson, S., Robertson, B., Claesson, G., and Wikstad, I., Experimental obstructive hydronephrosis in newborn rats. I. Surgical technique and long-term morphologic effects, *Investigative Urology*, 17, 478–483, 1980.

149. Nagle, R.B., Bulger, R.E., Cutler, R.E., Jervis, H.R., and Benditt, E.P., Unilateral obstructive nephropathy in the rabbit. I. Early morphologic, physiologic, and histochemical changes, *Laboratory Investigation*, 28, 456–467, 1973.

150. Nagle, R.B. and Bulger, R.E., Unilateral obstructive nephropathy in the rabbit. II. Late morphologic changes, *Laboratory Investigation*, 38, 270–278, 1978.

151. Steinhardt, G.F., Vogler, G., Salinas-Madrigal, L., and LaRegina, M., Induced renal dysplasia in young pouch opossum, *Journal of Pediatric Surgery*, 23, 1127–1130, 1988.

152. Steinhardt, G.F., Liapis, H., Phillips, B., Vogler, G., Nag, M., and Yoon, K.-W., Insulin-like growth factor improves renal architecture of fetal kidneys with complete ureteral obstruction, *The Journal of Urology*, 154, 690–693, 1995.

153. Steinhardt, G.F., Salinas-Madrigal, L., deMello, D., Farber, R., Phillips, B., and Vogler, G., Experimental ureteral obstruction in the fetal opossum: histologic assessment, *The Journal of Urology*, 152, 2133–2138, 1994.

154. Niimura, F., Labosky, P.A., Kakuchi, J., Okubo, S., Yoshida, H., Oikawa, T., Ichiki, T., Naftilan, A.J., Fogo, A., Inagami, T., Hogan, B.L.M., and Ichikawa, I., Gene targetting in mice reveals a requirement for angiotensin in the development and maintenance of kidney morphology and growth factor regulation, *Journal of Clinical Investigation*, 96, 2947–2954, 1995.

155. Hilgers, K.F., Norwood, V.F., and Gomez, R.A., Angiotensin's role in renal development, *Seminars in Nephrology*, 17, 492–501, 1997.

156. Horton, C.E., Jr., Davisson, M.T., Jacobs, J.B., Bernstein, G.T., Retik, A.B., and Mandell, J., Congenital progressive hydronephrosis in mice: a new recessive mutation, *The Journal of Urology*, 140, 1310–1315, 1988.
157. Reimschuessel, R., A fish model of renal regeneration and development, *ILAR Journal*, 42, 285–291, 2001.

CHAPTER 5

Animal Models for Xenotransplantation

David Whiting and Abbas Ardehali

CONTENTS

INTRODUCTION

    Organ transplantation is acceptable medical therapy for end-stage liver, kidney, heart, lung, small bowel, and pancreatic diseases. The major limitation to more widespread utilization of this procedure is a shortage of available organs. Improvements in peri-operative care have expanded the indications for organ transplantation, and consequently the waiting time for solid organs has increased. A clinical xenotransplant program, with proper selection of donor species, could provide a near limitless supply of transplantable organs. Transplantation requires the recipient organ to be physiologically comparable and immunologically compatible with the human host. These remain the major obstacles in the field of xenotransplantation. Rodents, large domesticated animals, and primates provide experimental models to examine the physiologic comparability and pathogenesis of xenotransplant rejection.

HISTORY

The first modern xenotransplant in a clinical situation occurred in 1963 when Dr. Keith Reemsta transplanted 13 chimpanzee kidneys into 13 patients with end-stage renal disease. Previous recorded accounts of xenotransplantation related to largely unsuccessful attempts at transplantation of bone, skin, and soft tissues from animals to injured humans. One of Dr. Reemsta's patients received two donor chimpanzee kidneys and lived for 9 months; the longest recorded survival of a xenotransplant recipient. The woman died because of an electrolyte imbalance believed to be caused by physiologic differences between chimpanzee and human kidneys. In 1964, Dr. Thomas Starzl performed baboon-to-human kidney transplants, but these patients succumbed to infection and organ failure within 60 days. The first heart xenotransplant was performed by Dr. James Hardy in 1964. The gravely ill patient received a chimpanzee heart that failed within 2 hours of grafting. Baby Fae's baboon heart xenotransplant in 1984 by Dr. Leonard Bailey is the last recorded xenotransplant in the United States. Born premature, her naïve immune system was thought to be less likely to reject the baboon organ. The heart was rejected, and she died 20 days after the transplant.

In 1970, Dr. Roy Calne extended the Swedish biologist Linnaeus' classification of animal taxonomy by labeling species as *discordant* and *concordant*. This classification is based on the severity of the immunologic response when a donor species organ is grafted into a recipient. The classification is not based on phylogenetic class, order, family, genus, or species, and is entirely a clinical classification. Calne's classification was based on the notion that concordant animals could be matched and graft viability could be achieved with immunosuppression, while in discordant animals this was not possible. He wrote, "Certain constituents of the recipient's blood react immediately and violently with the grafted organ, damaging the capillary walls leading to hemorrhage and failure of the circulation through the graft."[10] In his system, concordant xenotransplantation resulted in a functional organ (if only temporarily), while discordant xenotransplantation resulted in immediate graft rejection. The immediate and violent reaction noted by Dr. Calne refers to hyperacute rejection and remains one of the key concerns in xenotransplantation.

REJECTION IN XENOTRANSPLANTATION

Hyperacute Rejection

Hyperacute xenograft rejection begins within minutes to hours and is characterized pathologically by interstitial hemorrhage and diffuse thrombosis, and clinically by graft loss. Both xenografts and allografts are susceptible to ischemia and reperfusion injury related to surgical transplantation. This ischemic injury primes the graft to immunologic response. The interstitial hemorrhage and diffuse thrombosis of hyperacute rejection is initiated by the binding of xenoreactive antibodies (XNAs) and complement to the endothelial cells of the graft.[65] Pathologic examination of the rejected organ reveals deposits of immunoglobulin and classical complement factors on the vascular endothelial cells.[66] Depletion of XNAs from the recipient prolongs xenograft survival.[66] Similarly, immunologically naïve recipients of xenotransplants do not undergo hyperacute rejection.[41] Greater than 80% of XNAs recognize the oligosaccharide galactose α-(1,3)galactose epitope expressed on endothelial cells of the graft. The enzyme α-(1,3)galactosyltransferase catalyzes the transfer of the oligosaccharide to transmembrane proteins on the endothelial cells. All lower mammals and New World monkeys possess this enzyme and express this oligosaccharide. Humans, apes, and Old World monkeys do not possess this enzyme, and express naturally occurring antibodies reactive to this oligosaccharide.[29,30] The galactose α-(1,3)galactose epitope and the α-(1,3)galactosyltransferase that catalyzes its transfer to endothelial cells have been extensively studied and have emerged as targets for therapeutic intervention.

The presence of the XNAs is a key factor in the initiation of hyperacute rejection in xenotransplants. Humans, Old World monkeys, and apes are likely sensitized to the galactose α-(1-3) galactose epitope by exposure to gastrointestinal bacteria expressing similar epitopes.[26] Once XNAs are bound to the galactose α-(1-3)galactose epitope on the graft endothelial cell, recipient and donor complement is activated. Antibody-dependent or classical complement activation initiates hyperacute rejection. The exact pathogenesis is unknown; what is known is that the integrity of the blood vessels is disrupted leading to extravasation of vessel contents, and subsequent thrombosis and hemorrhage. The disruption of the endothelium is either caused by complement-mediated endothelial cell destruction (via the membrane-attack complex) or the formation of intercellular gaps caused by the assembly of the C57b678 complex and accelerated by the membrane-attack complex.[65,72] In addition, experimental models of discordant xenotransplantation, such as guinea pig-to-rat, pig-to-dog, indicate that complement can be activated without the presence of XNA via the alternative pathway.[63,65]

Two strategies have been developed to overcome hyperacute rejection; the first investigates ways to prevent interaction between XNAs and epitopes on xenograft epithelium, and the second investigates the activation of complement.[26] XNA can be depleted from the recipient by passing recipient blood through immunoadsorption columns containing the oligosaccharide galactose α-(1,3)galactose.[33] The XNA binding site in the donor organ can be presaturated by infusing the donor with synthetic carbohydrates containing the galactose α-(1-3) linkage.[86] Experimental evidence with animal models indicates that hyperacute rejection can be prevented with these techniques. Attempts to breed transgenic pigs with the α-(1,3)galactosyltransferase gene missing have not been successful. However, transgenic pigs expressing α-1,2-fucosyltransferase have been bred; these pigs have decreased activity of the α-(1,3)galactosyltransferase and consequently have decreased expression of the surface galactose α-(1-3)galactose epitope and are resistant to lysis in human serum *in vitro*.[48]

The activation and regulation of the complement system remain a focus of hyperacute rejection studies. Complement regulatory factors, or regulators of complement activity (RCAs) modulate complement-mediated reactions on cell surfaces. Complement regulatory proteins from different species may be ineffective when reacted together and may be responsible for unregulated complement destruction in the xenograft resulting in hyperacute rejection. Porcine RCAs are inefficient inactivators of human complement bound to xenograft endothelium. Specifically, the glycoprotein decay-activating factor (DAF/CD54), membrane co-factor (MCF/CD46), CD39, and homologous restriction factor (HRF) are species specific and have decreased effectiveness when combined with RCAs from different species. Transgenic pigs expressing DAF and CD59 have been bred. *In vitro* studies (discussed later in the chapter) using organs from these transgenic pigs have been resistant to hyperacute rejection.

Experimental models of discordant xenotransplantation, such as guinea pig-to-rat and pig-to-dog, indicate that complement can be activated without the presence of XNA via the alternative pathway.[63,65] In this pathway, recipient C3 complement factor binds to graft endothelial cells and becomes active. Activated C3 in turn activates B complement factor, creating C3Bb, the alternative pathway activating factor. In this model, functional complement regulatory factors are necessary for regulation, and their absence or poor function may result in hyperacute rejection.

Acute Vascular Rejection

Acute vascular rejection (delayed vascular rejection) occurs in discordant species pairs if hyperacute rejection is averted by either removing or suppressing the XNAs or by inhibiting or depleting complement.[4] Xenotransplants are susceptible to acute vascular rejection in the days and weeks following the transplant. Acute vascular rejection is characterized pathologically by endothelial cell activation and infiltration of the graft with recipient monocytes and natural killer cells. Diffuse intravascular coagulation, thrombosis, and interstitial inflammation result in loss of the graft. Investigators have also considered that acute vascular rejection may be a part of a continuum of hyperacute rejection and may be initiated by xenoreactive antibody deposits on vascular endothelium. The depletion or inhibition of XNAs and complement that initially averted hyperacute rejection may be incomplete, resulting in a "delayed hyperacute" rejection.[4] This theory is supported by four observations.[67] Acute vascular rejection is commonly associated with antibody deposits on vascular endothelium, levels of xenoreactive antibodies are elevated following exposure of primates to porcine tissue,[19] acute vascular rejection can be induced by infusion of anti-donor antibodies, and depletion of antibodies either by removal or inhibition of synthesis delays or averts acute vascular rejection.[54]

T-Cell-Mediated Rejection

The mechanisms of T-cell-mediated xenograft rejection have been difficult to study because of early graft loss from hyperacute and acute vascular rejection. As the obstacles of hyperacute and acute vascular rejection are beginning to be overcome, the importance of T-cell-mediated immune responses is being realized. T-cell-mediated rejection is similar in principle to acute rejection in allotransplantation, involving both the direct and indirect pathway of T-cell recognition.[67] In the direct pathway, xenoantigens are presented to the recipient T-cells by the donor antigen-presenting cells; this pathway is known to occur in porcine-to-human xenotransplants.[66,85] Direct T-cell-mediated responses are strong because porcine antigen-presenting cells are able to interact with human T-cells.[26] The indirect pathway involves the presentation of xenoantigens to recipient T-cells by recipient T-cells. Given the antigenic disparity in xenotransplantation, the role of the indirect pathway is likely to be substantial.[67] In addition, the indirect T-cell-mediated responses are also likely to be strong because porcine B7 molecules are able to deliver a co-stimulatory signal through human CD28.[70] The role of indirect vs. direct T-cell activation is important because genetic modifications of responding antigen-presenting cells may be an avenue for therapy.[67] Murine skin and pancreatic islet cell xenografts may be acceptable models of T-cell-mediated rejection because these grafts are not immediately vascularized, and consequently do not undergo hyperacute and acute vascular rejection.

Chronic Rejection

The problems of hyperacute and acute vascular rejection in xenotransplantation have been substantial. The role of chronic rejection in xenotransplantation has not been extensively studied because the xenografts, so far, have not survived long enough to develop chronic rejection. Chronic rejection in allografts is characterized by progressive T-cell-mediated arteriosclerosis of the graft arteries, and the resulting loss of the graft. It is expected that once the problems of hyperacute and acute vascular rejection are controlled long enough for long-term graft survival, the shift in research will be to establish models of chronic rejection in xenotransplantation.

SMALL ANIMAL MODELS

Small animals are used to study the pathogenesis of xenotransplant rejection. Animal models are used to study hyperacute rejection, acute vascular rejection, acute cellular rejection, and chronic rejection. Small animal models have the benefits of low cost, easy breeding, and the ready availability of transgenic animals, antibodies, and proteins. The relative ease in manipulation of genes and gene products in small animals (particularly mice) allows for the elucidation of molecular pathways in the pathogenesis of rejection. The primary disadvantage of small animals is the difficulty in extrapolating findings in small animal models to large animals and humans. It is generally believed that the large animal with the most potential for human xenotransplantation is the pig. The pig is easily bred in a short period of time, and the organs are similar in size and function. However, pigs are expensive and smaller animal models must be used for more basic xenotransplantation studies.

Xenotransplant research is primarily focused on elucidating and overcoming the problems of hyperacute, acute vascular, and chronic rejection. Difficulties with the physiology of the transplanted organ can only be addressed once the rejection processes are controlled long enough to create a functional xenotransplant model. The heart is the ideal organ for the study of xenotransplantation because graft function can be assessed by palpation of a second heartbeat. The procedure for heterotopic intra-abdominal heart transplantation has been well described.[18] The donor heart is arrested with heparinized saline, explanted, and placed on ice. Through a midline abdominal incision, the donor aorta is anastomosed to the recipient infrarenal abdominal aorta, and the donor pulmonary artery is anastomosed to the inferior vena cava. In this model, the left side of the heart is perfused, but remains non-functional.

Hyperacute Rejection

Discordant species pairs are used to study hyperacute rejection. The guinea pig-to-rat, mouse-to-rabbit, and guinea pig-to-mouse models are three small animal models that are being used for xenotransplantation research today. Concordant species pairs can also be used to study hyperacute rejection if the recipient has been pre-sensitized to the donor species by injection of donor splenocytes 14 days prior to transplantation.[88] These splenocytes stimulate the production of donor-directed antibodies. In this model, the donor heart was rejected in 14 minutes with pathologic features of hyperacute rejection. Flow cytometry revealed markedly elevated levels of serum xenoantibody.[88] These pre-sensitized concordant animal models for hyperacute rejection are particularly useful because rats and mice (two concordant species) can be used to study pathogenesis. Mice and rats are two species that have a particularly large collection of available transgenic animals, isolated proteins, and antibodies, making the pair an ideal animal model to study. Transgenic mice are available and are used to study hyperacute rejection.

Xenotransplants undergo hyperacute rejection because of the presence of xenoantibodies directed against a galactose-based oligosaccharide expressed on endothelial cells. Anti-galactose antibodies account for 60% of human anti-mouse xenoantibodies, and 70 to 90% of human anti-pig antibodies.[16,29] The α-(1,3)galactosyltransferase gene encodes for the enzyme that synthesizes the oligosaccharide on endothelial cells of non-primate animals. A transgenic α-(1,3)galacostyltransferase knockout mouse expresses no endothelial cell galactose α-(1,3)galactose. These mice are viable, express substantially less xenoantibody when compared to wild-type controls, and have less activation of human complement.[21]

The *mouse-to-rabbit* small animal model closely mimics the clinically relevant pathogenesis of pig-to-primate hyperacute rejection. The hyperacute rejection process is known to occur by xenoantibody-mediated classical complement activation. In this model, mouse hearts are heterotopically transplanted into both weanling and adult rabbits, with mean survival of the graft of 37 minutes and 40 minutes, respectively.[45] Serum from the weanling and adult rabbits was examined, and both were found to have high titers of IgM xenoantibodies and strong classical complement activity with minimal alternative pathway activity toward mouse red cells.[45] The model has the advantages of the close similarity of the pathogenesis of hyperacute rejection to the pig-to-primate model, and the availability of transgenic mice. The primary disadvantage of this model is the limited availability of transgenic rabbits and rabbit reagents, as well as the difficult post-operative care of the rabbits.[88]

The *guinea pig-to-rat* heterotopic heart transplant model has been used to elucidate the pathogenesis of hyperacute rejection. The recipient rat heart develops histological interstitial hemorrhage and thrombosis, cessation of graft function, and hyperacute rejection in minutes. The pathogenesis of guinea pig-to-primate hyperacute rejection was thought to be absolutely dependent on xenoantibody-mediated classical complement activation.[20,47] However, Platt's group has identified that hyperacute rejection is initiated by xenoantibody-dependent activation of the classical complement depletion of cascade as well as xenoantibody-independent complement activation by the alternative pathway.[47] In a series of experiments, Platt's group identified that depletion of recipient xenoantibodies did not prevent hyperacute rejection. However, the depletion of recipient complement with cobra venom factor did prevent hyperacute rejection.[47] These experiments question the relevance of the guinea pig-to-rat model because pig-to-primate (the current gold standard xenotransplant model) is dependent only on the xenoantibody-dependent, classical complement pathway.[22,69,88]

A model for hyperacute rejection that is most clinically relevant would simulate hyperacute rejection that occurs in a porcine–primate xenotransplant, specifically involving the galactose-α-galactose directed XNAs. A murine small animal model was recently created using *galactose α-(1,3)galactose transferase knockout mice* as recipients and α-galactose expressing mice as donors.[21] The recipient mice, like humans, lack the α-galactose epitope and express the galactose-α-galactose directed XNAs. In this model a donor heart is heterotopically transplanted into the abdomen of the recipient mice. Of the grafts, 56% failed within 48 hours due to classical hyperacute rejection characterized by interstitial hemorrhage, polymorphonuclear infiltration, and intravascular occlusion.[21]

Acute Vascular Rejection

The acute phase of xenograft rejection is characterized by cell-mediated vascular rejection. Concordant species pairs may be used to study acute vascular rejection because, as explained in the previous section, discordant species pairs undergo graft-destroying hyperacute rejection. Examples of small concordant animal models include hamster-to-rat, rat-to-mouse, and mouse-to-rat species pairs. These so-called humanized transgenic mice have been bred to study acute vascular rejection. In these models, severe combined immunodeficient (SCID) and recombinase activating gene-1 (RAG-1) deficient mice are reconstituted with human peripheral blood cells.

Skin xenograft models can be used to study acute vascular rejection and the effects of immunosuppression. Skin grafts undergo vigorous, well-defined, and rapid acute vascular rejection within 24 to 28 hours.[78] Neither concordant nor discordant species pairs undergo hyperacute rejection because there is no direct vascular anastomosis. Instead, the skin grafts undergo a secondary neovascularization. In addition, there is a high concordance of skin xenograft survival and organ survival, thus permitting a rapid, inexpensive assay to test for rejection. The relative simplicity of rodent skin grafting allows immunosuppressive therapies to be tested, without the confounding variables of complex surgery and anesthesia.[78]

The *hamster-to-rat* small animal model is a classical model of acute vascular rejection in which hamster xenografts undergo rejection in 3 to 4 days. In this model, rejection is likely to be T-cell-independent, since both normal and nude rats undergo rejection,[52] and are dependent on the innate immune system since recipient treatment with lefonomide (T-cell inhibitor) also results in acute vascular rejection.[53] This model has also been used to study the effects of immunosuppression on xenotransplants. Experiments with immunosuppression, including total lymphoid irradiation, cyclosporine, and tacrolimus (FK-506), have been undertaken,[34,47] with prolonged survival. A *Chinese hamster-to-Lewis rat* heterotopic heart model has been described, with acute rejection consistently developing in 4.1 ± 0.1 days.[13]

The *rat-to-mouse* and *mouse-to-rat* models of acute vascular rejection have also been studied, and are particularly useful in elucidating the pathogenesis of rejection. There is a multitude of transgenic mice and rats, and the battery of information about these two species is extensive. Of note, acute vascular rejection occurs in species pairs with MHC class-I and class-II matched antigens, suggesting that the process is MHC independent.[79] The rat-to-mouse model has been used with donor hearts, kidneys, and small bowel;[46] however, the heterotopic heart model remains most popular due to its technical simplicity. [88]

Chronic Rejection

Chronic rejection in xenografts has remained difficult to study because of the short graft survival secondary to hyperacute and acute rejection. Thus, few models of xenotransplant chronic rejection exist. One group has described a model of chronic rejection in heart xenotransplantation with histologic changes that closely resemble chronic rejection in human cardiac transplantation, or cardiac allograft vasculopathy. In this model, of *hamster-to-Lewis rat* xenotransplantation, a 1-cm section of *hamster aorta* is anastomosed to the aorta of a *Lewis rat*. Intimal graft arteriosclerosis developed at day 21 and was reduced in those rats receiving cyclosporin.[74]

LARGE ANIMAL MODELS

Current efforts in developing a pre-clinical model for xenotransplantation are focused on the porcine donor model. It is believed that pigs will serve as the best donor because they are easily bred, their organ size and physiology are similar to humans, and the chance of zoonosis (the spread of a pig virus to human) is unlikely given their extensive exposure to humans.[17] Baboons were previously considered to be the ideal donor species for human xenotransplantation because of their phylogenetic proximity to humans. There is a shortage of monkeys; the chimpanzee, for example, is considered an endangered species and the available animals are used for virological research.[36] The *baboon-to-cynomolgus monkey* was a popular pre-clinical animal model. The survival of cynomolgus monkey-to-baboon xenografts has approached that of allografts. The ethical debate of using primates for organ donation is also eliminated, as there is unlikely to be strong ethical debate regarding the sacrifice of pigs for organ transplant.

Hyperacute and Acute Vascular Rejection

Ex vivo models involving the isolated perfusion of porcine heart, liver, or kidney provide additional information about hyperacute rejection. In particular, continuous monitoring of the graft function and graft rejection is possible, allowing for the correlation of physiologic changes in the graft with rejection. However, the *ex vivo* models must be carefully considered. Isolated models of perfusion, for example, have the advantage of being able to use human blood as a perfusate. In addition, the perfusate may be altered experimentally; however, the human blood that perfuses the organ has a limited amount of bioactive antibodies, complement, and platelets that may adversely affect the rejection.[75,88] *Ex vivo* models where the organ is in circuit with an animal, as in an extracorporeal circuit, may avoid this drawback.

The *pig-to-monkey* and *pig-to-baboon* animal models are two large animal models that closely approximate the transplantation of a pig organ into a human. Pigs are discordant to monkeys, baboons, and humans. Currently, the baboon is the favored recipient. Compared to the monkey, the adult baboon is larger (10 to 15 kg vs. 3 to 5 kg). While the larger size increases the cost of breeding, the larger size of the baboons allows mature pigs to be used as donors, allows for the safer administration of anesthesia, and a large enough blood volume to allow for post-operative studies.[88] In addition, the pig xenografts do not universally undergo hyperacute rejection in all monkeys. Although all apes and Old World monkeys produce anti-αGal antibodies, certain cynomolgus monkeys do not undergo uniform hyperacute rejection.[82] Baboon recipients of porcine xenotransplants universally undergo hyperacute rejection, suggesting that this model may more closely approximate a pig-to-human transplant.[88] Baboons have anti-αGal IgM levels similar to those of humans but lower levels of anti-αGal IgG.[49]

Three approaches have been explored in pig-to-primate experimental models in an effort to overcome hyperacute rejection, including the depletion or neutralization of anti-αGal antibody, the depletion or inhibition of complement, and the use of organs from genetically engineered pigs that express human complement regulatory proteins.[49] It is unlikely that an animal model with inactivated or absent complement systems would be viable. Instead, efforts have been made to encode the grafts with recipient (human) complement regulatory proteins. Hearts from transgenic pigs constructed with CD59/DAF genomic clones do not undergo humoral rejection and demonstrate improved survival in primates.[12,59] In a heterotopic pig-to-baboon model of heart xenotransplantation, the addition of the human complement regulatory protein CD46 with mini-gene constructs to the pig results in a mean graft survival of 23 days and histologic absence of C5b and MAC vascular deposition.[24]

A *rat-to-monkey* model of discordant xenotransplantation has also been established. In this model, the rat heart is heterotopically transplanted into the groin of a cynomolgus monkey by anastomosing the rat aorta and monkey iliac artery and rat pulmonary artery with monkey iliac vein.[3] The rat heart was found to undergo hyperacute rejection in 5.4 ± 1.4 minutes with pathological examination revealing classic hyperacute rejection with pathogenesis similar to porcine–primate hyperacute rejection. The primary advantage of this model is the availability and low cost of transgenic donor rats, and the similarity to hyperacute rejection in pig-to-primate rejection. The primary disadvantage is the confounding variable of the non-functioning, non-physiologic heterotopic placement of the heart. In addition, this similarity assumes that the mechanisms of hyperacute rejection in the rat-to-monkey model can be extrapolated to the more clinically relevant pig-to-primate model.

The *pig-to-primate vein graft* model is a convenient model to study the molecular interactions of the xenoantibody with the endothelial cell in a large animal. In this model, femoral veins from the legs of a donor pig are removed, and anastomosed end-to-end to one of the femoral veins of a recipient monkey.[57] The advantages of this model are the simplicity of the operation and the ease in obtaining biopsies and samples for analysis.

Chronic Rejection

The *pig-to-monkey cartilage* model is a potential large animal model of chronic rejection. The development of a model for chronic rejection in xenotransplantation has been particularly onerous because of graft failure caused by hyperacute and acute vascular rejection. A model has been proposed where porcine and bovine meniscal cartilage is transplanted into the suprapatellar pouches of cynomolgus monkeys.[76] Cartilage does not undergo hyperacute and acute vascular rejection because of its limited vascular, neural, and lymphatic supply, and low expression of α-galactosyl epitopes.[76] Dr. Stone's group describes a form of chronic rejection in the explanted cartilage that developed after 1 month, characterized by T-lymphocyte, macrophage, and eosinophil migration. It is not known whether this model of chronic rejection is pathogenically similar to the chronic rejection of a pig xenograft.

CELLULAR XENOTRANSPLANTATION

The transplantation of animal cells into humans may provide treatments for certain diseases that are caused by deficiency of a cell or cell product. Experiments are currently under way to studying the feasibility of the transplantation of porcine pancreatic islet cells as treatment for insulin-dependent diabetes mellitus, hepatocytes for acute liver failure, and dopaminergic brain cells as treatment for refractory Parkinson's disease. The possibility of successful xenotransplantation of cells is particularly optimistic because, unlike vascularized organ xenografts, classic hyperacute rejection does not occur. The blood supply is from the recipient and the primary immunologic hurdle is T-cell-mediated rejection, for which many immunosuppressive drugs have been developed.[88]

Pancreatic Islet Cells

The reversal of experimental diabetes by fetal pancreas transplantation has been achieved in small and large animal models. The *non-obese diabetic mouse (NOD)* is an appropriate model for studying the feasibility of pancreatic islet cell xenotransplantation. These mice develop diabetes at 12 weeks.[62,81] The pathogenesis of diabetes in the non-obese diabetic mouse appears to be similar to human diabetes mellitus. In this model, there is a strong association of diabetes with gene loci on the major histocompatibility complex;[58,77] an autoimmune pathogenesis is suggested in both species by the presence of lymphocytic inflammation in the pancreatic islets, the presence of anti-islet cell antibodies, and the modulating effect of cyclosporin A.[62,81] Of interest, splenocytes from NOD mice can be adoptively transferred into wild-type mice, and the wild-type mice will develop diabetes.

A *pig-to-mouse* model has been used to study mechanisms of islet encapsulation. This model utilizes C57/Bl6 mice and induces diabetes (defined by blood glucose >22mmol/L on at least 2 consecutive days) by intraperitoneal injection of 160 mg/kg streptozotocin, administered 7 to 10 days before xenotransplanation.[58] The pig pancreatic islet cells are implanted within the capsule of the donor kidney. This model has been used to study the effects of immunosuppression on cell-mediated rejection.

Hepatocytes

Chronic liver failure is particularly amenable to xenotransplantation if physiologically similar animal hepatocytes can be either transplanted or placed in an extracorporeal circuit. Clinical liver failure is characterized by coagulopathy, metabolic disorder, and toxic hepatic encephalopathy secondary to synthetic and metabolic dysfunction of the hepatocytes. Many attempts have been made to use functional animal hepatocytes to substitute for the non-functioning hepatocytes. Extracorporeal circulation of patient blood through a bed of porcine hepatocytes, as well as the transplantation of porcine hepatocytes is being actively investigated. Cell microencapsulation with a semi-permeable membrane has been necessary in animal models to shield the hepatocytes from the recipient's immune system. A group is investigating hepatocyte transplantation using a *pig-to-rat* model. In this model, hepatocytes are isolated from large white pigs using collagenase. The purified hepatocytes are then encapsulated in a dialysis membrane (acrylonitrile–methylallyl sulfonate) and grafted into the intraperitoneal cavity of Lewis rats. Using assays for albumen synthesis and cytochrome p450 function, the pig hepatocytes were found to be functioning after 15 days.[6]

Neural Tissue

Xenotransplantation of neural tissue for focal central nervous system disorders, including Parkinson's and Huntington's disease, remains a focus of research efforts. Parkinson's disease is characterized by the loss of dopaminergic neurons in the nigrostriatal pathway. Initially treated with dopaminergic drugs, the diseases eventually become refractory to medical treatment. In limited trials, the transplantation of dopaminergic porcine embryonic cells into primate recipients has restored the deficits associated with Parkinson's disease. It is estimated that a minimum of 100,000 dopaminergic neurons must survive in each half of the brain for clinical benefit to occur.[55] The physiology and rejection of the neural tissue xenotransplants have been studied in porcine-to-rodent models. In a *porcine embryo-to-rat* model, Parkinson's disease is induced by the stereotactic injection of 6-hydroxydopamine in the medial forebrain of Lewis rats. Embryonic dopaminergic neurons are harvested from pig embryos at day 27, and transplanted in the striatum of the Lewis rats. Anatomically correct neural connections were observed, as well as restoration of induced Parkinson's-like deficits.[31] Despite the evidence of rejection on autopsy, these xenotransplants are particularly promising because the brain is, at least in part, immunologically segregated by the blood–brain barrier.[9]

ETHICAL CONCERNS

The current trend in xenotransplantation research is to overcome the challenges of hyperacute, acute vascular, and T-cell-mediated rejection, in hopes of developing a clinically feasible xenotransplant program. This program will most likely involve the transplantation of pig organs into humans. Previously, xenotransplantation programs were expected to involve the transplantation of primate organs into humans. Significant ethical issues were raised, including the appropriateness of using engaging, sociable primates for "spare parts." The realities of establishing a clinical xenotransplant program quickly shifted attention to other animals as sources of organs. It was found that Old World monkeys, baboons, and chimpanzees were in too short supply to provide a reasonable source of organs. Focus quickly shifted to the pig — an animal that has been bred for food for centuries, with millions slaughtered each year for food. Research efforts advanced quickly, with breeding colonies being established to produce transgenic pigs that would fit, both immunologically and physiologically, into humans better. However, there still remain significant ethical concerns with the current plans for clinical xenotransplantation.

The primary ethical concern that needs to be addressed before the implementation of a clinical xenotransplant program is the risk of disease transmission (known and unknown) to the transplant patient and to the population as a whole. This phenomenon is called zoonosis, and refers to disease transmission between species. With regard to the pig, many viruses including the porcine endogenous retrovirus (PERV) are known to exist; however, concern is that the zoonotic agent (in this case the PERV) may undergo genetic changes that make it more dangerous to humans. Investigators believe that zoonotic agents in transplanted organs are at particularly high risk for mutation because of the large viral load in the graft and the continuous exposure of the agent to the host. They also fear the poor resistance of the host to infection secondary to the immunosuppression and underlying disease process, and the possible immunologic seclusion of the zoonotic agent in the animal graft because of incompatibility of the donor T-cell-mediated repertoire and graft MHC antigens.[67] Dr. Platt summarizes the questions that must be answered with regard to zoonosis: (1) Can the agent infect human subjects *in vivo*? (2) Can the agent cause disease? (3) Can the agent be transferred from one individual to another?[67]

Xenotransplantation has the potential to provide life-saving treatment for patients suffering from many end-stage diseases. It is clear that xenotransplantation involves significant risks to the patient, including rejection, physiologic incompatibility, and spread of animal diseases to the patient. The latter risk of zoonosis may be extended to close contacts and the population as a whole. The U.S. government has established regulatory commissions under the auspices of the Public Health Service (PHS) and the Food and Drug Administration. Here, xenotransplantation has been defined as transplantation, or infusion into a human recipient live cells, tissues, or organs from a non-human animal source, or human body fluid, cells, tissues, or organs that have had *ex vivo* contact with live non-human animal cells, tissues, or organs.[7] One document outlines a series of regulations including the implementation of a federal xenotransplantation advisory committee, the requirement that all proposed non-human primate xenotransplantation proposals be submitted only after the scientific community has deliberated the risks of the proposal. The document concludes by saying that the U.S. government has not yet established the safety and ethics of non-human primate xenotransplantation.

CONCLUSION

Xenotransplantation could provide a near limitless supply of organs to patients with end-stage diseases. A xenotransplant must be physiologically and immunologically compatible with the human recipient. Animal models are necessary for the study of xenotransplantation, and have provided considerable insight into hyperacute, acute, and chronic rejection. Small animal models have the advantages of low cost, easy breeding, and availability of transgenic animals. Large animals are necessary to study the physiology of the xenotransplant and perform immunologic studies that can be more easily extrapolated to humans. The pig has emerged as the most viable source of transplantable organs for humans because of the similar organ size and low breeding cost. With the advent of pigs that express human genes, the reality of a clinical xenotransplant program is closer than ever. However, the ethics of breeding animals for human transplantation, as well as the risk of transmission of animal diseases to human population, has to be considered by society.

REFERENCES

1. Auchinloss, H. Xenogeneic transplantation. *Transplantation*. 45, 1, 1988.
2. Auchincloss, H. et al. Xenograft rejection of class I-expressing transgenic skin is CD4-dependent and CD8-independent. *Transplant. Proc*. 5, 2335, 1990.
3. Azimzadeh, A. et al. Assessment of hyperacute rejection in a rat-to-primate cardiac xenoraft model. *Transplantation*. 61, 1305, 1996.
4. Bach, F.H. et al. Delayed xenograft rejection. *Immunol. Today*. 17, 379, 1996.
5. Benhamou, P.Y. et al. Fetal pancreas transplantation in miniature swine. *Transplantation*. 59, 1660, 1995.
6. Benoist, S. et al. Survival and differentiation of porcine hepatocytes encapsulated by semiautomatic device and allotransplanted in large number without immunosuppression. *J. Hepatol*. 2, 208, 2001.
7. Bloom, E.T. Xenotransplantation: regulatory challenges. *Curr. Opin. Biotechnol*. 3, 312, 2001.
8. Boehle, A.S. et al. An improved orthotopic xenotransplant procedure for human lung caner in SCID mice. *Ann. Thorac. Surg*. 69, 1010, 2000.
9. Brevig, T., Holgersson, J., and Widner, H. Zoonosis in xenotransplantation. *Transplant. Proc*. 7, 1551, 2000.
10. Calne, R.Y. Organ transplantation between widely disparate species. *Transplant. Proc*. 2, 550, 1970.
11. Chen, R.H., Kadner, A., Tracy, J., Santerre, D., and Adams, D.H. Differential expression of α-gal and human CD59 molecules on pig-to-primate cardiac xenotransplantation: a marker of delayed xenograft rejection. *Transplantation*. 33, 732, 2001.
12. Chen, R.H. et al. Hearts from transgenic pigs constructed with CD59/DAF genomic clones demonstrate improved survival in primates. *Xenotransplantation*. 6, 1994, 1999.
13. Chong, A.S. et al. Delayed xenograft rejection in the concordant hamster heart into Lewis rat model. *Transplantation*. 62, 90, 1996.
14. Chong, S.J. et al. Histological characterization and pharmacological control of chronic rejection in xenogeneic and allogeneic heart transplantation. *Transplantation*. 66, 692, 199.
15. Collignon, P. and Purdy, L. Xenografts: are the risks so great that we should not proceed? *Microbes and Infection*. 3, 341, 2001.

16. Collins, B.H. et al. Mechanisms of injury in porcine livers perfused with blood of patients with fulminant hepatic failure. *Transplantation.* 58, 1162, 1994.

17. Cooper, D.K.C. The safety of xenotransplantation. *Transplant. Proc.* 5, 2461, 1998.

18. Corry, R., Winn, H., and Russell, P. Primarily vascularized allografts of hearts in mice. The role of H-2D, H-2K, and non-H-2 antigens in rejection. *Transplantation.* 16, 643, 1973.

19. Cotterell, A.H. et al. The humoral immune response in humans following cross-perfusion of porcine organs. *Transplantation.* 60, 861, 1995.

20. Dalmasso, A. et al. Mechanism of complement activation in the hyperacute rejection of porcine organs transplanted into primate recipients. *Am. J. Pathol.* 140, 1157, 1992.

21. d'Apice, A., Nottle, M., and Cowan, P.J. Genetic modification for xenotransplantation: transgenics and clones. *Transplant. Proc.* 33, 3053, 2001.

22. Delriviere, L.D. et al. Basic anatomical and physiological differences between species should be considered when choosing combinations for use in models of hepatic xenotransplantation: an investigation of the guinea pig-to-rat combination. *Transplantation.* 66, 112, 1998.

23. Deodhar, S.D. Review of xenografts in organ transplantation. *Transplant. Proc.* 18, 83, 1986.

24. Diamond, L. et al. A human CD46 transgenic pig model system for the study of discordant xenotransplantation. *Transplantation.* 71, 132, 2001.

25. DiCarlo, A. et al. Activation of porcine hepatic microvascular sinusoidal endothelial cells in pig-to-human liver xenotransplantation.*Transplant. Proc.* 33, 759, 2001.

26. Dorling, A., Riesbeck, K., Warrens, A., and Lechler, R. Clinical xenotransplantation of solid organs. *Lancet.* 349, 867, 1997.

27. Faustman, D. and Coe, C. Prevention of xenograft rejection by masking donor HLA class I antigens. *Science.* 252, 1700, 1991.

28. Fischel, R.J., Bolman, R.M., Platt, J.L., Najarian, J.S., Bach, F.H., and Matas, A.J. Removal of IgM anti-endothelial antibodies results in prolonged cardiac xenograft survival. *Transplant. Proc.* 22, 1077, 1990.

29. Galili, U. et al. Human natural anti-alpha galactosyl IgG. II. The specific recognition of alpha (1,3)-linked galactose residues. *J. Exp. Med.* 162, 573, 1985.

30. Galili, U. et al. Man, apes, and Old World monkeys differ from rat hearts expressing human decay accelerating factor (DAF) transplanted into primates. *J. Biol. Chem.* 263, 17755, 1988.

31. Galpern, W.R. Xenotransplantation of porcine fetal ventral mesencephalon in a rat model of Parkinson's disease: functional recovery and graft morphology. *Exp Neurology.* 140, 1, 1996.

32. Gock, H. et al. Anti-α1,3 galactose-mediated hyperacute rejection of vascularized transplants in a small animal model. *Transplant. Proc.* 32, 2075, 2000.

33. Good, A.H. et al. Identification of carbohydrate structures that bind human antiporcine antibodies: implications for discordant xenografting in humans. *Transplant. Proc.* 24, 559, 1992.

34. Goto, T., Kino, T., Hatanaka, H. et al. Discovery of FK-506, a novel immunosuppressant isolated from *Streptomyces tsukubaensis. Transplant. Proc.* 19: 4, 1987.

35. Grant, D., Mendicino, M., and Levy, G. Xenotransplantation: just around the corner. *Surgery.* 129, 243, 2000.

36. Gridelli, et al. Experimental concordant liver xenotransplantation, in *Xenotransplantation,* 2nd ed. Cooper, D.K.C. et al. Eds. 1997.

37. Halperin, E.C. Non-human to human organ transplantation: its biologic basis and a potential role for radiation therapy. *Int. J. Cancer.* 96, 76, 2001.

38. Hasan, R., Van Den Bogaerde, J.B., Wallwork, J., and White, D.J. Evidence that long-term survival of concordant xenografts is achieved by inhibition of anti-species antibody production. *Transplantation.* 54, 408, 1992.

39. Johnsson, C. et al. Successful retransplantation of mouse-to-rat cardiac xenografts under immunosuppressive monotherapy with cyclosporine. *Transplantation.* 63, 652, 1997.

40. Kanai, N. et al. Delayed hyperacute xenograft rejection in porcine to canine fetal liver transplantation. *Transplant. Immunol.* 2, 95, 1999.

41. Kaplan, E. et al. Total lymphoid irradiation and discordant cardiac xenografts. *J Heart Transplant.* 1, 11, 1990.

42. Karlson-Parra, A. et al. Xenograft rejection of porcine islet-like cell clusters in normal and natural killer cell-depleted mice. *Transplantation.* 61, 1313, 1992.

43. Keefe, E.B. Liver transplantation: current status and novel approaches to liver replacement. *Gastro-enterology.* 120, 749, 2001.

44. Kellersmann, K.H. et al. Rat-to-mouse small bowel xenotransplantation: a novel model for studying acute vascular and hyperacute xenograft rejection and xenogeneic cell migration. *Xenotransplantation.* 6, 28, 1999.

45. Kerr, S.R. et al. Mouse-to-rabbit xenotransplantation. *Transplantation.* 67, 360, 1999.

46. Kiyochi, H. et al. Pathology and cell migration in a novel rat-to-mouse small bowel xenotransplant model. *Transplant. Proc.* 31, 587, 1999.

47. Knechtle, S., Halperin, E., and Bollinger, R. Xenograft survival in two species combinations using total-lymphoid irradiation and cyclosporine. *Transplantation.* 43, 173, 1987.

48. Koike, K. et al. How can human DAF and HRF20 prevent HAR in transgenic mice? *Transplant. Proc.* 28, 599, 1996.

49. Lambrights, D., Sachs, D., and Cooper, D. Discordant organ xenotransplantation in primates-world experience and current status. *Transplantation.* 66, 547, 1998.

50. Leventhal, J.R. et al. The immunopathology of cardiac xenograft rejection in the guinea pig-to-rat model. *Transplantation.* 56, 1, 1993.

51. Levental, J.R. et al. Prolongation of cardiac xenograft survival by depletion of complement. *Transplantation.* 4, 857, 1994.

52. Lim, S.M. et al. Both concordant and discordant heart xenografts are rejected by athymic (nude) rats with the same tempo as in T cell competent animals. *Transplant. Proc.* 23, 581 1991.

53. Lim, T,, Vandeputte, M., and Waer, M. Natural killer cell and macrophage mediated rejection of concordant xenografts in the absence of T and B cell responses. *J. Immunol.* 158, 5658, 1997.

54. Lin, S.S., Weidner, B.C., Byrne, G.W. et al. The role of antibodies in acute vascular rejection of pig-to-baboon cardiac transplants. *J. Clin. Invest.* 101, 175, 1998.

55. Lindvall, O. Neural transplantation: a hope for patients with Parkinson's disease. *Neuroreport.* 8, iii-x, 1997.

56. Logan, J.S. Prospects for xenotransplantation. *Curr. Opin. Immunol.* 12, 563, 2000.

57. Luo, Y. et al. Pig xenogeneic antigen modification with green coffee bean alpha-galactosidase. *Xenotransplantation.* 6, 238, 1999.

58. Marchetti, P. et al. Prolonged survival of discordant porcine islet xenografts. 61, 1100, 1996.

59. McCurry, K. et al. Human complement regulatory proteins protect swine to primate cardiac xenografts from humoral injury. *Nature Medicine.* 1, 423, 1995.

60. Merten, S. et al. The cellular basis of cardiac allograft recognition. *Transplantation.* 65, 1152, 1998.

61. Micheler, R., McManus, R., Smith, R., Sadeghi, A.N., and Rose, E.A. Technique for primate hetero-topic cardiac xenotransplantation. *J. Med. Primatol.* 14, 357, 1985.

62. Miller, B.J., Appel, M.C., O'Neil, J.J., and Wicker, L.S. Both the LYT-2+ and L3T4+ T cell subsets are required for the transfer of diabetes in nonobese diabetic mice. *J Immunol.* 40, 52, 1988.

63. Miyagawa, S. et al. The mechanism of discordant xenograft rejection. *Transplantation.* 46, 825, 1988.

64. Onion, D. et al. An approach to the control of disease transmission in pig-to-human xenotransplan-tation. *Xenotransplantation.* 2, 143, 2000.

65. Parker, W. et al. Transplantation of discordant xenografts: a challenge revisited. *Immunol. Today.* 17, 373, 1996.

66. Platt, J.L. et al. Immunopathology of hyperacute xenograft rejection in a swine-to-primate model. *Transplantation.* 52, 214, 1991.

67. Platt, J.L. Physiologic barriers to xenotransplantation. *Transplant. Proc.* 32, 1547, 2000.

68. Platt, J.L. Zoonosis in xenotransplantation. *Transplant. Proc.* 32, 1551, 2000.

69. Pruit, S.K. et al. The effect of xenoreactive antibody and B cell depletion on hyperacute rejection of guinea pig-to-rat cardiac allografts. 56, 1318, 1993.

70. Rogers, N.J., Mirenda, V., Jackson, I., Dorling, A., and Lechler, R.I. Immunosuppression of direct T-cell-mediated xenorecognition *in vitro. Transplant. Proc.* 33, 697, 2001.

71. Rosengard, A.M. et al. Tissue expression of human complement inhibitor, decay-accelerating factor, in transgenic pigs. *Transplantation.* 59, 1325, 1995.

72. Saadi, S. and Platt, J. Transient perturbation of endothelial integrity induced by natural antibodies and complement. *J. Exp. Med.* 181, 21, 1995.

73. Sandler, S. et al. Assessment of insulin secretion *in vitro* from microencapsulated fetal porcine islet-like cell clusters and rat, mouse, and human pancreatic islets. *Transplantation*. 63, 1712, 1997.
74. Scheringa, M. et al. Chronic rejection of concordant aortic xenografts in the hamster in the hamster-to-rat model. *Transplant. Immunol*. 4, 1992, 1996.
75. Schmoekel, M. et al. Orthotopic heart transplantation in a transgenic pig-to-primate model. *Transplantation*. 65, 1570, 1998.
76. Stone, K.R. et al. Porcine and bovine cartilage transplants in cynomolgus monkey: I. A model for chronic xenograft rejection. *Transplantation*. 63, 640, 1997.
77. Stone, K.R. et al. Porcine cartilage transplants in the cynomolgus monkey. III. transplantation of α-galactosidase-treated porcine cartilage. *Transplantation*. 27, 1577, 1998.
78. Thomas, F.T. et al. Reversal of naturally occurring diabetes in primates by unmodified islet xenografts without chronic immunosuppression. *Transplantation*. 67, 846, 1999.
79. Torgersen, K.M. et al. Major histocompatibility complex class I-independent killing of xenogeneic targets by rat allospecific natural killer cells. *Transplantation*. 63, 119, 1997.
80. van Denderen, B. et al. Decay-accelerating factor transgenic mouse hearts are protected from human complement-mediated attack. *Transplant. Proc*. 28, 583, 1996.
81. Weber, C.J., Safley, S., Hagler, M., and Kapp, J. Evaluation of graft–host response for various tissue sources and animal models. *Ann. NY Acad. Sci*. 875, 233, 1999.
82. White, D.J. and Yannoutsos, N. Production of pigs transgenic for human DAF to overcome complement mediated hyperacute rejection in man. *Res. Immunol*. 147, 88, 1996.
83. White, D.G. hDAG transgenic pig organs: are they concordant for human transplantation? *Xenotransplantation*. 4, 50, 1996.
84. Xiao, F. et al. Leflunamide controls rejection in hamster to rat cardiac xenografts. *Transplantation*. 58, 28, 1994.
85. Yamada, K., Sachs, D.H., and Dersimonian, H. Human anti-porcine xenogeneic T-cell response. Evidence for allelic specificity of mixed leukocyte reaction and for both direct and indirect pathways of recognition. *J. Immunol*. 155, 5249, 1995.
86. Ye, Y. et al. Evidence that intravenously administered alpha-galactosyl carbohydrates reduce baboon serum cytotoxicity to pig kidney cells (PK15) and transplanted pig hearts. *Transplantation*. 58, 330, 1994.
87. Ye, Y. et al. The pig as a potential organ donor for man. A study of potentially transferable disease from donor pig to recipient man. *Transplantation*. 5, 694, 1994.
88. Zhang, Z. et al. Animal models in xenotransplantation. *Exp. Opin. Invest. Drugs*. 9, 2051, 2000.

CHAPTER 6

Animal Models in Neuroscience

Jesper Mogensen

CONTENTS

INTRODUCTION

The human brain is almost certainly the least understood of our organs. Consequently, when facing the diseases affecting the brain, the medical sciences are often in the unfortunate situation of studying and attempting to prevent or cure relatively unknown pathological processes within an organ in which even the normal conditions are poorly understood. On such a background, it can be no surprise that within psychiatry and neurology, numerous diseases are in a desperate need of both an improved understanding and more adequate methods of intervention (pharmacological and otherwise). The changing age composition of the population makes the human, as well as financial problem of increasing occurrence of Alzheimer's dementia, a constantly growing issue. The schizophrenias continue to be an immense problem in terms of individual suffering as well as social impact. And focal brain damage on vascular incidence and various types of accidents demand improved methods of posttraumatic functional rehabilitation (in turn calling for an improved understanding of the mechanisms of such functional recoveries). These and numerous other examples stress the need for continued and expanding neuroscientific research. And despite the growing number of methods that allow a more detailed study of the living human brain (e.g., various neuroimaging techniques), the necessity for well-controlled studies using manipulations of living brains continues to require the use of neuroscientific animal models.

All scientific studies involving animal models are plagued by problems of a theoretical, practical, and ethical nature. Some of these problems, such as the ethical question of whether human use of subhuman species in the fight against human disease is "speciesism"[1] and whether such speciesism is acceptable or not,[2] are common to all branches of animal model research and will not be dealt with in this chapter. Other issues are more specific to the neuroscientific area and its clinical subdisciplines, neurology and psychiatry. A number of these problems are linked to the assumed uniqueness of the human brain and its functions and dysfunctions. Although few may challenge that the livers of human and subhuman species are essentially similar, the neuroscientific community is far from reaching consensus about the level of similarity between the brains and "minds" of humans and other species. The question of similarities between structures and functions of the brains of various species is often considered the most basic problem for the use of animal models in studies of diseases of the human brain. However, such endeavors are often impaired by the lack of detailed and objective methods within the areas of clinical and animal experimentation. Finally, some of the confusion and contradiction within experimental neuroscience may spring from uncertainties about the definition of an optimal neuroscientific animal model.

SPECIES COMPARISONS

The major task of comparative neuroscience is to go beyond the superficial species differences and identify the basic differences and similarities between species. Many structural differences (e.g., the pattern of cortical sulci and gyri) may be of little or no consequence for the organization of brains. Although anatomical analysis has revealed some basic species differences, there seems to be a growing body of evidence indicating a common "bauplan" for the brains of a broad spectrum of species.

A number of features have traditionally been believed to mark the major differences between human and subhuman brains. Although some such features still appear to be rather unique to the human brain, other aspects of the human brain have been found to be shared with more species than originally believed. Although some aspects of the cortical areas believed to mediate production and perception of speech appear to be present in both humans and in certain non-human primates,[3,4] the presence of unilateral, cortical areas specialized in mediation of linguistic functions, including the Broca area, appears likely to be a privilege of the human brain. Animal models of traumatic aphasias are unlikely ever to be developed — even in non-human primates; see, however, the arguments of Noback.[5] Another aspect of the human brain originally believed to be rather specifically "human" is the fact that the prefrontal cortex constitutes approximately one third of the total neocortical surface. The prefrontal cortex has long been believed to be a privilege of mammals, and some data seem to indicate that "higher" mammals, such as primates, have a relatively larger prefrontal cortex compared with "lower" mammals, such as rodents.[6] Partly on the basis of such observations and partly on the basis of the fact that the prefrontal cortex of some species (rodents) differs cytoarchitectonically from the prefrontal area of primates, it has been argued that studies on the functions of the prefrontal cortex should mainly be conducted in primates.[6] More recent studies of the prefrontal cortex have, however, indicated that this structure may be present in a broader variety of species. Histochemical,[7] biochemical,[8] and functional[9,10] studies have indicated that the posterodorsolateral neostriatum of the pigeon should be considered equivalent to the prefrontal cortex of mammals. Furthermore, the prefrontal cortex of the echidna (*Tachyglossus aculeatus*, an egg-laying mammal belonging to the subclass Prototheria) constitutes approximately 50% of the total cortical surface.[11-14] The prefrontal cortex appears to be present in mammals and in at least some non-mammals alike. The ratio between prefrontal and non-prefrontal cortical surface is not in itself an index of evolution.

Studies within the areas of comparative anatomy and physiology of the brain are of importance to the use of neuroscientific animal models in at least two ways. First, such studies may indicate the areas within which animal models are likely to be useful and the species that are likely to be acceptable for such studies. As indicated above, animal models of traumatic aphasias are hardly feasible. On the other hand, the prefrontal system seems to subserve functions of rather general survival value, and consequently a broad spectrum of species may be available for model experiments in which the focus is on the prefrontal system, its functions, and potential prefrontal involvement in pathological conditions. Motivation for developing animal models of aspects of normal and abnormal functions of the human prefrontal cortex may stem from repeated observations of the prefrontal cortex in patients with schizophrenia.[15-26]

The second way in which comparative neuroscience may contribute to the development of animal models is by providing the information necessary for making adequate comparisons between structural as well as functional aspects of human and non-human brains. In the case of rat models of processes involving the human prefrontal cortex, the subdivisions of which are functionally heterogeneous,[27,28] it is important that adequate choices are made about the cortical areas to be manipulated in the animal. Detailed analysis of the anatomy (primarily the afferent connections) of the rat prefrontal cortex[29-32] has modified such strategies by redefining the boundaries of subdivisions of the prefrontal cortex.[33] Despite the progress that is being made in the attempts to delineate adequate boundaries between subareas of the prefrontal cortex of the rat (and to establish adequate comparisons to such areas in primates), a number of somewhat dissimilar maps are presently being offered to those who attempt to use rat models in the studies of the prefrontal system. The delineations of Divac et al.,[29] Krettek and Price[32] (used in the atlas of Paxinos and Watson),[34] and Groenewegen et al.[30,31] are only in partial agreement. Even the feasibility of using cortical projections of the mediodorsal thalamic nucleus (MD) as a basis for definition and delineation of the rat prefrontal cortex has been questioned and consequently subjected to an experimental scrutiny that concluded that although extraprefrontal cortical projections of the MD do exist, such projections are sufficiently rare to allow the MD-based definition of the prefrontal cortex of the rat.[35] A subcortical example of the ways in which model studies depend on comparative neuroanatomy is found in studies of the neostriatum. The neostriata of both rodents and primates are frequently the focus of studies that attempt to model aspects of the extrapyramidal diseases such as Huntington's chorea, in which the primary cell loss seems to be within the neostriatum, and Parkinson's disease, in which a presumed primary cell loss in the pars compacta of substantia nigra causes a drastic reduction in the striatal concentration of the neurotransmitter dopamine. Although pathological changes may be found in non-striatal brain regions of even early parkinsonian cases, it can hardly be doubted that essential aspects of both conditions can be studied in animal models in which the neostriatum has been affected by mechanical lesion, toxins, or local injection of drugs. However, studies on functional aspects of the neostriatum frequently pay insufficient attention to the connectivity and consequent regional specialization within this structure. The neostriatum of all species studied is subdivided into regions, each of which receives input from a specific cortical area with which it is functionally yoked in such a way that lesions of a neostriatal region and its associated cortical area are both accompanied by similar patterns of postlesion symptoms.[36,37] A possible exception to this rule may be found in the "motor" part of the neostriatum.[36] Because the neostriatum is heterogeneous and its regions may indeed be as functionally specialized as the areas of the cortex, knowledge about neostriatal organization is of primary importance when one is to construct or evaluate animal models in which parts of the neostriatum have been manipulated.

FUNCTIONAL ANALYSES

Within psychiatry, and to some extent even neurology, most of the symptoms defining the diseases are aspects of behavior or introspection and, in the case of introspection, mainly those that are reflected in verbal behavior. The nature of the symptoms defining such diseases is an obvious problem for the construction of animal models within clinical neuroscience.

Traditionally, the situation in this field has been that the condition of the patient is characterized by subjective and often poorly defined symptoms and that the behavior of the subjects of animal modeling is analyzed in a rather crude manner. Such a state of affairs strongly impairs comparisons between the conditions of patient and animal.

Similar Tests in Patient and Animal

An important step toward the solution of this problem has been the trend toward applying more detailed behavioral and physiological analyses to not only neurological but even psychiatric patients. Such studies may in themselves provide important information about the structural and functional basis of a certain disease, for instance, the indication by various neuroimaging and functional methods of an association between schizophrenia and dysfunction of the prefrontal system. Additionally, the gathering of objective information about the condition of patients may allow more direct comparisons between patients and animal models. Studies of the prepulse acoustic startle paradigm in individuals with schizophrenia exemplify this type of progress. When exposed to a burst of strong noise, humans with schizophrenia, as well as those without, display an objectively measurable startle response. If a prestimulus in the form of a weak tone precedes the startle-eliciting noise by 60 to 120 msec, the startle response of healthy controls is significantly reduced, and the degree to which the presentation of the (warning) prepulse is able to inhibit the startle response can be measured as the percentage reduction of startle. Patients with schizophrenia appear to have a significantly less reduced startle response in the presence of the prestimulus when compared with the case of healthy controls.[38] Because the acoustic startle paradigm can be applied to non-human species — and the prestimulus-associated reduction in startle response can be seen in healthy subjects from such non-human species — this technique allows essentially identical testing methods to be applied to both patients with schizophrenia and animal models. The dominating theory about the neural substrate of schizophrenia is the *dopamine hypothesis*,[39–42] which postulates an association between increased activity of dopamine neurotransmission and the schizophrenic disease (or diseases). The major lines of evidence supporting the dopamine hypothesis are as follows:

- Direct or indirect dopaminergic agonists, such as D-amphetamine, aggravate the symptomatology of patients with schizophrenia and can, even in healthy controls, induce a temporary, psychosis-like condition that is indistinct from acute paranoid schizophrenia.[39]
- There is a strong positive correlation between the clinical efficacy of antipsychotic drugs and their ability to act as antagonists at the dopamine receptor.[43]
- Postmortem studies of patients with schizophrenia indicate an increased concentration of receptors.[44] The up-regulation of the receptors may, however, be the consequence of medication rather than a true aspect of a primary disease. Positron emission tomography studies (PET) have indicated that young, nonmedicated patients with schizophrenia show no measurable change in the concentration of receptors.[45]

Almost all current animal models of schizophrenia spring from one or another aspect of the dopamine hypothesis. The rat model focusing on the acoustic startle paradigm[46] accomplishes either regional or global dopamine receptor hypersensitivity by injecting the dopaminergic neurotoxin 6-hydroxydopamine into either a limited target area or the cerebral ventricles. The toxin causes destruction of presynaptic dopaminergic neurons and, consequently, a postsynaptic up-regulation of dopamine receptors. In animals treated this way, systemic injection of the dopamine agonist apomorphine will cause stimulation of all dopamine receptors and, consequently, dopamine receptor hyperactivity in the region or regions treated with 6-hydroxydopamine. In this rat model, it appears that global dopamine receptor hypersensitivity is associated with an impaired warning effect of the prestimulus tone in the acoustic startle paradigm — a pattern similar to that observed for patients with schizophrenia. Furthermore, local receptor hypersensitivity in both the substantia nigra and the nucleus accumbens (but not in the frontal cortex) seems to be associated with a similar symptom.[46] Such results lend support to theories associating part of the schizophrenic symptomatology and hyperactivity within the dopaminergic system, and the outcome of these studies may even indicate the regional distribution of such dopaminergic abnormalities. On the other hand, it should be remembered that the acoustic startle paradigm focuses on only one aspect of the disease and that manipulating other neurochemical or regional systems might have provoked similar symptoms.

Although variations of the animal models based on the dopamine hypothesis of schizophrenia have almost completely dominated the animal model-based studies of schizophrenia for many years (and to some extent continue to do so), a number of more recent animal models of schizophrenia have been developed as well. One such model uses a disruption of fetal neurogenesis by administration of methylazoxymethanol (MAM). The MAM model of schizophrenia is inspired by indications that some of the cytoarchitectonical abnormalities seen in patients with schizophrenia appear to be associated with developmental abnormalities.[47,48] Prenatal administration of MAM to rats induces cytoarchitechtonical as well as functional and behavioral abnormalities that appear to be comparable to some of the abnormalities associated with schizophrenia.[49,50] Another animal model of schizophrenia focusing primarily on neuroanatomical (rather than neurochemical or pharmacological) aspects of the disease is the *ventral hippocampal lesion* model.[51] Structural changes within the hippocampus[52,53] and the entorhinal cortex[54,55] have been found in patients with schizophrenia, and consequently, early (but postnatal) lesions within the ventral hippocampus are seen as a potential model of schizophrenia.[51] What seems particularly interesting about this model is that rats subjected to such an intervention demonstrate increased locomotor activity in response to stress, D-amphetamine, or novelty when tested in adulthood — while showing no such symptoms before puberty.[51] Such a pattern of symptoms is particularly interesting because patients with schizophrenia normally only exhibit symptoms in early adulthood or later (despite the indications that at least some aspects of the neural abnormalities accompanying schizophrenia are present at or even before birth). Some symptoms seen in the ventral hippocampal lesion model of schizophrenia, however, appear to be present even before puberty. Impaired social interaction is one such symptom.[56]

Interpretation of Behavioral Tests

Although clinicians need to provide more objective information about patients, it is equally important that experimenters working with animal models improve the methods of behavioral analysis. Such analysis must be performed at a level of sophistication that allows the experimenter to establish a detailed and broad-spectrum functional profile of the animal. Only such a profile will make it possible to determine the nature of functions that are impaired by a certain neural manipulation (and potentially reinstated by therapy). In determining areas of impairment, it is equally important to establish the integrity of functional spheres that are assumed to be spared by the manipulation under investigation. Alternatively, the observed impairments might be secondary to more basic — but unnoticed — dysfunctions. One example is the observation that prolonged thiamine deficiency in the rat (a potential model for the Wernicke–Korsakoff syndrome), which is associated with impaired acquisition, and retention of an active, step-through shock-avoidance test[57–59] might not reflect a cognitive impairment but rather might be secondary to a motor impairment. This possibility is emphasized by the observation that thiamine-deficient rats are impaired in tests of locomotion. The motor impairment of thiamine-deficient rats does not in itself invalidate the model because patients suffering Wernicke-Korsakoff syndrome may demonstrate ataxia.[60] To establish whether thiamine-deficient rats model the learning and memory impairment that is central to the Wernicke-Korsakoff syndrome, it will be necessary to analyze the performance of such rats in a learning task that is able to reflect acquisition or retention in ways that are rather independent of the motor performance of the animal. Such a task could be a place-learning task administered in a water maze (a circular pool of water).[61] In this task, the animal's latency to find a submerged platform may be heavily influenced by the rat's motor abilities. However, the distance swum and other test parameters (such as the degree to which the animal initially swims directly toward the target position) are rather unaffected by motoric abilities and — if sensory impairment such as blindness can be ruled out — reflect rather truthfully the cognitive aspects of the test.

Method Dependence of Behavioral Tests

The necessity of multiple, well-selected, and detailed behavioral tests was emphasized by Sanberg,[62] who compared three animal models: lesions of the neostriatum obtained via the neurotoxin kainic acid, a model of Huntington's disease;[63] AF64A, which destroys cholinergic neurons selectively[64,65] and is consequently used in animal models of Alzheimer's disease; and cortical as well as neostriatal maldevelopment after fetal administration of the toxin MAM.[66,67] The combined analysis of daytime activity and passive avoidance behavior was unable to discriminate among any of the three models, whereas a subsequent and detailed analysis of aspects of nocturnal locomotion in the same three models allowed discrimination between the MAM model and the two other models. Furthermore, the nocturnal-locomotion analysis was able to discriminate between the MAM model and a model including subpial aspiration lesions of the cortex.

The importance of an awareness of the characteristics of the behavioral tests employed is underlined by results demonstrating that various measures of what is commonly described as locomotion, exploration, or "general activity" reflect the activity of only partly overlapping neural systems;[68] that the nature of the apparatus in which the "delayed alternation" behavior of the rat is tested determines whether this behavior, which is often considered the "Babinski sign" of the prefrontal system, is able to reflect massive destruction of prefrontal structures;[69] and that although lesions of the parietal association cortex of the rat impair the place-learning behavior in a big water maze,[70] similar animals in a smaller water maze do not behave in a way significantly different from that of sham-operated controls.[71]

Often, the quality of the water maze-based place-learning ability of rats is considered a reliable measure of the functional integrity of the hippocampal system. Repeated demonstrations of significantly impaired place learning in water mazes after lesions of the hippocampus, the fimbria-fornix, or both seem to support such a notion.[72-76] The neural substrate that mediates place learning in water mazes in the rat is, however, significantly dependent on the details of the experimental setup. Not only the size of the water maze[70,71] but even the number and arrangement of the extramaze cues offered to the animal during task solution are of critical importance.[77,78] When fewer and less three-dimensionally arranged cues are offered, normal place learning can be demonstrated by animals subjected to transections of the fimbria-fornix[78] or to scopolamine-induced inhibition of the cholinergic system.[79] Using the same water maze and identical place-learning procedures, Mogensen et al.[80] have demonstrated significantly impaired place learning after fimbria-fornix transections when an abundance of three-dimensionally arranged cues is offered around the water maze. Although being associated with a diminished importance of the hippocampal and cholinergic task mediation, the *restricted-cue task* seemed to be mediated by a neural substrate more heavily dependent on the prefrontal cortex.[77] Place-learning procedures in water mazes are often used in the behavioral testing of rat models addressing various "cognitive" functions, and consequently the danger of misinterpretation of experimental results because of unnoticed or even unrecorded differences between experimental setups is likely to become a growing problem.

A final example of significant functional differences between behavioral tasks that could formally be seen as identical is found in the report of Lepore et al.[81] In this study, cats subjected to a split-brain operation were tested for interhemispheric transfer of relevant visual information acquired monocularly. No interhemispheric information transfer was found if the animals were tested in a classic two-choice discrimination box in which food was offered as reinforcement. However, when trained and tested in a Lashley-type jumping stand, animals suffering identical lesions demonstrated relatively good interhemispheric transfer of information. Although such conflicting results should ultimately be able to provide a deeper understanding of the relevant neural mechanisms, the immediate conclusion has to be that direct comparison between apparently similar behavioral tests should only be conducted with major caution. Frequently, functionally relevant aspects of a behavioral test remain neglected and unreported, or results are generalized across tests, which are superficially but not fully identical.

Species Selection

Although comparative neuroanatomy is probably the best indicator of which species are available for the creation of a certain animal model, ethical, practical, and financial considerations[82] are likely to determine the species that is actually selected. In the case of the 1-methyl-4-phenyl-1,2,3,6-tetrahydropyridine (MPTP) model of Parkinson's disease, which indicates destruction of the dopaminergic cells of substantia nigra by the neurotoxin MPTP,[83] the choice between primates and rodents may be determined by several factors. Originally, MPTP-induced destruction of nigral neurons was believed to be possible only in primates,[84,85] but this model has been found to be feasible even in rodents.[86,87] The MPTP concentration necessary for achieving nigral damage in rodents is, however, substantially higher than that required in primates. Although neither this species difference nor the relative lack of Parkinson-like symptoms in MPTP-treated rodents necessarily invalidates the rodent MPTP model of Parkinson's disease (or at least of the disease variant, which in humans can be induced by MPTP), a number of practical problems remain. The toxicity of MPTP necessitates that substantial precautions be taken whenever the substance itself, injected animals, or the cages of such animals are handled.[88] The higher MPTP dosage required if a rodent model is chosen calls for even stricter laboratory procedures than those required for the primate model.

General Strategies

Once decisions about species selection have been made, all available knowledge about the comparative anatomy of the neural systems under consideration will have to be consulted. As much as possible of the available knowledge about the pathological condition being modeled should be taken into account — especially important are data about objectively measurable conditions. Although the majority of studies dealing with animal models in neuroscience have dealt adequately with these issues, more frequent shortcomings are found in the area of animal behavioral analysis. It is essential to the future of neuroscientific animal models that more precise and detailed methods of analyzing behavior are developed. Progress in the area of animal models of *global amnesia,* including the development of monkeys with combined bilateral lesions of hippocampus and amygdala as a model of this condition, and the subsequent development of theories about the division of the memory systems into those subserving memories and those subserving habits,[89–91] have been emphasized as an example of the importance of selecting non-human primates for certain modeling purposes. However, the selection of adequate behavioral tests may have been an even more crucial factor for this successful interaction among clinical observations, animal modeling, and basic neuroscientific studies. Even for non-primates, such as rats, available tests can reflect both habits and memories, the latter being impaired by lesions within some of the same neural systems as those necessary for mediation of such tasks in primates.[92,93]

THE ROLE OF ANIMAL MODELS IN NEUROSCIENCE

What should be required of an animal model within neurology or psychiatry? Is what is now considered the optimal neuroscientific animal model realistically obtainable? And what kind of models should be striven for? The answers to some of these questions may reside with one additional question: what do we want to get out of such models?

Homologous, Isomorphic, and Partial Models

An animal model can, if certain conditions are met, be either *homologous* or *isomorphic*.[94] To be considered homologous, the symptoms displayed by the animal and the cause of the condition in the animal should be identical to the human symptoms and the cause of the human disease. Given our relative lack of knowledge of the etiology of most psychiatric and many neurological diseases, such models within neuroscience are only possible in the case of well-defined lesion syndromes.[95] Even for isomorphic models, it is demanded that the symptoms displayed by patient and animal must be similar, but the animal condition need not be provoked by the same events as those that cause the human condition. If, in a theoretical disease, a specific population of neurons died for unknown reasons, such as genetic predisposition, and it would be possible by injection of a neurotoxin into regions of the rat brain to eliminate a neuron population similar to the one lost in humans, the rats lesioned in such a manner might constitute an isomorphic model of the disease. In this case, the final test of whether or not the model could be considered isomorphic would be the degree of similarity between the symptoms displayed by model and disease. As stressed by several authors,[2,95] numerous, if not most, neuroscientific animal models are neither homologous nor isomorphic but could be more adequately described as "partial." Such projects make no attempt at modeling the entire disease but focus on more limited aspects of the human condition.

Many systems have been developed to evaluate the quality or validity of animal models. Although the classification of a model as homologous, isomorphic, or partial constitutes a rather simple and crude system, examples of more elaborate models are those of McKinney[96] and Leonard.[97] McKinney[96] demands the following of the optimal model: comparable symptomatology, comparable etiology, comparable neurophysiological background, and concordant effects of drugs. Leonard[97] emphasizes the need for comparable symptomatology and normalization of the model condition by drug therapy similar to the pharmacological therapy effective against the human condition and stresses that the time course of a drug-induced normalization, for instance, beneficial effects of chronic but not acute medication, should be similar to what is seen in patients. Although a number of the issues stressed by McKinney[96] and Leonard[97] are similar to the demands that a model would have to fulfill to be considered homologous, the most important additional issue taken into account in these systems is the necessity for the model to respond to a given therapy in ways similar to the clinical response to therapy. As emphasized by Willner,[98] the therapies against which neuroscientific models can be tested need not be pharmacological but could include such methods as electroconvulsive stimulation and behavioral therapy. Willner[98] and others have even included separate evaluations of predictive validity, face validity, and construct validity (concepts initially used in the area of psychological testing) in the systems against which neuroscientific animal models are tested.

Given our present level of knowledge, it would be futile to use any of the evaluation systems as a checklist on which every animal model was expected to meet every single demand. The result would, in most if not all cases, be a rejection of the model. Rather, the evaluation systems should be seen as guidelines to the directions in which both partial and more complete models should develop. Furthermore, the evaluation systems may highlight the relative strengths and weaknesses of various models of a given condition.

Application of Animal Models in Neuroscience

Neuroscientific animal models mainly serve in two capacities: they are used as a testing ground during early and intermediate phases of the development of new therapies (frequently drugs), and they are used in the process of developing and testing hypotheses about the neurological and psychiatric diseases in general and about their neural substrates in particular. For the purpose of testing whether a particular therapy is efficient in preventing, relieving, or eliminating the symptoms of a disease and whether administration of the therapy is associated with side effects, one should ideally employ an animal model that mimics as closely as possible all aspects of the disease. A homologous, or at least isomorphic, model is likely to be the optimal choice for evaluation of potential therapies. Given the rareness of such complete models, evaluation of drugs and other therapies is frequently performed in models that are only partial. Some such models may, as Willner[98] has argued in the case of some of the models used in the testing of antidepressive drugs, be little more than "behavioral receptor assays." Although some of the partial models are far from being a reasonable substitute for the actual disease, valuable preclinical evaluation of drugs and other therapies may be achieved through the use of such models — especially if the same therapeutic method is evaluated against a number of different partial models, each of which focuses on a different aspect of the disease.

Although a homologous or isomorphic model may be optimal for the purpose of therapy evaluation, the models most helpful to the process of studying the mechanisms of diseases are those that lead the experimenter to suspect and eventually realize previously undiscovered processes and relationships. Important aspects of a disease may be discovered in a simple animal model, which focuses on only a single aspect of the human condition. In fact, such a simple model may provide a better environment for discovery than a model that tries simultaneously to mimic all aspects of the disease. As pointed out elsewhere,[2,95] the models most beneficial to the studies of neuropathological conditions are those of the greatest heuristic value, irrespective of whether such models are partial or of a more "complete" nature. The decision of whether to select or develop a partial or more complete model must depend on which purpose the model in question is supposed to serve. Partial models may be of substantial value in the gradual process of building a more complete image of the disease and its mechanism, whereas more complete models, which usually are only possible in case of better understood diseases, may be ideal for the purpose of testing and evaluating drugs or other therapies.

When developing neuroscientific animal models, the experimenter most frequently chooses as the point of departure the dominant theory about the disease under consideration. Although such an approach may seem logical, it involves a risk of unwanted conservatism. Clinical studies of the organic substrate of schizophrenia indicate four major areas of abnormalities: dopaminergic hyper-transmission, dysfunction of the prefrontal cortex and system, cerebral ventricular enlargement,[99,100] and structural changes in parts of the temporal lobe.[52–55,101–104] Because the prefrontal cortex contains the highest cortical amount of dopamine and has the highest cortical concentration of dopamine receptors,[105,106] both the prefrontal abnormalities and the abnormalities in dopaminergic transmission may be covered by the dopamine hypothesis of schizophrenia. Most animal models of schizophrenia — such as chronic administration of D-amphetamine,[39–42,107] administration of apomorphine after 6-hydroxydopamine-induced lesions of dopaminergic neurons, or repeated electrical stimulation ("kindling") of the ventral tegmental area in which dopaminergic neurons project to the prefrontal cortex and nucleus accumbens[108] — focus one way or another on the association between schizophrenia and various parts of the dopaminergic system. Part of the logic of the dopamine hypothesis is that the most potent of the known anti-schizophrenia drugs appear to have a major action on the dopaminergic system. The use of dopaminergic animal models in the search for anti-schizophrenia medication may, in this respect, be a self-fulfilling hypothesis. Such models may favor drugs oriented toward the dopaminergic system and neglect non-dopaminergic medication, regardless of its potential effects on the actual disease. Furthermore, the process of developing a more complete understanding of the neural substrate of schizophrenia may be seriously impaired by the rather one-sided focus of the dopaminergic animal models. An aspect often ignored by such models is the repeated observation of temporal lobe pathology in patients with schizophrenia. Schmajuk[109] has suggested the hippocampally lesioned rat as an animal model of schizophrenia. Although such a model is in itself highly partial and ignores important aspects of the disease, it represents a step toward widening the focus of animal models of schizophrenia. A number of more recently developed animal models attempt more specifically to address various aspects of the developmental nature of the schizophrenias. Such models include the above-mentioned MAM model[47,48] and the ventral hippocampal lesion model.[51]

An example of the seemingly successful widening of the focus of an animal model comes from work on Alzheimer's disease. This dementia has traditionally been associated with dysfunction (and assumed cell death) within the neural system that uses acetylcholine as its neurotransmitter, because cholinergic markers are reduced in the brains of patients with Alzheimer's and the degree of cholinergic reduction seems to correlate with the extent of the cognitive impairment.[110–112] However, it has even been found that in such patients, minor changes are present in a number of other neurotransmitter-defined systems, such as the serotonergic system.[113,114] Most animal models of Alzheimer's disease have dealt extensively with the cholinergic system, such as using the cholinergic toxin AF64A to destroy cholinergic projections from the medial septum and basic forebrain to hippocampus and cortex.[64,65,115,116] In an attempt to establish whether the serotonergic changes seen in the brains of patients with Alzheimer's contribute significantly to the development of the strongly disabling dementia of Alzheimer's disease, Nilsson et al.[117] studied rats in which the activity of both the cholinergic and the serotonergic systems had been blocked. These animals exhibited a dementia that, in comparison to the symptoms of rats subjected to cholinergic blockade alone, appeared to be more similar to the human condition in being both chronic and more severe. It appears that the addition of a serotonergic manipulation brought the cholinergic rat model of Alzheimer's disease closer to the human condition and, consequently, a partial model evolved in the direction of more completeness and validity.

As already emphasized, so-called partial animal models may in many instances be as valuable as those models of a particular disease or condition that are considered more complete. It is, however, important to keep the partiality of a particular model in mind when interpreting results and using the model relative to the human condition in question. Within any area of interest, the research endeavors should ideally include detailed scrutiny of individual processes (using partial models) and various types of more holistic approaches (using more complete models to evaluate interaction between individual systems and functions). And obviously, the entire animal model-based research program needs to be continually evaluated against all available data from clinical and human experimental sources. Only when the mysteries of the normal and the diseased brain are approached in such a multifactorial program can there be any hope of a significant progress that may ultimately benefit the patients suffering the combined effects of our ignorance and of devastating diseases.

REFERENCES

1. Ryder, R.D., *Victims of Science,* Davis-Poynter, London, 1975.
2. Bond, N.W., Animal models in psychopathology: an introduction, in *Animal Models in Psychopathology,* Bond, N.W., Ed., Academic Press, Sydney, 1984, 1.
3. LeMay, M. and Geschwind, N., Hemispheric differences in the brains of great apes, *Brain Behav. Evol.,* 11, 48, 1975.
4. Petersen, M.R., Beecher, M.D., Zoloth, S.R., Moody, D.B., and Stebbins, W.C., Neural lateralization of species-specific vocalizations by Japanese macaques (*Macaca fuscata*), *Science,* 202, 324, 1978.
5. Noback, C.R., Neurobiological aspects in the phylogenetic acquisition of speech, in Armstrong, E., and Falk, D., Eds., *Primate Brain Evolution. Methods and Concepts,* Plenum Press, New York, 1982, 279.
6. Fuster, J.M., *The Prefrontal Cortex. Anatomy, Physiology, and Neuropsychology of the Frontal Lobe,* Raven Press, New York, 1980.
7. Divac, I. and Mogensen, J., The prefrontal "cortex" in the pigeon. Catecholamine histofluorescence, *Neuroscience,* 15, 677, 1985.

8. Divac, I., Mogensen, J., and Björklund, A., The prefrontal "cortex" in the pigeon. Biochemical evidence, *Brain Res.,* 332, 365, 1985.

9. Mogensen, J. and Divac, I., The prefrontal "cortex" in the pigeon. Behavioral evidence, *Brain Behav. Evol.,* 21, 60, 1982.

10. Mogensen, J. and Divac, I., Behavioural effects of ablation of the pigeon-equivalent of the mammalian prefrontal cortex, *Behav. Brain Res.,* 55, 101, 1993.

11. Divac, I., Holst, M.-C., Nelson, J., and McKenzie, J.S., Afferents of the frontal cortex in the echidna *(Tachyglossus aculeatus).* Indication of an outstandingly large prefrontal area, *Brain Behav. Evol.,* 30, 303, 1987.

12. Divac, I., Pettigrew, J.D., Holst, M.-C., and McKenzie, J.S., Efferent connections of the prefrontal cortex of echidna *(Tachyglossus aculeatus), Brain Behav. Evol.,* 30, 321, 1987.

13. Regidor, J. and Divac, I., Architectonics of the thalamus in the echidna *(Tachyglossus aculeatus):* search for the mediodorsal nucleus, *Brain Behav. Evol.,* 30, 328, 1987.

14. Welker, W. and Lende, R.A., Thalamocortical relationships in echidna *(Tachyglossus aculeatus),* in Ebbesson, S.O.E., Ed., *Comparative Neurology of the Telencephalon,* Plenum Press, New York, 1980, 449.

15. Buchsbaum, M.S., Positron emission tomography in schizophrenia, in Meltzer, H.Y., Ed., *Psychopharmacology: The Third Generation of Progress,* Raven Press, New York, 1987, 783.

16. Buchsbaum, M.S. and Haier, R.J., Functional and anatomical brain imaging: impact on schizophrenia research, *Schizoph. Bull.,* 13, 115, 1987.

17. Buchsbaum, M.S., Nuechterlein, K.H., Haier, R.J., Wu, J., Sicotte, N., Hazlett, E., Asarnow, R., Potkin, S., and Guich, S., Glucose metabolic rate in normals and schizophrenics during the continuous performance test assessed by positron emission tomography, *Br. J. Psychiatr.,* 156, 216, 1990.

18. Goldberg, T.E., Berman, K.F., Mohr, E., and Weinberger, D.R., Regional cerebral blood flow and cognitive function in Huntington's disease and schizophrenia. A comparison of patients matched for performance on a prefrontal-type task, *Arch. Neurol.,* 47, 418, 1990.

19. Goldberg, T.E., Weinberger, D.R., Berman, K.F., Pliskin, N.H., and Podd, M.H., Further evidence for dementia of the prefrontal type in schizophrenia? A controlled study of teaching the Wisconsin Card Sorting Test, *Arch. Gen. Psychiat.,* 44, 1008, 1987.

20. Ingvar, D.H. and Franzén, G., Abnormalities of cerebral blood flow distribution in patients with chronic schizophrenia, *Acta Psychiatr. Scand.,* 50, 425, 1974.

21. Karson, C.N., Coppola, R., Morihisa, J.M., and Weinberger, D.R., Computed electroencephalographic activity mapping in schizophrenia. The resting state reconsidered, *Arch. Gen. Psychiatr.,* 44, 514, 1987.

22. Mathew, R.J. and Wilson, W.H., Chronicity and a low anteroposterior gradient of cerebral blood flow in schizophrenia, *Am. J. Psychiatr.,* 147, 211, 1990.

23. Meltzer, H.Y., Biological studies in schizophrenia, *Schizoph. Bull.,* 13, 77, 1987.

24. Morice, R., Cognitive inflexibility and pre-frontal dysfunction in schizophrenia and mania, *Br. J. Psychiatr.,* 157, 50, 1990.

25. Paulman, R.G., Devous Sr., M.D., Gregory, R.R., Herman, J.H., Jennings, L., Bonte, F.J., Nasrallah, H.A., and Raese, J.D., Hypofrontality and cognitive impairment in schizophrenia: dynamic single-photon tomography and neuropsychological assessment of schizophrenic brain functions, *Biol. Psychiat.,* 27, 377, 1990.

26. Westphal, K.P., Grözinger, B., Diekmann, V., Scherb, W., Reess, J., Leibing, U., and Kornhuber, H.H., Slower theta activity over the midfrontal cortex in schizophrenic patients, *Acta Psychiat. Scand.,* 81, 132, 1990.

27. McAndrews, M.P. and Milner, B., The frontal cortex and memory for temporal order, *Neuropsychologia,* 29, 849, 1991.

28. Milner, B., Petrides, M., and Smith, M.L., Frontal lobes and the temporal organization of memory, *Hum. Neurobiol.,* 4, 137, 1985.

29. Divac, I., Kosmal, A., Björklund, A., and Lindvall, O., Subcortical projections to the prefrontal cortex in the rat as revealed by the horseradish peroxidase technique, *Neuroscience,* 3, 785, 1978.

30. Groenewegen, H.J., Organization of the afferent connections of the mediodorsal thalamic nucleus in the rat, related to the mediodorsal-prefrontal topography, *Neuroscience,* 24, 379, 1988.

31. Groenewegen, H.J., Berendse, H.W., Wolters, J. G., and Lohman, A.H.M., The anatomical relationship of the prefrontal cortex with the striatopallidal system, the thalamus and the amygdala: evidence for a parallel organisation, *Prog. Brain Res.,* 85, 95, 1990.

32. Krettek, J.E. and Price, J.L., The cortical projections of the mediodorsal nucleus and adjacent thalamic nuclei in the rat, *J. Comp. Neurol.,* 171, 157, 1977.

33. Mogensen, J. and Divac, I., Sequential behavior after modified prefrontal lesions in the rat, *Physiol. Psychol.,* 12, 41, 1984.

34. Paxinos, G. and Watson, C., *The Rat Brain in Stereotaxic Coordinates,* 3rd ed., Academic Press, San Diego, 1997.

35. Divac, I., Mogensen, J., Petrovic-Minic, B., Zilles, K., and Regidor, J., Cortical projections of the thalamic mediodorsal nucleus in the rat. Definition of the prefrontal cortex, *Acta Neurobiol. Exp.,* 53, 425, 1993.

36. Divac, I., The neostriatum viewed orthogonally, in *Ciba Foundation Symposium 107: Functions of the Basal Ganglia,* Pitman, London, 1984, 201.

37. Divac, I. and Mogensen, J., Modularity of the prosencephalon: the vertical systems, in Will, B., Schmitt, P., and Dalrymple-Alford, J., Eds., *Brain Plasticity, Learning, and Memory,* Plenum Press, New York, 1985, 205.

38. Braff, D., Stone, C., Callaway, E., Geyer, M., Glick, I., and Bali, L., Prestimulus effects on human startle reflex in normals and schizophrenics, *Psychophysiology,* 15, 339, 1978.

39. Randrup, A. and Munkvad, I., Special antagonism of amphetamine-induced abnormal behaviour. Inhibition of stereotyped activity with increase of some normal activities, *Psychopharmacologia,* 7, 416, 1965.

40. Randrup, A. and Munkvad, I., Role of catecholamines in the amphetamine excitatory response, *Nature,* 211, 540, 1966.

41. Randrup, A. and Munkvad, I., Evidence indicating an association between schizophrenia and dopaminergic hyperactivity in the brain, *Orthomol. Psychiatr.,* 1, 2, 1972.

42. Scheel-Krüger, J. and Randrup, A., Stereotyped hyperactive behaviour produced by dopamine in the absence of noradrenaline, *Life Sci.,* 6, 1389, 1967.

43. Creese, I., Burt, D.R., and Snyder, S.H., Dopamine receptor binding predicts clinical and pharmacological potencies of antischizophrenic drugs, *Science,* 192, 481, 1976.

44. Seeman, P., Ulpian, C., Bergeron, C., Riederer, P., Jellinger, K., Gabriel, E., Reynolds, G., and Tourtellotte, W., Bimodal distribution of dopamine receptor densities in brain of schizophrenics, *Science,* 225, 728, 1984.

45. Farde, L., Wiesel, F.-A., Hall, H., Halldin, C., Stone-Elander, S., and Sedvall, G., No receptor increase in PET study of schizophrenia, *Arch. Gen. Psychiatr.,* 44, 671, 1987.

46. Swerdlow, N., Braff, D., Geyer, M., and Koob, G., Central dopamine hyperactivity in rats mimics abnormal acoustic startle response in schizophrenics, *Biol. Psychiatr.,* 21, 23, 1986.

47. Akbarian, S., Bunney, W.E., Potkin, S.G., Wigal, S.B., Hagman, J.O., Sandman, C.A., and Jones, E.G., Altered distribution of nicotinamide-adenine dinucleotide phosphate-diaphorase cells in frontal lobe of schizophrenics implies disturbances of cortical development, *Arch. Gen. Psychiatr.,* 50, 169, 1993.

48. Akbarian, S., Vinuela, A., Kim, J.J., Potkin, S.G., Bunney, W.E., and Jones, E.G., Distorted distribution of nicotinamide-adenine dinucleotide phosphate-diaphorase neurons in temporal lobe of schizophrenics implies anomalous cortical development, *Arch. Gen. Psychiatr.,* 50, 178, 1993.

49. Johnston, M.V. and Coyle, J.T., Cytotoxic lesions and the development of transmitter systems, *Trends Neurosci.,* 5, 153, 1982.

50. Thalamini, L.M., Koch, T., Ter Horst, G.J., and Korf, J., Methylazoxymethanol acetate-induced abnormalities in the entorhinal cortex of the rat: parallels with morphological findings in schizophrenia, *Brain Res.,* 789, 293, 1998.

51. Lipska, B.K., Jaskiw, G.E., and Weinberger, D.R., Postpubertal emergence of hyperresponsiveness to stress and to amphetamine after neonatal exitotoxic hippocampal damage: a potential animal model of schizophrenia, *Neuropsychopharmacology,* 9, 67, 1993.

52. Bogerts, B., Lieberman, J.A., Ashtari, M., Bilder, R.M., Degreef, G., Lerner, G., Hohns, B., and Masiar, S., Hippocampus-amygdala volumes and psychopathology in chronic schizophrenia, *Biol. Psychiatr.,* 33, 236, 1933.

53. Shenton, M.E., Kikinis, R., Jolesz, F.A., Pollak, S.D., LeMay, M., Wible, C.G., Hokama, H., Martin, J., Metcalf, D., and Coleman, M., Abnormalities of the left temporal lobe and thought disorder in schizophrenia. A quantitative magnetic resonance imaging study, *N. Engl. J. Med.,* 327, 604, 1992.

54. Jacob, J. and Beckmann, H., Prenatal developmental disturbances in the limbic allocortex in schizophrenics, *J. Neural Transm.*, 65, 303, 1986.

55. Jacob, J. and Beckmann, H., Circumscribed malformation and nerve cell alterations in the entorhinal cortex of schizophrenics, *J. Neural Transm.*, 98, 83, 1994.

56. Sams-Dodd, F., Lipska, B.K., and Weinberger, D.R., Neonatal lesions of the rat ventral hippocampus result in hyperlocomotion and deficits in social behaviour in adulthood, *Psychopharmacology*, 132, 303, 1997.

57. Hemmingsen, R., Mogensen, J., Laursen, H., Barry, D., and Ulrichsen, J., Behavioral effects of thiamine deficiency and ethanol intoxication in rats without structural brain lesion, *Scand. J. Lab. Anim. Sci.*, 16(Suppl. 1), 63, 1989.

58. Ulrichsen, J., Laursen, H., Mogensen, J., Clemmesen, L., and Hemmingsen, R., Impaired active avoidance performance in thiamine deficient rats without detectable neuropathological changes, *Neurosci. Res. Commun.*, 1, 65, 1987.

59. Ulrichsen, J., Mogensen, J., Lauersen, H., Barry, D., and Hemmingsen, R., Behavioral impairment during thiamine deficiency and ethanol intoxication in rats without detectable neuropathological changes, *Neurosci. Res. Commun.*, 9, 99, 1991.

60. Victor, M., Adams, R.D., and Collins, G.H., *The Wernicke-Korsakoff Syndrome*, F.A. David, Philadelphia, 1971.

61. Morris, R., Developments of a water-maze procedure for studying spatial learning in the rat, *J. Neurosci. Methods*, 11, 47, 1984.

62. Sanberg, P.R., Neurobehavioral aspects of some animal models of age-related neuropsychiatric disorders, in Fisher, A., Hanin, I., and Lachman, C., Eds., *Alzheimer's and Parkinson's Diseases. Strategies for Research and Development*, Plenum Press, New York, 1986, 479.

63. McGeer, P.L. and McGeer, E.G., Kainic acid: the neurotoxic breakthrough, *CRC Crit. Rev. Toxicol.*, 10, 1, 1982.

64. Chrobak, J.J., Hanin, I., and Walsh, T.J., AF64A (ethylcholine aziridinium ion), a cholinergic neurotoxin, selectively impairs working memory in a multiple component T-maze task, *Brain Res.*, 414, 15, 1987.

65. Chrobak, J.J., Hanin, I., Schmechel, D.E., and Walsh, T.J., AF64A-induced working memory impairment: behavioral, neurochemical and histological correlates, *Brain Res.*, 463, 107, 1988.

66. Beaulieu, M. and Coyle, J.T., Effects of fetal methylazoxymethanol acetate lesion on the synaptic neurochemistry of the adult rat striatum, *J. Neurochem.*, 37, 878, 1981.

67. Johnston, M.V. and Coyle, J.T., Ontogeny of neurochemical markers for noradrenergic, GABAergic, and cholinergic neurons in neocortex lesioned with methylazoxymethanol acetate, *J. Neurochem.*, 34, 1429, 1980.

68. Geoffroy, M. and Mogensen, J., Differential recovery in measures of exploration/locomotion after a single dosage of reserpine in the rat, *Acta Neurobiol. Exp.*, 48, 263, 1988.

69. Mogensen, J., Iversen, I.H., and Divac, I., Neostriatal lesions impaired rats' delayed alternation performance in a T-maze but not in a two-key operant chamber, *Acta Neurobiol. Exp.*, 47, 45, 1987.

70. Kolb, B. and Walkey, J., Behavioural and anatomical studies of the posterior parietal cortex in the rat, *Behav. Brain Res.*, 23, 127, 1987.

71. Kolb, B., Sutherland, R.J., and Whishaw, I.Q., A comparison of the contributions of the frontal and parietal association cortex to spatial localisation in rats, *Behav. Neurosci.*, 97, 13, 1983.

72. DiMattia, B.D. and Kesner, R.P., Spatial cognitive maps: differential role of parietal cortex and hippocampal formation, *Behav. Neurosci.*, 102, 471, 1988.

73. Morris, R.G.M., Garrud, P., Rawlins, J.N.P, and O'Keefe, J., Place navigation impaired in rats with hippocampal lesions, *Nature*, 297, 681, 1982.

74. Morris, R.G., Hagan, J.J., and Rawlins, J.N., Allocentric spatial learning by hippocampectomised rats: a further test of the "spatial mapping" and "working memory" theories of hippocampal function, *Q. J. Exp. Psychol.*, 38, 365, 1986.

75. Sutherland, R.J., Kolb, B., and Whishaw, I.Q., Spatial mapping: definitive disruption by hippocampal or medial frontal cortical damage in the rat, *Neurosci. Lett.*, 31, 271, 1982.

76. Sutherland, R.J., Whishaw, I.Q., and Kolb, B., A behavioural analysis of spatial localization following electrolytic, kainate- or colchicine-induced damage to the hippocampal formation in the rat, *Behav. Brain Res.*, 7, 133, 1983.

77. Mogensen, J., Pedersen, T.K., Holm, S., and Bang, L.E., Prefrontal cortical mediation of rats' place learning in a modified water maze, *Brain Res. Bull.,* 38, 425, 1995.
78. Wörtwein, G., Saerup, L.H., Charlottenfeld-Starpov, D., and Mogensen, J., Place learning by fimbria-fornix transected rats in a modified water maze, *Int. J. Neurosci.,* 82, 71, 1995.
79. Mogensen, J., Christensen, L.H., Johansson, A., Wörtwein, G., Bang, L.E., and Holm, S., Place learning in scopolamine-treated rats: the roles of distal cues and catecholaminergic mediation, *Neurobiol. Learn. Memory,* 78, 139, 2002.
80. Mogensen, J., Lauritsen, K.T., Elvertorp, S., Hasman, A., Moustgaard, A., and Wörtwein, G., Place learning and object recognition by rats subjected to transection of the fimbria-fornix and/or ablation of the prefrontal cortex, submitted.
81. Lepore, F., Ptito, M., Provencal, C., Bedard, S., and Guillemot, J.-P., Interhemispheric transfer of visual training in the split-brain cat: effects of the experimental set-up, *Can. J. Psychol.,* 37, 527, 1985.
82. Kolb, B., Functions of the frontal cortex of the rat: a comparative review, *Brain Res. Rev.,* 8, 65, 1984.
83. Burns, R.S., Phillips, J.M., Chiueh, C.C., and Parisi, J.E., The MPTP-treated monkey model of Parkinson's disease, in Markey, S.P., Castagnoli, N., Trevor, A.J., and Kopin, I.J., Eds., *MPTP: A Neurotoxin Producing a Parkinsonian Syndrome,* Academic Press, Orlando, FL, 1986, 23.
84. Jenner, P., Rupniak, N.M. J., Rose, S., Kelly, E., Kilpatrick, G., Lees, A., and Marsden, D., Methyl-4-phenyl-1,2,3,6-tetrahydropyridine-induced parkinsonism in the common marmoset, *Neurosci. Lett.,* 50, 85, 1984.
85. Langston, J.W., Forno, L.S., Rebert, C.S., and Irwin, I., Selective nigral toxicity after systemic administration of 1-methyl-4-phenyl-1,2,5,6-tetrahydropyridine (MPTP) in the squirrel monkey, *Brain Res.,* 292, 390, 1984.
86. Heikkila, R.E., Cabbat, F.S., Manzino, L., and Duvoisin, R.C., Effects of 1-methyl-4-phenyl-1,2,5,6-tetrahydropyridine on neostriatal dopamine in mice, *Neuropharmacology,* 3, 711, 1984.
87. Jenner, P., Marsden, C.D., Costall, B., and Naylor, R.J., MPTP and MPP$^+$ induced neurotoxicity in rodents and the common marmoset as experimental models for investigating Parkinson's disease, in Markey, S.P., Castagnoli, N., Trevor, A.J., and Kopin, I.J., Eds., *MPTP: A Neurotoxin Producing a Parkinsonian Syndrome,* Academic Press, Orlando, FL, 1986, 45.
88. Pitts, S.M., Markey, S.P., Murphy, D.L., Weisz, A., and Lunn, G.., Recommended practices for the safe handling of MPTP, in Markey, S.P., Castagnoli, N., Trevor, A.J., and Kopin, I.J., Eds., *MPTP: A Neurotoxin Producing a Parkinsonian Syndrome,* Academic Press, Orlando, FL, 1986, 703.
89. Mishkin, M., A memory system in the monkey, *Philosoph. Trans. Royal Soc., London, B,* 298, 85, 1982.
90. Mishkin, M., Malamut, B., and Bachevalier, J., Memories and habits: two neural systems, in Lynch, G., McGaugh, J.L., and Weinberger, N.M., Eds., *Neurobiology of Learning and Memory,* Guilford Press, New York, 1984, 65.
91. Mishkin, M. and Petri, H.L., Memories and habits: some implications for the analysis of learning and retention, in Squire, L.R. and Butters, N., Eds., *Neuropsychology of Memory,* Guilford Press, New York, 1984, 287.
92. Thomas, G.J. and Gash, D.M., Mammillothalamic tracts and representational memory, *Behav. Neurosci.,* 99, 621, 1985.
93. Thomas, G.J. and Spafford, P.S., Deficits for representational memory induced by septal and cortical lesions (singly and combined) in rats, *Behav. Neurosci.,* 98, 394, 1984.
94. Kornetsky, C., Animal models: promises and problems, in Hanin, I. and Usdin, E., Eds., *Animal Models in Psychiatry and Neurology,* Pergamon Press, Oxford, United Kingdom, 1977, 1.
95. Mogensen, J. and Holm, S., Basic research and animal models in neuroscience — the necessity of "co-evolution," *Scand. J. Lab. Anim. Sci.,* 16(Suppl. 1), 51, 1989.
96. McKinney, W.T., Biobehavioural models of depression in monkeys, in Hanin, I. and Usdin, E., Eds., *Animal Models in Psychiatry and Neurology,* Pergamon Press, Oxford, 1977, 117.
97. Leonard, B.E., From animals to man: advantages, problems and pitfalls of animal models in psychopharmacology, in Hindmarch, I. and Stonier, P.D., Eds., *Human Psychopharmacology: Measures and Methods,* Vol. 2, John Wiley & Sons, New York, 1989, 23.
98. Willner, P., *Depression. A Psychobiological Synthesis,* John Wiley & Sons, New York, 1985.
99. Raz, S., Raz, N., Weinberger, D.R., Boronow, J., Pickar, D., Bigler, E.D., and Turkheimer, E., Morphological brain abnormalities in schizophrenia determined by computed tomography: a problem of measurement?, *Psychiatr. Res.,* 22, 91, 1987.

100. Weinberger, D.R., Computed tomography (CT) findings in schizophrenia: speculation on the meaning of it all, *J. Psychiat. Res.,* 18, 477, 1984.

101. Altshuler, L.L., Conrad, A., Kovelman, J.A., and Scheibel, A., Hippocampal pyramidal cell orientation in schizophrenia, *Arch. Gen. Psychiatr.,* 44, 1094, 1987.

102. Bogerts, B., Zur Neuropathologie der Schizophrenien, *Fortschr. Neurol. Psychiat.,* 52, 428, 1984.

103. Falkai, P. and Bogerts, B., Cell loss in the hippocampus of schizophrenics, *Eur. Arch. Psychiatr. Neurol. Sci.,* 236, 154, 1986.

104. Scheibel, A.B. and Kovelman, J.A., A neurohistological correlate of schizophrenia, *Biol. Psychiatr.,* 19, 1601, 1984.

105. Divac I., Björklund, A., Lindvall, O., and Passingham, R.E., Converging projections from the mediodorsal thalamic nucleus and mesencephalic dopaminergic neurons to the neocortex in three species, *J. Comp. Neurol.,* 180, 59, 1978.

106. Divac, I., Braestrup, C., and Nielsen, M., Distribution of dopamine and serotonin receptors in the monkey cerebral cortex, *Neurosci. Lett.,* Suppl. 5, S99, 1980.

107. Ellinwood, E.H. and Kilbey, M.M., Chronic stimulant intoxication models of psychosis, in Hanin, I. and Usdin, E., Eds., *Animal Models in Psychiatry and Neurology,* Pergamon Press, Oxford, United Kingdom 1977, 61.

108. Glenthøj, B., Mogensen, J., Laursen, H., Holm, S., and Hemmingsen, R., Electrical sensitization of the meso-limbic dopaminergic system in rats: a pathogenetic model for schizophrenia, *Brain Res.,* 619, 39, 1993.

109. Schmajuk, N.A., Animal models for schizophrenia: the hippocampally lesioned animal, *Schizoph. Bull.,* 13, 317, 1987.

110. Collerton, D., Cholinergic function and intellectual decline in Alzheimer's disease, *Neuroscience,* 19, 1, 1986.

111. Francis, P.T., Palmer, A.M., Sims, N.R., Bowen, D.M., Davison, A.N., Esiri, M.M., Neary, D., Snowden, J.S., and Wilcock, G.K., Neurochemical studies of early-onset Alzheimer's disease: possible influence on treatment, *N. Engl. J. Med.,* 313, 7, 1985.

112. Perry, E.K., Curtis, M., Dick, D.J., Candy, J.M., Atack, J.R., Bloxham, C.A., Blessed, G., Fairbairn, A., Tomlinson, B.E., and Perry, R.H., Cholinergic correlates of cognitive impairment in Parkinson's disease: comparisons with Alzheimer's disease, *J. Neurol. Neurosurg. Psychiatr.,* 48, 413, 1985.

113. Mann, D.M.A. and Yates, P.O., Serotonergic nerve cells in Alzheimer's disease, *J. Neurol. Neurosurg. Psychiatr.,* 46, 96, 1983.

114. Yamamoto, T. and Hirano, A., Nucleus raphe dorsalis in Alzheimer's disease: neurofibrillary tangles and loss of large neurons, *Ann. Neurol.,* 17, 573, 1985.

115. Fisher, A. and Hanin, I., Potential animal models for senile dementia of Alzheimer's type, with emphasis on AF64A-induced cholinotoxicity, *Annu. Rev. Pharmacol. Toxicol.,* 26, 161, 1986.

116. Walsh, T.J. and Emerich, D.R., Transplantation of fetal cholinergic neurons promotes recovery of AF64A-induced behavioral and neurochemical deficits, *Soc. Neurosci. Abstr.,* 15, 1094, 1989.

117. Nilsson, O.G., Strecker, R.E., Daszuta, A., and Björklund, A., Combined cholinergic and serotonergic denervation of the forebrain produces severe deficits in a spatial learning task in the rat, *Brain Res.,* 453, 235, 1988.

CHAPTER 7

Animal Models for Psychological Disorders

Robert Murison

CONTENTS

INTRODUCTION

It might surprise the lay reader to know that psychological disorders have been modeled in animals for over a century and that the studies of, for example, Pavlov have been crucial to our understanding of both basic psychological processes and psychopathology. A cursory examination of the index of almost any standard introductory text in psychology reveals how influential animal research and animal modeling have been for the development of the discipline. In more recent texts, authors often have chosen to omit the fact that the research findings are based on animal research, which belittles its contribution. One might surmise that this is done to avoid upsetting the student, out of ignorance, or out of political correctness.

Psychological disorders are generally associated with negative feelings and emotions (one rarely becomes depressed by being successful), and thus the models are generally associated with negative events for the animal. Therefore, it is not surprising that psychological studies have been particularly targeted by opponents of animal experiments. This is disappointing in view of the considerable beneficial consequences that much of this research has had on how we treat our fellow animals.

The issue of similarities between the mental lives of animals and humans is of course fundamental. Claims of animal *consciousness* or *unconsciousness* are difficult, if not impossible, to verify. However, for a model to be useful, it is sufficient that there are similarities along a phylogenetic

0-8493-1084-9/03/$0.00+$1.50

continuum. It is not necessary for the animal mind to be as complex as the human mind — anxiety occurs in both and indeed serves a crucial adaptive function. Perhaps Damasio's[1] differentiation between *core consciousness* (present in most if not all animals to varying extents) and *extended consciousness* (limited probably to humans and their closest relatives) may provide a useful framework. The latter is associated with the presence of theory of mind and awareness of mortality. Following this distinction, it would be fruitless to attempt to model disorders associated with extended consciousness, except in our closest relatives, whereas disorders concerned with core consciousness may be modeled.

To understand the use of animal models in studies of psychological disorders, it is necessary first to delineate the functions of models. This has been discussed extensively by several authors. Overmier[2] provides a useful framework for this field, listing the functions of models as *heuristic* (question generating), *evidential* (theory testing), and *representational*. It is perhaps the first of these that has had the most impact on psychological science by generating hypotheses that are of importance to both animal and human mental health. Models derive their usefulness by their ability to set up analogies between the animal and human domains. Relationships in the one domain help us generate hypotheses about potential relationships in the other domain.[3]

This chapter focuses on behavioral models of psychological disorders. Psychopharmacological research will only be touched on within this context. The themes to be discussed include models of anxiety, depression, posttraumatic stress, and schizophrenia, which are arguably the most pervasive psychological disorders. The discussion cannot be exhaustive but will cover those models considered to have high face validity with respect to human disorders. There has also, of course, been a rapid growth in the use of knockout animals in this field, for example in models of dementia and other cognitive deficits, but it is perhaps too early to provide a comprehensive review of such studies.

ANIMAL MODELS OF DEPRESSION

Does the behavioral state of depression have an adaptive value? Social withdrawal in the face of adversity will conserve the individual's energy until recovery from a perceived threat or stressor is possible. Lowering of anhedonic tone and increased neophobia will protect the organism from unidentified threats at a time of general danger. Depression as a phylogenetic adaptation is discussed at length by Nesse.[4] One of the key features of the depression models here is that they involve aversive experience and a component of uncontrollability over these events. Thus, cognitive factors are central — the organism must be able to perceive that responses and outcomes are independent. Furthermore, for a model of a psychological disorder to function, the disorder that is being modeled must be definable. This would appear to be easier in the case of the affective disorders than in psychoses (to be discussed below).

Learned Helplessness

Historically, there have been several animal models of depression that have proved useful in both the heuristic sense and in the development of behavioral and pharmacological treatments in humans. One of the most established of these, and the most cognitively oriented, is the so-called learned helplessness (LH) model of Seligman[5] and colleagues. The model arose from the finding that naive dogs exposed to a series of inescapable electric footshocks (IS) developed a pattern of behaviors that included a failure to learn to avoid shocks, passivity, and resignation.[6] A parallel phenomenon could be produced in humans using uncontrollable noise.[7] The key to inducing helplessness is that the organism must learn that its responses and their consequences are independent — that whatever the animal does, the outcome is unpleasant. This is also a key concept in later theories of human stress, well-being, and disease.[8] In the animal model, it is crucial that the amount of aversive stimulation (shock) is of a certain intensity and number; in rats, this is typically 70+ 1-mA shocks, each of 5-sec duration and with semirandomized intershock intervals. Provision of signals either for danger (shock) or for "safe" periods modulates the behavioral effects. As we shall see later, qualitatively different effects are produced by a smaller number of shocks.

Helplessness is seen in several species, including rats, although the criteria for helplessness might not be the same. Significantly, induction of helplessness is preventable by "immunization" (previous experience with controllable shock) and, in fact, Seligman[5] found it almost impossible to induce helplessness in "streetwise" animals. The importance of developmental and earlier experiential factors is thus highlighted. Learned helplessness as first demonstrated has a limited time span, but recent studies have shown that the state is subject to classical conditioning.[9] Significantly, the helplessness condition in animals may be treated by procedures also effective in humans, and it is also related to nonsuppression in the Dexamethasone suppression test,[10] paralleling human clinical depression.

In the rat model, helplessness is not generally manifest as a failure to avoid shock or in increased escape latencies under simple fixed-ratio 1 (FR1) contingencies.[11] Rather, it is manifest as increased latency to escape under FR2 contingencies; that is, the rat seems only to be impaired in relatively complex situations. Furthermore, it seems that not all animals develop the syndrome and that the escape deficit dissipates over time without further testing. No deficit is found if the period between inescapable shock and testing is more than 4 d. The temporal dissipation is parallel to neurochemical changes induced by the inescapable shock procedures.[12]

Clearly, a method that induces a short-lived "depression" has little face value for those primarily interested in human clinical depression. However, new results from Maier[9] show that the escape deficit in helpless rats may be prolonged by reexposure to the cues associated with IS but that the effect of reexposure also dissipates over time. Furthermore, the exposure to the cues must occur within a time period during which the escape deficit normally is manifest. Repeated reexposure to the cues of inescapable shock prolongs the deficit for up to 18 d. However, if the animals are exposed to IS cues for long periods of time, apparently they eventually learn that shock will not occur, and the deficit recedes. Elicitation of a nonspecific stress response by reexposure to cues does not explain the deficit because using other stressors has no "reminding" effect.

A PubMed search reveals more than 1000 references to the LH model since 1967, suggestive of a substantial influence on depression research. The model has been exploited for the development of both behavioral and pharmacological approaches to the human disorder and has clearly been successful in this regard. However, in recent years, the use of the model has been constrained by ethical considerations and in some countries has come to be regarded as too extreme,[13] stimulating explorations of other potential models. Other criticisms of the model have included the "unnaturalness" of the induction procedures, but within a cognitive perspective it matters not what the organism is unable to control, so long as the animal develops negative outcome expectancies.[8]

As with any animal model of any disorder, there are considerable interstrain differences in susceptibility. As just one example, WKY rats seem particularly prone.[14] Early experience also affects vulnerability, a phenomenon of increasing interest not only with respect to depression research. Early handling of animals appears to be protective against later helplessness induction,[15] whereas prenatal stress renders the animal more susceptible.[16]

Chronic Unpredictable Stress and Anhedonia

Anhedonia — a general lack of interest in the pleasures of life — is a core symptom of human depression and can easily be tested in animals. The most common methods for measuring hedonic tone include avidity for sucrose or saccharine consumption.[17,18]

Whereas the LH model generally relies on one exposure to a stressor, the chronic unpredictable stress (CUS) model used by Katz[19] uses a series of different uncontrollable stressors (inescapable shock, forced swim, periods of deprivation of food or water or both, and heat stress, to name but a few) over a period of weeks. After the final stress exposure, the animals exhibit anhedonia, as indexed by lowered sucrose or saccharine consumption and preference. Significantly, stress-induced anhedonia found in this model is sensitive to the antidepressant imipramine (given during the chronic stress phase). It is reasonable to claim that the LH and CUS models are tapping a common condition. Exposure to inescapable shock leads to a reduction of intracranial self-stimulation in the mesocorticolimbic system, a critical brain area for reward mechanisms,[20] and, conversely, experience with chronic stress procedures enhances the helplessness behavior in rats.[21]

Chronic Mild Stress

The logic underlying the Katz model was followed up in the chronic mild stress (CMS) model originally developed by Willner and colleagues.[22] The measure of depression was the same — anhedonia — but the procedures used to induce the state were reduced significantly in severity in comparison with the Katz procedures. The logic is that depression is the consequence of daily, mild, nonspecific hassles rather than of exposure to one or more traumatic stressors. As with the Katz model, the animals (rats or mice) are exposed over some weeks to uncontrollable events, but none of these by themselves are regarded as particularly stressful. These include periods of deprivation of food or water or both, rehousing with strange animals, soiling of the cage bedding, changes from normal light–dark cycles, periods of stroboscopic lighting, and cage tilt. The hedonic deficit is first observed after 1 to 2 weeks of the CMS procedures and is sensitive to a variety of antidepressant treatments, including electroconvulsive therapy and various clinically effective pharmacological agents, including serotonin reuptake inhibitors. The hedonic changes are not limited to sucrose and saccharine consumption but also include sexual behavior,[23] sleep patterns[24,25] (similar to human depressives), and intracranial self-stimulation.[26]

The CMS procedure is finding increasing popularity because it avoids the use of strongly aversive treatments. However, the effect of the procedures is not always apparent, and both its robustness and validity have been questioned.[27] It seems unclear exactly which if any of the elements of CMS procedures are necessary to produce the anhedonic effect, and some workers have chosen to include non-mild stressors such as intraperitoneal saline injections.[28] In our own studies, we have observed both increases and decreases in hedonic tone using the sucrose test (Murison and Hansen, in preparation). Although a decrease in hedonic tone might be a useful index of depression (but see Argyropoulos and Nutt[29]), an increase might be the consequence of environmental enrichment.[30] Because CMS-induced anhedonia is not completely robust, researchers using the model with other dependent measures should ensure that an anhedonic state has been achieved. Failure to do so will lead to misleading results and interpretations. Notwithstanding the criticisms concerning the robustness of the CMS model, it should not be discarded. Detailed parametric studies are needed to identify which components of the procedure are either necessary or sufficient to induce anhedonia, as well as whether there are interactions with early life events and genetic influences.

One interesting principal question attached to the CMS model is whether the *mild* refers to the procedures or the outcome. If CMS produces an effect similar to the more severe CUS and LH methods, can it really be regarded as mild?

Developmental Models

One of the most renowned studies in animal psychology involved the separation of monkeys from their mothers during infancy, performed by Harlow and colleagues.[31] The result of this manipulation was dramatic, involving social withdrawal, fear, and a condition with parallels to anaclitic depression that is seen in human infants.[32] The studies provoked strong criticism and are often cited as exemplars by those who are particularly opposed to psychological animal experiments.[33]

For work with rodents, there is a considerable literature on the effects of early manipulations. As long ago as 1956, Levine showed that early handling or maternal separation of rats permanently altered their emotional and endocrinological state in adulthood.[34–38] Generally, brief daily early handling rendered animals less emotional and stress resistant as adults, whereas either a single long or several shorter separations from the mother rendered the animals stress sensitive as adults. Problems with the reliability of this paradigm have arisen from the multiplicity of procedures used — age at separation, length of separation, and maintenance of body temperature, to name but a few critical factors.[39] The more recent studies of Meaney and colleagues have tied these effects to specific mother–pup interactions[40] and have shown that the effects may also be transmitted across generations.[41]

ANXIETY AND ANXIETY-RELATED DISORDERS

Within its normal range, anxiety clearly represents an adaptive phenomenon, protecting the animals against unknown threats. This is in contrast to fear (and phobias), which is targeted against known threats. Anxiety becomes nonadaptive, or a state of disorder, when it interferes with normal function. Anxiety in animals can be measured by a number of techniques, all with high face validity, but the indices do not always correlate well, probably because of procedural differences.

The oldest and arguably most reliable measurement technique is that of open-field exploration, which might be of either the *forced* or *free* type. In the former, the animal (rat or mouse, generally) is placed in the center of an empty arena (typically of the order of 1×1 m^2) and its behavior recorded over a chosen period (from 3 to 15 min). Behaviors typically recorded are activity around the peripheral walls of the arena (*thigmotaxis*), crossings of the central area, vertical activity, grooming, and defecation. In some studies, defecation has been used as the cardinal measure of anxiety. The disadvantage with the method, as well as the advantage, is the potential for collecting vast amounts of data. Free exploration involves placing the animal in a start box attached to the test arena. As well as those measures mentioned above, the most important score for anxiety is the latency to emerge from the start box into the open-field area. In principle, this latter test is similar to the dark–light two-chamber test. The advantages and disadvantages of this measure have been discussed at length elsewhere,[42,43] but the test remains popular.

A second popular method is the elevated plus maze.[44] Here, a four-armed maze is placed on legs approximately 1 m above the floor. Two arms are enclosed by high walls, whereas the remaining two are open. Anxiety is measured by the ratio of the amount of time that the animal spends in the closed and open arms, and the number of entrances that are made into the open arms.

A third and more recent method is the defensive-burying situation developed by Treit and colleagues.[45] Many rodent species have a natural tendency to bury objects that they perceive to be aversive. The defensive-burying test entails presenting animals with an aversive object, such as a shock probe, a discrete source of an aversive odor (e.g., ammonia), or a flashbulb. Treit and colleagues[45] have argued that the intensity of burying is an index of anxiety and that this response is modulated by anxiolytic agents. However, it could be argued that this is a test of fear rather than anxiety.

An interesting and simple method is implicitly based on the association between anxiety and increased vigilance. The *audiogenic immobility reaction* is induced by first habituating an animal to a test chamber with a background of white noise of a given intensity, typically on the order of 80 dB. The habituation session is for a given period of 6 min. On the subsequent test session, the background noise is abruptly turned off after the first 3 min, and the animal's behavior is observed for the remaining 3 min of silence. The index of anxiety here includes both the time spent immobile after noise is turned off and the amount of vertical activity (rearing). The animal is not totally immobile. Typically, the animal will remain in one position but with head movements indicative of increased vigilance. This method is easy and cheap to perform and has proven useful (see below).

A final method is the acoustic-startle response. Animals are exposed to a semirandom series of brief acoustic stimuli of varying intensities (for example, 95, 105, and 115 dB), and the startle response is measured by movement sensors under the tube in which the animal has been placed. This method has been highly standardized and elaborated. For example, the response is potentiated by fear conditioning[46] and sensitized by earlier shock.[47] It is debatable whether the pure acoustic-startle response is a measure of anxiety or fear, although as we shall see, anxiety disorders are related to increased startle. In humans, the startle response may be measured using the eye-blink reflex to an air puff.

Nonpharmacological methods of raising anxiety levels in rodents again involve the use of aversive stimulation. An important series of studies with regard to this was performed by van Dijken.[48–50] Briefly, rats exposed to a small number of shocks (ten, well below the number required to induce a state of learned helplessness) exhibited a long-lasting reduction in exploratory behavior in a forced exploration (open-field) test up to 21 d after shock. Interestingly, the effect was least 1 d after shock and grew over increasing postshock intervals (note that these were independent groups of animals), and a later study showed no differences in locomotion 1 or 4 h after shock. A marked increase in the auditory immobility response was seen 21 d after shock. Significantly, the long-lasting behavioral changes were sensitive to anxiolytic but not antidepressant drugs. The progressively increasing effects of the short shock regimen over time differ fundamentally from the transient effects of LH procedures, which are, in contrast, sensitive to antidepressant drugs. In a direct comparison of the effects of a short shock exposure with the effects of LH induction, we have shown that the LH shock failed to produce an increase in the auditory immobility response 14 d after shock, in contrast to the ten-shock paradigm,[51] whose effects we have observed up to 3 months after shock.

Animal models are potentially highly useful in studies of one particular anxiety disorder, post-traumatic stress disorder (PTSD), and it could be argued that both the LH and the short shock methods described above are indeed modeling PTSD. In humans, PTSD is characterized by increased startle reactivity, flashbacks, and avoidance as a consequence of exposure to unusual traumatic events, and some have reported lower than normal levels of plasma cortisol.[52] Significantly, not all individuals exposed to trauma develop the disorder, the incidence varying from 20 to 60%. It would clearly be useful to develop a model that would allow us to identify risk factors for PTSD.

SCHIZOPHRENIA

Animal modeling of human psychoses such as schizophrenia poses a much more difficult problem than do the affective disorders, for a number of reasons. First, anyone with even limited experience with animals recognizes the face validity of such constructs as fear, anxiety, and even depression, at least in mammalian species; but with schizophrenia there is a lack of the "initial analogy"[3] so that one must resort to conceptual equivalence rather than material equivalence. Second, there is clearly an element of learning involved in acquisition of anxiety and depression, which facilitates animal modeling. Third, the affective disorders seem to reflect that a normally adaptive phenomenon has become maladaptive. Fourth, schizophrenia seems to affect higher cognitive processes — a disturbance in thinking[53] — and may become apparent only in species capable of these processes. Crow[54] argues that the condition is human specific and related to the development of the capacity for language. And finally, the term *schizophrenia* and the diagnosis of the condition may be insufficiently delineated to model. In summarizing a recent Nobel Symposium on the subject, Terenius[55] cautions us that "schizophrenia may eventually be shown to be elicited by a large number of mechanisms at a fundamental level…with a final common outcome." That is, there may be several etiologies leading to a common proximal process responsible for the condition. This is reflected in the multitude of factors found to be of epidemiological importance in schizophrenia, such as seasonal effects, relationship to infections during pregnancy, drug abuse, etc. It is also important to note that schizophrenia is characterized by two sets of symptoms — so-called positive symptoms and negative symptoms, which are differentially responsive to the so-called typical and atypical antipsychotic drugs.

Even given these limitations, models of schizophrenia serve several purposes. First, they may be heuristic, providing a framework in which to ask questions about etiology. Second, they may be predictive, for example, used to test potential antipsychotic treatments.

Schizophrenia is often regarded as a cluster of symptoms reflecting thought disorders that are consequent to a brain dysfunction. Because we do not have access to the animals' mind, researchers have developed animal models based on (1) epidemiological findings and (2) known therapeutic effects in man. The latter is represented by the fact that antipsychotic agents are antagonists of dopaminergic function and that dopaminergic agents induce psychotic symptoms. It has been argued that models based on this have high predictive validity but no construct validity.[56]

The key issue is what aspect of schizophrenia one should choose to model as the dependent variable in an animal model. On the behavioral level, perhaps the most promising at present involves the phenomenon of prepulse inhibition (PPI) of the startle response.[57] The logic underlying this model is that schizophrenia is associated with a deficit in sensory gating, by which the animal is normally able to filter out most of the information available and that allows attention to be directed to salient stimuli. The startle response mentioned above is sensitive to a number of manipulations that will affect intensity and habituation. One of these, PPI, involves presenting a lower intensity acoustic stimulus immediately preceding the normal high-intensity startle stimulus. When this occurs, the normal response to the startle stimulus is modulated. In human schizophrenics, there is a deficit in PPI, suggestive of a weakening of sensory gating.[58] It is important to note that the phenomenon of PPI is not restricted to any one sensory modality. Deficits in PPI correlate with thought disorders of people with schizophrenia.[57] However, deficits in PPI are not specific to schizophrenia but are also found in other disorders associated with deficits in sensory, motor, or cognitive gating.

Etiological models of schizophrenia have either focused on direct pharmacological manipulations, particularly of the dopaminergic and glutamate systems, which seem to directly mimic the abnormalities of the human schizophrenic brain, or on nonpharmacological manipulations aimed at exploring etiological factors. With respect to the former, dopamine agonists reduce PPI in rats, including apomorphine, primarily through acting at the D2 receptor, and the effect can be blocked by haloperidol. The effect is also blocked by both typical and atypical antipsychotic agents. The PCP model in rats involves glutamate antagonist action and again is associated with deficits in PPI. This effect is not reversed by typical antipsychotics such as haloperidol. However, these models, although having high predictive validity (and therefore useful in development of therapeutic strategies), have little to say about the natural etiology of the disorder. Given that it is well established that schizophrenia is associated with dopaminergic abnormalities, it should not be surprising that pharmacological manipulation of the dopaminergic system will induce changes paralleling schizophrenia.

Currently there is considerable interest in the role of early environmental factors in schizophrenia. Schizophrenia is often seen as a neurodevelopmental disorder that only becomes fully manifest after puberty. Candidates for the induction of the disorder include prenatal infections[59] and early stress.[60] With respect to the former, several studies have shown how viral infections disrupt normal neurodevelopment (for review, see Lipska and Weinberger[56]). With respect to early stress and environmental manipulations, research has focused in particular on effects of early handling, maternal separation, and isolation rearing on PPI in the adult rat. Ellenbroek and Cools[61] studies using rat lines selected for high or low sensitivity to apomorphine suggest that a single 24-h maternal separation on day 7 or 10 induces a deficit in PPI. In a recent critical review, Weiss and Feldon[62] claimed no evidence of either early handling or maternal separation effects on PPI but indicated substantial evidence for PPI deficits in adult animals that had been socially isolated in the period from weaning to adulthood. This effect was reversed by both typical and atypical drugs.

"PSYCHOSOMATIC" AND FUNCTIONAL DISORDERS

The term *psychosomatic* in its original form means that psychological factors may influence the initiation and development of somatic dysfunction. In contrast to earlier thinking, few today would argue that a disease state is caused by psychological factors. However, most disease states are multifactorial and accessible to psychological influences through either direct nervous control or psychoendocrine influences.

Perhaps the most studied of these is stress-induced gastric erosions. Although these local bleeding areas of the stomach are induced by "physical" stress such as cold or electric shock, the severity is strongly influenced by psychological conditions. Weiss[63] showed in a series of studies that severity of ulceration was modulated by providing the animals with control over a physical stressor, in this case electric shock. The Weiss studies provided a framework for later models of the relationship between effort, feedback, and human disease.[8,64] In rats, exposure to uncontrollable shock stress renders the animal more sensitive to stress gastric erosions, an effect that is related to induction of LH and is blocked by naloxone and mimicked by morphine.[65] Prior experience with controllable stress and coping, however, appears to reduce the animals' vulnerability to stress erosions.[66,67]

As a model for ulcer, one has to be careful in considering these stress erosion studies. Since the discovery of *Helicobacter pylori,* ulcer disease in humans has been regarded as primarily an infectious disease. However, most clinicians and basic researchers agree that other factors are involved, as evidenced by the fact that so few infected individuals develop ulcers.[68–70] And both older experimental and newer field studies on primates clearly implicate a role for psychological factors in gastric pathology in our closer relatives.[71,72] Others have suggested that gastric erosions of the kind seen in these studies might better be models of erosive prepyloric changes sometimes observed in patients with functional (non-ulcer) dyspepsia.[73]

Other studies of psychological influences on gastrointestinal pathology have focused on animal models of inflammatory bowel disease. The models employed have included 2,4,6-trinitrobenzene sulfonic acid (TNBS)- and dinitrobenzene sulfonic acid (DNBS)-induced colitis and, more recently, dextran sulfate sodium (DSS)-induced colitis. Evidence is emerging that vulnerability to and recovery from such chemically induced ulcerative colitis may be influenced by stress.[74–76] In primates, the cotton-topped tamarin shows spontaneous colitis, a phenomenon that again has been ascribed to stress.[77]

In the 1970s, evidence began to mount for brain–immune interactions. In particular, the studies by Ader and Cohen[78] of conditioning of the immune response attracted considerable attention. Little credence was given to the phenomenon until mechanisms were identified, both endocrine and nervous.[79,80] Even then, there remained doubt as to whether the so-well-demonstrated interactions had a biological significance either in animals or humans. Although stress clearly impinges on the immune system, and vice versa, implications of classical conditioning have been little explored. Exton and colleagues[81] have convincingly shown that classical conditioning of cyclosporin-induced immunosuppression in the rat has dramatic effects on longevity after transplant surgery. Such findings, together with the enormous efforts being made to identify molecular mechanisms, will inevitably lead eventually to a recognition of the importance of the animal work. In a related area, it is also known that conditioning procedures are effective in altering mast cell function in the gut, a finding that will have implications for, among other things, colon disease.[82]

Functional disorders are less easy to model in animals, purely because they are defined by the absence of identifiable organic changes. However, studies by Stam and colleagues[83] have made use of gut-recording techniques in rats to investigate how prior life events might affect intestinal motility, a potential model for irritable bowel syndrome, which is a disorder also associated with significant levels of psychopathology. This functional disorder in humans is also sometimes associated with prior infections that might sensitize the perception of autonomic signals. There clearly are great potentials for pursuing animal models in this field. Other functional disorders, such as fibromyalgia and lower back pain, will be more difficult to model but not necessarily impossibly so.

CONCLUSION

It is clear that animal models have provided insight into the etiology and mechanisms underlying affective psychological disorders such as depression and anxiety, and that these have had an impact on the development of theories and treatment of human disorders. The animal-based cognitive theories of depression have led to an understanding that behavioral therapies may replace or at least provide an important supplement to pharmacological strategies.[84] Similarly, cognitive behavioral approaches are proving useful in the treatment of anxiety disorders such as PTSD.[85]

For human psychosis, the implications of the animal models are less clear. But when schizophrenia is seen as a neurodevelopmental disorder, the models at least provide us with an understanding of its risk factors and putative mechanisms. The impact on treatment strategies for the future lies most likely within the psychopharmacological domain.

For the classical psychosomatic conditions, in which organic alterations are identifiable, the impact of the animal models is in emphasizing the need for combining psychological and medical treatments, the latter to remedy the physical symptoms and the former to prevent relapse. Both for these and for the functional disorders, an important lesson from the basic research concerns the importance of changing the individual's core beliefs concerning personal control over the environment.

Animal models have been developed for several other psychological disorders not discussed here, including alcoholism,[86] memory disorders,[87] attention deficit hyperactivity disorder, aggression,[88] and fears and phobias,[89] and the reader is directed to recent reviews that deal with these in greater detail than is possible here.

In all animal model research, consideration must be given to genotype–environment interactions. Different strains of animals may be more suitable than others, depending on the disorder that one wishes to address; and the rapidly developing field of functional genetics will provide us, one hopes, with a much richer picture of these interactions. In the meantime, however, even a cursory examination of the basis of the various models reveals extraordinary variations in the strains of animals used and the exact procedures employed. If we are serious in our use of animal models, greater emphasis should be placed on parametric studies, both with respect to strains and species and to procedures, including husbandry.

REFERENCES

1. Damasio, A., *The Feeling of What Happens,* William Heinemann, London, 1999.
2. Overmier, J.B., On the nature of animal models of human behavioral dysfunction, in *Animal Models of Human Emotion and Cognition,* Haug, M. and Whalen, R.E., Eds., American Psychological Association, Washington, D.C., 1999, 15.
3. Overmier, J.B. and Patterson, J., Animal models of human psychopathology, in *Selected Models of Anxiety, Depression and Psychosis,* Vol. 1, Simon, P., Soubrié, P., and Wildlocher, D., Eds., Karger, Basel, Switzerland, 1988, 1.
4. Nesse, R.M., Is depression an adaptation?, *Arch. Gen. Psychiatr.,* 57, 14, 2000.
5. Seligman, M.E.P., *Helplessness: On Depression, Development and Death,* W.H. Freeman, San Francisco, 1975.

6. Overmier, J.B. and Seligman, M.E., Effects of inescapable shock upon subsequent escape and avoidance responding, *J. Comp. Physiol. Psychol.*, 63, 28, 1967.

7. Miller, W.R. and Seligman, M.E., Depression and learned helplessness in man, *J. Abnorm. Psychol.*, 84, 228, 1975.

8. Ursin, H., Expectancy and activation: an attempt to systematize stress theory, in *Neurobiological Approaches to Human Disease*, Hellhammer, D.H., Florin, I., and Weiner, H., Eds., Hans Huber, Toronto, 1988, 313.

9. Maier, S.F., Exposure to the stressor environment prevents the temporal dissipation of behavioral depression/learned helplessness, *Biol. Psychiatr.*, 49, 763, 2001.

10. Haracz, J.L., Minor, T.R., Wilkins, J.N., and Zimmermann, E.G., Learned helplessness: an experimental model of the DST in rats, *Biol. Psychiatr.*, 23, 388, 1988.

11. Maier, S.F., Role of fear in mediating shuttle escape learning deficit produced by inescapable shock, *J. Exp. Psychol. Anim. Behav. Process.*, 16, 137, 1990.

12. Weiss, J.M., Goodman, P.A., Losito, B.G., Corrigan, S., Charry, J.M., and Bailey, W.H., Behavioral depression produced by an uncontrollable stressor: relationship to norepinephrine, dopamine, and serotonin levels in various regions of rat brain, *Brain Res. Rev.*, 3, 167, 1981.

13. Brain, P.F. and Brain, V.F., Using animals to study human neuroses and psychoses: practices and problems, *Scand. J. Lab. Anim. Sci.*, 25, 29, 1998.

14. Paré, W.P., Open field, learned helplessness, conditioned defensive burying, and forced-swim tests in WKY rats, *Physiol. Behav.*, 55, 433, 1994.

15. Costela, C., Tejedor-Real, P., Mico, J.A., and Gibert-Rahola, J., Effect of neonatal handling on learned helplessness model of depression, *Physiol. Behav.*, 57, 407, 1995.

16. Secoli, S.R. and Teixeira, N.A., Chronic prenatal stress affects development and behavioral depression in rats, *Stress*, 2, 273, 1998.

17. Willner, P., Benton, D., Brown, E., Cheeta, S., Davies, G., Morgan, J., and Morgan, M., "Depression" increases "craving" for sweet rewards in animal and human models of depression and craving, *Psychopharmacology (Berl.)*, 136, 272, 1998.

18. Dess, N.K., Raizer, J., Chapman, C.D., and Garcia, J., Stressors in the learned helplessness paradigm: effects on body weight and conditioned taste aversion in rats, *Physiol. Behav.*, 44, 483, 1988.

19. Katz, R., Animal model of depression: pharmacological sensitivity of a hedonic deficit, *Pharmacol. Biochem. Behav.*, 16, 965, 1982.

20. Zacharko, R.M. and Anisman, H., Stressor-induced anhedonia in the mesocorticolimbic system, *Neurosci. Biobehav. Rev.*, 15, 391, 1991.

21. Murua, V.S. and Molina, V.A., Effects of chronic variable stress and antidepressant drugs on behavioral inactivity during an uncontrollable stress: interaction between both treatments, *Behav. Neural Biol.*, 57, 87, 1992.

22. Willner, P., Towell, A., Sampson, D., Sophokleous, S., and Muscat, R., Reduction of sucrose preference by chronic unpredictable mild stress, and its restoration by a tricyclic antidepressant, *Psychopharmacology*, 93, 358, 1987.

23. D'Aquila, P.S., Brain, P., and Willner, P., Effects of chronic mild stress on performance in behavioural tests relevant to anxiety and depression, *Physiol. Behav.*, 56, 861, 1994.

24. Cheeta, S., Ruigt, G., van Proosdij, J., and Willner, P., Changes in sleep architecture following chronic mild stress, *Biol. Psychiatr.*, 41, 419, 1997.

25. Moreau, J.-L., Scherschlicht, R., Jenck, F., and Martin, J.R., Chronic mild stress-induced anhedonia model of depression: sleep abnormalities and curative effects of electroshock treatment, *Behav. Pharmacol.*, 6, 682, 1995.

26. Moreau, J.L., Jenck, F., Martin, J.R., Mortas, P., and Haefely, W.E., Antidepressant treatment prevents chronic unpredictable mild stress-induced anhedonia as assessed by ventral tegmentum self-stimulation behavior in rats, *Eur. Neuropsychopharmacol.*, 2, 43, 1992.

27. Broekkamp, C., Predictive validity and the robustness criterion for animal models, *Psychopharmacology (Berl.)*, 134, 341, 1997.

28. Moreau, J.L., Bourson, A., Jenck, F., Martin, J.R., and Mortas, P., Curative effects of the atypical antidepressant mianserin in the chronic mild stress-induced anhedonia model of depression, *J. Psychiatr. Neurosci.*, 19, 51, 1994.

29. Argyropoulos, S.V. and Nutt, D.J., Anhedonia and chronic mild stress model in depression, *Psychopharmacology (Berl.)*, 134, 333, 1997.

30. Fernandez-Teruel, A., Escorihuela, R.M., Castellano, B., Gonzalez, B., and Tobena, A., Neonatal handling and environmental enrichment effects on emotionality, novelty/reward seeking, and age-related cognitive and hippocampal impairments: focus on the Roman rat lines, *Behav. Genet.*, 27, 513, 1997.

31. Suomi, S.J. and Harlow, H.F., Production and alleviation of depressive behaviors in monkeys, in *Psychopathology: Experimental Models,* Maser, J.D. and Seligman, M.E.P., Eds., W.H. Freeman, San Francisco, 1977, 131.

32. Spitz, R.A. and Wolf, K.M., Anaclitic depression: an enquiry into the genesis of psychiatric conditions in early childhood, II, *Psychoanal. Stud. Child*, 2, 313, 1946.

33. Blum, D., *The Monkey Wars,* Oxford University Press, New York, 1996.

34. Levine, S., Chevalier, J.A., and Korchin, S.J., The effects of shock and handling in infancy on later avoidance learning, *J. Personality,* 24, 475, 1956.

35. Levine, S., Maternal and environmental influences on the adrenocortical response to stress in weanling rats, *Science,* 156, 258, 1967.

36. Rots, N.Y., de Jong, J., Workel, J.O., Levine, S., Cools, A.R., and De Kloet, E.R., Neonatal maternally deprived rats have as adults elevated basal pituitary-adrenal activity and enhanced susceptibility to apomorphine, *J. Neuroendocrinol.*, 8, 501, 1996.

37. van Oers, H.J., de Kloet, E.R., and Levine, S., Persistent effects of maternal deprivation on HPA regulation can be reversed by feeding and stroking, but not by dexamethasone, *J. Neuroendocrinol.*, 11, 581, 1999.

38. Weinberg, J. and Levine, S., Early handling influences on behavioral and physiological responses during active avoidance, *Dev. Psychobiol.*, 10, 161, 1977.

39. Lehmann, J. and Feldon, J., Long-term biobehavioral effects of maternal separation in the rat: consistent or confusing?, *Rev. Neurosci.*, 11, 383, 2000.

40. Caldji, C., Tannenbaum, B., Sharma, S., Francis, D., Plotsky, P.M., and Meaney, M.J., Maternal care during infancy regulates the development of neural systems mediating the expression of fearfulness in the rat, *Proc. Natl. Acad. Sci. U.S.A.*, 95, 5335, 1998.

41. Francis, D., Diorio, J., Liu, D., and Meaney, M.J., Nongenomic transmission across generations of maternal behavior and stress responses in the rat, *Science,* 286, 1155, 1999.

42. Archer, J., Tests for emotionality in rats and mice: a review, *Anim. Behav.*, 21, 205, 1973.

43. Ivinski, A., The reliability of behavioural measures obtained in the open-field, *Aust. J. Psychol.*, 20, 173, 1968.

44. Pellow, S., Chopin, P., File, S.E., and Briley, M., Validation of open:closed arm entries in an elevated plus-maze as a measure of anxiety in the rat, *J. Neurosci. Methods,* 14, 149, 1985.

45. Treit, D., Pinel, J.P., and Fibiger, H.C., Conditioned defensive burying: a new paradigm for the study of anxiolytic agents, *Pharmacol. Biochem. Behav.*, 15, 619, 1981.

46. Davis, M., Pharmacological and anatomical analysis of fear conditioning using the fear-potentiated startle paradigm, *Behav. Neurosci.*, 100, 814, 1986.

47. Richardson, R., Shock sensitization of startle: learned or unlearned fear?, *Behav. Brain Res.*, 110, 109, 2000.

48. Van Dijken, H.H., Mos, J., van der Heyden, J.A., and Tilders, F.J., Characterization of stress-induced long-term behavioural changes in rats: evidence in favor of anxiety, *Physiol. Behav.*, 52, 945, 1992.

49. Van Dijken, H.H., Tilders, F.J., Olivier, B., and Mos, J., Effects of anxiolytic and antidepressant drugs on long-lasting behavioural deficits resulting from one short stress experience in male rats, *Psychopharmacology*, 109, 395, 1992.

50. Van Dijken, H.H., Van der Heyden, J.A., Mos, J., and Tilders, F.J., Inescapable footshocks induce progressive and long-lasting behavioural changes in male rats, *Physiol. Behav.*, 51, 787, 1992.

51. Murison, R. and Overmier, B.J., Comparison of different animal models of stress reveals a non-monotonic effect, *Stress,* 2, 227, 1998.

52. Yehuda, R., Giller, E.L., Southwick, S.M., Lowy, M.T., and Mason, J.W., Hypothalamic-pituitary-adrenal dysfunction in posttraumatic stress disorder, *Biol. Psychiatr.*, 30, 1031, 1991.

53. Andreasen, N.C., Schizophrenia: the fundamental questions, *Brain. Res. Rev.*, 31, 106, 2000.

54. Crow, T.J., Schizophrenia as the price that *Homo sapiens* pays for language: a resolution of the central paradox in the origin of the species, *Brain Res. Rev.,* 31, 118, 2000.

55. Terenius, L., Schizophrenia: pathophysiological mechanisms — a synthesis, *Brain Res. Rev.,* 31, 401, 2000.

56. Lipska, B.K. and Weinberger, D.R., To model a psychiatric disorder in animals: schizophrenia as a reality test, *Neuropsychopharmacology,* 23, 223, 2000.

57. Geyer, M.A., Krebs-Thomson, K., Braff, D.L., and Swerdlow, N.R., Pharmacological studies of prepulse inhibition models of sensorimotor gating deficits in schizophrenia: a decade in review, *Psychopharmacology (Berl.),* 156, 117, 2001.

58. Braff, D., Stone, C., Callaway, E., Geyer, M., Glick, I., and Bali, L., Prestimulus effects on human startle reflex in normals and schizophrenics, *Psychophysiology,* 15, 339, 1978.

59. Mednick, S.A., Machon, R.A., Huttunen, M.O., and Bonett, D., Adult schizophrenia following prenatal exposure to an influenza epidemic, *Arch. Gen. Psychiatr.,* 45, 189, 1988.

60. Feldon, J. and Weiner, I., From an animal model of an attentional deficit towards new insights into the pathophysiology of schizophrenia, *J. Psychiatr. Res.,* 26, 345, 1992.

61. Ellenbroek, B.A. and Cools, A.R., The neurodevelopment hypothesis of schizophrenia: clinical evidence and animal models, *Neurosci. Res. Commun.,* 22, 127, 1998.

62. Weiss, I.C. and Feldon, J., Environmental animal models for sensorimotor gating deficiencies in schizophrenia: a review, *Psychopharmacology (Berl.),* 156, 305, 2001.

63. Weiss, J.M., Effects of coping responses on stress, *J. Comp. Physiol. Psychol.,* 65, 251, 1968.

64. Ursin, H., Murison, R. and Knardahl, S., Sustained activation and disease, in *Biological and Psychological Basis of Psychosomatic Disease,* Ursin, H. and Murison, R., Eds., Pergamon Press, Oxford, 1983, 269.

65. Overmier, J.B. and Murison, R., Anxiety and helplessness in the face of stress predisposes, precipitates, and sustains gastric ulceration, *Behav. Brain. Res.,* 110, 161, 2000.

66. Murison, R. and Isaksen, E., Gastric ulceration and adrenocortical activity after inescapable and escapable pre-shock in rats, *Scand. J. Psychol.,* Suppl. 1, 133, 1982.

67. Sandbak, T., Murison, R., Sarviharju, M., and Hyytia, P., Defensive burying and stress gastric erosions in alcohol-preferring AA and alcohol-avoiding ANA rats, *Alcohol Clin. Exp. Res.,* 22, 2050, 1998.

68. Murison, R., Is there a role for psychology in ulcer disease?, *Integr. Physiol. Behav. Sci.,* 36, 75, 2001.

69. Levenstein, S., Peptic ulcer at the end of the 20th century: biological and psychological risk factors, *Can. J. Gastroenterol.,* 13, 753, 1999.

70. Weiner, H. and Shapiro, A.P., Is *Helicobacter pylori* really the cause of gastroduodenal disease?, *Q. J. Med.,* 91, 707, 1998.

71. Brady, J.V., Porter, R.W., Conrad, D.G., and Mason, J.W., Avoidance behavior and the development of gastroduodenal ulcers, *J. Exp. Anal. Behav.,* 1, 69, 1958.

72. Tarara, E.B., Tarara, R.P., and Suleman, M.A., Stress-induced gastric ulcers in vervet monkeys (*Cercopithecus aethiops*): the influence of life history factors. Part II, *J. Zoo Wildl. Med.,* 26, 72, 1995.

73. Berstad, A. and Nesland, A., Erosive prepyloric changes (EPC) — a new entity, *Scand. J. Gastroenterol. Suppl.,* 128, 94, 1987.

74. Gué, M., Bonbonne, C., Fioramonti, J., More, J., Del Rio-Lacheze, C., Comera, C., and Bueno, L., Stress-induced enhancement of colitis in rats: CRF and arginine vasopressin are not involved, *Am. J. Physiol.,* 272, G84, 1997.

75. Collins, S.M., McHugh, K., Jacobson, K., Khan, I., Riddell, R., Murase, K., and Weingarten, H.P., Previous inflammation alters the response of the rat colon to stress, *Gastroenterology,* 111, 1509, 1996.

76. Million, M., Taché, Y., and Anton, P., Susceptibility of Lewis and Fischer rats to stress-induced worsening of TNB-colitis: protective role of brain CRF, *Am. J. Physiol.,* 276, G1027, 1999.

77. Wood, J.D., Peck, O.C., Tefend, K.S., Stonerook, M.J., Caniano, D.A., Mutabagani, K.H., Lhotak, S., and Sharma, H.M., Evidence that colitis is initiated by environmental stress and sustained by fecal factors in the cotton-top tamarin (*Saguinus oedipus*), *Dig. Dis. Sci.,* 45, 385, 2000.

78. Ader, R. and Cohen, N., Behaviorally conditioned immunosuppression, *Psychosom. Med.,* 37, 333, 1975.

79. Felten, D.L., Felten, S.Y., Carlson, S.L., Olschowka, J.A., and Livnat, S., Noradrenergic and peptidergic innervation of lymphoid tissue, *J. Immunol.,* 135(Suppl. 2), 755s, 1985.

80. Dunn, A.J., Interactions between the nervous system and the immune system., in *Psychopharmacology: The Fourth Generation of Progress,* Bloom, F.E. and Kupfer, D.J., Eds., Raven Press, New York, 1995, 719.

81. Exton, M.S., von Auer, A.K., Buske-Kirschbaum, A., Stockhorst, U., Göbel, U., and Schedlowski, M., Pavlovian conditioning of immune function: animal investigation and the challenge of human application, *Behav. Brain. Res.,* 110, 129, 2000.

82. MacQueen, G., Marshall, J., Perdue, M., Siegel, S., and Bienenstock, J., Pavlovian conditioning of rat mucosal mast cells to secrete rat mast cell protease II, *Science,* 243, 83, 1989.

83. Stam, R., Croiset, G., Akkermans, L.M., and Wiegant, V.M., Psychoneurogastroenterology: interrelations in stress-induced colonic motility and behavior, *Physiol. Behav.,* 65, 679, 1999.

84. Schwartz, A. and Schwartz, R.M., *Depression: Theories and Treatments: Psychological, Biological, and Social Perspectives,* Columbia University Press, New York, 1993.

85. Foa, E.B., Psychological processes related to recovery from a trauma and an effective treatment for PTSD, *Ann. N.Y. Acad. Sci.,* 821, 410, 1997.

86. McBride, W.J. and Li, T.K., Animal models of alcoholism: neurobiology of high alcohol-drinking behavior in rodents, *Crit. Rev. Neurobiol.,* 12, 339, 1998.

87. Overmier, J.B., Savage, L.M., and Sweeney, W.A., Behavioral and pharmacological analyses of memory offer new behavioral options for remediation, in *Animal Models of Human Emotion and Cognition,* Haug, M. and Whalen, R., Eds., American Psychological Association, Washington, D.C., 1999.

88. Koolhaas, J., de Boer, S.F., de Ruiter, A.J.H., and Bohus, B., Animal aggression: a model for stress and coping, in *Animal Models of Human Emotion and Cognition,* Haug, M. and Whalen, R.E., Eds., American Psychological Association, Washington, D.C., 1999, 259.

89. Mineka, S., The frightful complexity of the origin of fears, in *Affect, Conditioning, and Cognition: Essays on the Determinants of Behavior,* Brush, F.R. and Overmier, J.B., Eds., Lawrence Erlbaum Associates, Hillsdale, NJ, 1985, 55.

CHAPTER 8

Animal Models in Mycology

Henrik Elvang Jensen

CONTENTS

INTRODUCTION

The development and application of experimental animal models in mycology are indispensable and used extensively in the study of a wide range of aspects such as pathogenesis, pathology, virulence, transformative properties, defense mechanisms (immunity), therapy, and prophylaxis. For diagnostic purposes, animal models are important for the isolation and identification of some fungi from both clinical and environmental materials and in the standardization of immunodiagnostic assays. Although some fungi are almost host specific — such as the anthropophilic dermatophytes that only very rarely infect animals, *Histoplasma capsulatum* var. *farciminosum,* which naturally is restricted to equines, and *Pneumocystis carinii* — fungi are generally not host specific in contrast to many other invasive microorganisms. Therefore, a variety of different animal species are suitable for infection with most of the fungi that are of importance in both human and veterinary medicine.

For the establishment of experimental mycotic infections in animals, a number of different routes for challenge are used. The route of choice is strictly dependent on the goal of the study, which also must reflect the animal, fungus, and disease model applied. In general, disseminated infections are produced after intravascular administration, usually intravenous (i.v.), or by intraperitoneal (i.p.) and per-oral (p.o.) challenge. For a number of fungi, the latter two routes will only produce localized mycosis, but they are more regularly established subsequent to intracerebral (i.cer.), intranasal (i.n.), intratracheal (i.t.), intratesticular (i.test.), intracorneal, intramuscular (i.m.), intramammary, intracutaneous (i.c.), subcutaneous (s.c.), or intravaginal (i.vag.) inoculation.

In addition to causing infection, a number of fungi are deleterious to human and animal health because of their formation of mycotoxins, some of which are among the most toxic (e.g., ocratoxin) and carcinogenic (e.g., aflatoxin) substances known. Moreover, fungi are potent sources of antigens, and some of these (allergens) are the cause of immediate hypersensitivity response (type I allergy). Fungal allergy is usually characterized by respiratory diseases and a high serum level of immunoglobin E (IgE) to the allergens. The most important source of fungal allergens seems to be spores of especially *Cladosporium* and *Alternaria,* but allergy may also result from exposure to hyphae, as seen in, for example, allergic bronchopulmonary aspergillosis.

In the present chapter, only the infective aspects of animal models in mycology are covered.

ANIMAL MODELS OF DERMATOPHYTOSIS

In dermatophytosis, the fungi are usually superficially located in keratinized layers of skin, hair, and nails. In severe cases, however, the infection may lead to granuloma formation in the subcutis or become disseminated to internal organs.[1,2] Animal models of dermatophytosis are used especially in the evaluation of new therapeutic agents, but are also applied in the study of pathogenicity, immune responses, and pathology.

Experimental animal infections in a variety of animal species have been performed with zoophilic dermatophytes, especially *Trichophyton mentagrophytes* var. *mentagrophytes* and var. *granulare, Trichophyton verrucosum,* and *Microsporum canis.*[3,4] Infections with the geophilic and anthropophilic dermatophytes, e.g., *Microsporum gypseum* and *Trichophyton rubrum,* are generally difficult to establish in laboratory animals. *T. rubrum,* the fungus most often isolated from human ringworm, unfortunately has a rather low ability to induce experimental ringworm in laboratory animals.[1,3] However, certain strains with a high virulence, selected, for example, by passage in animals, produce exothrix as well as endothrix infection in guinea pigs.[4,5] Infection of rabbits with *T. rubrum* has also been reported, but the lesions produced were not homogeneous; and before inoculation, the animals were exposed to irradiation or were castrated.[6] Models using the natural ringworm dermatophyte of mice, *T. mentagrophytes* var. *quinckeanum,* are also used in the study of infection and immunity because of the close resemblance to human dermatophytosis.[7,8]

Generally, in the study of experimental dermatophytes, guinea pigs are the animal of choice over mouse, rat, hamster, rabbit, and dog because these animals make their toilet by licking or scratching, and they bite itching or irritated lesions intensively.[9] In the study of skin lesions caused by dermatophytosis, hairless strains of guinea pigs are preferred because the lesions produced are more like those seen in humans.[10] Moreover, hairless animals are more suitable for the application of topical antifungal agents. Studies of infections in dogs are few, but dermal inoculations by zoophilic and geophilic dermatophytes produce uniform and long-lasting infections (3 to 4 months), with mongrels presumably being more sensitive to infection than beagles.[9]

Epidermal inoculation of dermatophytes is the classic method of inoculation and may be done in a number of ways, such as by abrasion with sandpaper, a scalpel, or a lancet, after which the inoculum is applied. Repeated putting on and pulling off tape on a hair-cut area in guinea pigs has also been used to make the skin more suitable for inoculation.[4] Depilation with sodium sulfide (36%) for 30 min is also useful.[9] Prick inoculation is performed with a needle smeared with inoculum. An advantage of this method is that the enlargement of the process can be expressed numerically, which is important when testing the effect of therapeutic agents.[4] A disadvantage, however, is that the rate of positive infections is less in comparison with the results of the abrasive methods. A nontraumatizing method used on guinea pigs is the occlusive-dressing method, where the area is kept moist after plucking off the hair and the inoculum is applied under a polyethylene film and an elastic bandage.[11,12] In this model, the severity of lesion increases proportionally with the time of occlusion.

A general disadvantage of the experimental dermatophytosis models is that they are not long-lasting. However, a prolonged infection in guinea pigs can be maintained using highly virulent strains of *T. mentagrophytes* or by transplantation of their skin, which subsequently is infected, into athymic nude mice.[4,13] However, administration of steroids and other immunosuppressants and the use of germ-free animals are not effective for prolonging an infection.[14]

The i.v. route for the establishment of dermatophytosis is also widely used, especially as a model in the testing of new therapeutic agents.[9,15–17] As in skin inoculations, the zoophilic dermato-phytes especially exhibit a trophism for infecting the skin after i.v. inoculation (Figure 8.1). A disadvantage of the i.v. route for dermatophytes is that internal organs, especially the lungs, also are regularly invaded. Moreover, in these models, relapse of ringworm in animals that were cured is often seen and is thought to originate from lesions in internal organs.[9] Concerning reproductivity of skin lesions after i.v. inoculation with *T. mentagrophytes* as an example, the guinea pig is also the animal of choice, with the rabbit and dog being of intermediate value, and the chicken, mouse, and rat being considered useless due to a very low susceptibility.[4,9] Intravenous inoculation of non-dermatophytes, such as *Candida albicans, Cryptococcus neoformans, Rhizopus* spp., and *Absidia corymbifera*, may also result in mycotic folliculitis and skin eruptions.[9,18–20]

Routes of infection other than the cutaneous and intravenous are usually not successful or only sporadically successful. However, intraperitoneal inoculation of mice with *T. rubrum* may result in the development of granulomatous lesions.[21]

Apart from laboratory animals, domestic animals, such as goats, pigs, cattle, and horses, are also used for experimental inoculations.[4] However, the course of infection in these animals are often too short to be compared with the chronic spontaneous infections found in humans and animals. Particular attention has been paid to the development of a vaccine against trichophytosis in cattle based on a killed or an attenuated strain of *T. verrucosum*.[22,23] However, in humans, the results of vaccination against different types of superficial mycoses, including dermatophytosis, have been rather disappointing.[24] Experimental dermatophytosis has also been produced in volunteers, and when their course of infection is compared with spontaneous infections, it always resolves quickly, like experimental infections in most animals.[25]

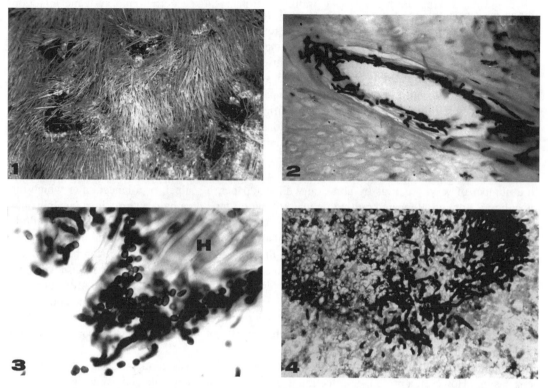

Figure 8.1   Experimental trichophytosis in the guinea pig by intravenous challenge with *Trichophyton menta-grophytes*. (1) Ringworm lesions on the back 3 weeks after infection. (2) Fungi in the hair root sheath. (3) Fungal elements are seen in the hair shaft (H). (4) Granulomatous mycotic pneumonia has formed. (Parts 1 and 2, from Van Cutsem, *J. Curr. Top. Med. Mycol.*, 3, 1, 1989. With permission.)

When dealing with laboratory animals with ringworm, whether received experimentally or naturally, one must always pay attention to the risk of being infected, as many of the zoophilic dermatophyte species also easily cause ringworm in humans.

ANIMAL MODELS OF SUBCUTANEOUS MYCOSES

In this group of mycoses, a number of heterogeneous fungi are responsible for infection. In general, the infections are the result of traumatic implantation of the fungus into the skin, and the infection is only slowly spreading into surrounding tissues.[26] In some infections, extension by lymph vessels is frequent (sporotrichosis); in other diseases, hematogenous spread may also be seen (chromoblastomycosis).

Chromomycosis

Chromoblastomycosis encompasses a specific clinical entity (verrucous dermatitis) and is caused by a limited series of soil-inhabiting dematiaceous fungi, showing sclerotic cells as the parasitic form, of which *Fonsecaea* spp. are the most important.[4,26,27] Other clinical types of infection with dematiaceous fungi are termed phaeohyphomycosis (hyphal forms in infected tissue) and may be manifested in a variety of clinical types. In humans, the infection may be caused by a variety of fungi belonging to several genera, such as *Wangiella* spp. and *Cladosporium* spp.[4,26] Chromoblastomycosis and phaeohyphomycosis are collectively referred to as chromomycosis. Mice, rats, rabbits, hamsters, guinea pigs, and monkeys are susceptible to experimental chromomycosis, with mice and rats having the highest susceptibility.[28] Both localized dermal and systemic infections with reactions that resemble those observed in humans have been produced in a number of animal models by inoculation by different routes, such as s.c., i.v., and i.p.[4,26,29] Moreover, animal inoculations are used to distinguish *Cladosporium carrionii* from *Cladosporium bantianum,* the latter being highly neurotropic.[26]

Lobomycosis

Lobomycosis is caused by a yeast-like organism referred to as *Loboa loboi*, which has not been cultured *in vitro*.[26] Clinically, lobomycosis is a chronically localized subepidermal infection. Experimental infections have been successfully established in hamsters by inoculation of clinical material, resulting in a clinical picture similar to that seen in humans.[30] In turtles, tortoises, and armadillos, the lesions develop more rapidly and are accompanied by liquefactive necrosis.[26] In mice, i.p., i.c., and i.test. inoculations have been unsuccessful, whereas transfer of the infection through generations of mice is feasible by using the hind footpad as the inoculum site.[26,30]

Mycetoma

Mycetoma s. *maduromycosis* is a clinical syndrome of localized indolent, deforming, swollen lesions and sinuses, involving cutaneous and subcutaneous tissues, facia, and bone.[31] The infection is established by a variety of bacteria (actinomycetoma) and true fungi (eumycetoma). Experimental actinomycotic granules caused by *Norcardia* spp. and *Actinomadura* spp. have been produced in a variety of animals: mice, hamsters, rabbits, goats, and guinea pigs.[4] Subcutaneous lesions are generally produced after s.c. inoculations, whereas granules in internal organs and on the abdominal wall are produced after i.v. and i.p. inoculation, respectively. With eumycotic agents, establishment of animal models has had limited success, and reports of experimental animal inoculations are few.[4,31] Inoculation of eumycotic fungi i.p. into mice only produces granules in a small number of the animals challenged.[32,33] However, s.c. nodules with granules similar to those in patients are formed in rabbits inoculated s.c. with *Exophiala jeanselmei*.[34] Only rarely are fungi such as *Aspergillus fumigatus* and *T. rubrum* the causative agents in mycetomas. However, i.p. inoculation of mice with these fungi may also result in the formation of granules.[35,36]

Rhinosporidiosis

Rhinosporidiosis is a chronic granulomatous disease of the nasal mucocutaneous tissue and is caused by *Rhinosporidium seeberi*. Although many attempts to transfer the disease to experimental animals have been done, a model for prolonged and chronic disease has not yet been developed.[26] In a few instances, granulomata have been produced, but sustained and progressive disease as seen in humans has not occurred.[26]

Sporotrichosis

Sporotrichosis is caused by the dimorphic fungus *Sporothrix schenckii*. Clinical types of sporotrichosis are cutaneous, lymphocutaneous, extracutaneous, and disseminated.[26,37] In laboratory animals, infection with *S. schenckii* may be established in mice, rats, gerbils, hamsters, rabbits, guinea pigs, dogs, cats, and monkeys.[4,26] The disease is seen after challenge by the i.p., i.v., i. test., s.c., and i.m. routes. Mice and rats are particularly susceptible, and a systemic infection is established after, for instance, i.p. inoculation, a course of infection only rarely seen in humans.[37] In rabbits and guinea pigs, the course of disease is more variable than in mice and rats.[4] A lymphatic infection that in many aspects resembles the course of human infection is produced in cats, hamsters, and monkeys after s.c. footpad inoculation.[38–41] Histopathologically, characteristic asteroid bodies surrounding the fungal cells are sometimes seen in testicular tissue of mice, rats, hamsters, and guinea pigs.[26] Furthermore, differences in thermophilia for colony formation (35°C and 37°C) of *S. schenckii* isolate the fungus and, depending on the temperature under which the animals are kept, the fungus will grow in different organs of mice and rats.[42] Therefore, when working with experimental infections due to *S. schenckii*, it is mandatory that the temperature under which the animals are kept is fully controlled. Some investigators recommend that the animals be kept at 20°C as the rate of infection is higher at this temperature.[43,44]

ANIMAL MODELS OF MYCOSES DUE TO OBLIGATE PATHOGENIC FUNGI

Mycoses in this group are caused by species that have the ability to elicit disease in normal hosts when the inoculum is of a sufficient size.[45] Therefore, cultures of these fungi should be handled in the most rigorous of containment facilities, and by experienced personnel only. The mycoses are usually systemic and occur in restricted geographic areas, primarily in North and South America and Africa.[45] The obligate pathogenic fungi are dimorphic and exhibit a morphological transition from a mycelial (saprophytic) form to a budding yeast-like (parasitic) form in infected tissue in which chronic granulomatous processes are formed.[45,46]

Blastomycosis

Blastomycosis is caused by *Blastomyces dermatitidis* and is characterized by having a primary pulmonary stage that may be followed by dissemination to other body sites, especially the skin and bones.[45] Mice are highly susceptible to yeasts of *B. dermatitidis,* but the maturity of mice (body weight and age) is a critical factor in resistance, as is the strain of mice used, because they influence both the course of infection and the lethality in mice when challenged with *B. dermatitidis.*[47,48] Mice are preferably infected by the aerogene route because it is the natural portal of entry in humans. After i.n. challenge, an acute to chronic pulmonary infection is established, and dissemination to other organs may be seen.[48,49] In this model, the course of infection and the pathological reactions seen are comparable with human blastomycosis.[50] By experiments in hamsters, which are more susceptible to infection than mice, a female:male lethal ratio of 1:7 is observed, which corresponds to the 1:9 ratio in humans.[46,51,52] Moreover, treatment of ovariectomized hamsters with testosterone will render them as susceptible as male hamsters, and castrated males are more resistant than normal ones.[51] These results with experimental blastomycosis strongly point to the importance of always giving full information on the model used. More rarely, guinea pigs and dogs are also used as models of blastomycoses.[46]

Coccidioidomycosis

Coccidioidomycosis is usually a mild respiratory infection due to *Coccidioides immitis*. Rarely, the infection is an acute or chronic disseminating and fatal mycosis.[45,46]

Experimental disease can be produced in most laboratory animals. Mice are usually used, and according to inoculum, port of entry, and strain, the course of disease may vary from acute fatal to chronic.[46] In the i.p. and i.n. model of coccidioidomycosis, as in blastomycosis, a marked difference in susceptibility has been found in a variety of genetically different but defined mice.[53,54] Also, the course of coccidioidomycosis in mice is highly age dependent but not sex dependent.[54] The pulmonary model in mice mimics the infection of humans with a characteristic formation of granulomas.[46] As immunized mice restrict extrapulmonary dissemination,[55,56] which is seldom seen in human cases, this model should be considered in, for example, pathogenicity studies. Apart from mice, guinea pigs, dogs, and monkeys are also applicable in the study of different aspects of coccidioidomycosis.[46]

Histoplasmosis

Histoplasmosis capsulati, a granulomatous disease, is caused by *Histoplasma capsulatum* var. *capsulatum* and has worldwide distribution. Clinically, the disease may vary from subclinical or completely benign to a chronic progressive lung disease, a chronic cutaneous or systemic disease, or an acute fulminant and fatal systemic infection.[57]

While there may be no good animal model of the more chronic forms of infection by *H. capsulatum* var. *capsulatum,* reproductive animal models of acute pulmonary, disseminated, and ocular forms have been developed and are applied extensively in studies concerning therapy.[45,46] Experimental histoplasmosis is easily produced in mice and dogs by i.v. and i.n. challenge, whereas guinea pigs, hamsters, rabbits, and rats vary considerably in their susceptibility to infection.[45] The self-resolving infection of the murine lung after i.t. inoculation of yeast cells is an essential model for the most frequent human form of subclinical infection.[58] Because as few as one to ten yeast cells or even a single macroconidium will infect a mouse, it is a useful means of isolation of the fungus from patient material and soil samples, for which a standardized procedure is devised.[45] Also, monkeys and poikilothermic animals have been used as experimental models of histoplasmosis.[45] In the latter group, it was found that the lesions of animals kept at 25°C contained mycelium, and those housed at 37°C contained yeast cells regardless of the infectious material.

Histoplasmosis farciminosi is caused by a variant called *Histoplasma capsulatum* var. *farciminosum* and is the cause of epizootic lymphangitis in horses, donkeys, and mules. Experimental disease by i.d. and i.p. inoculation of mice and rabbits has been produced.[59,60] However, in these animals, the disease had not caused what is seen in equines, that is, formation of lymphangitis.

Histoplasmosis duboisii (African histoplasmosis) is caused by *Histoplasma capsulatum* var. *duboisii,* and the disease evoked by this fungus is characterized by granulomatous and suppurative lesions, primarily of the cutaneous, subcutaneous, and osseous tissues.[45] Because the space of time between infection and clinical symptoms in natural infection with *H. capsulatum* var. *duboisii* is long, the disease sometimes has been imported through primates to countries outside the African continent.[61,62] Experimental infections in animals have been studied in a number of species, such as mice, hamsters, guinea pigs, rabbits, and pigeons; and in comparison with *H. capsulatum* var. *capsulatum,* the *duboisii* variant is of relatively low virulence.[45,63] In laboratory animals, the course of infection is comparable to that in human cases.[45,63] Histologically, the reaction is initially histiocytic, which is later replaced by giant cells. These are also dominant in the human granulomatous lesions of African histoplasmosis.

Paracoccidioidomycosis

Paracoccidioidomycosis is caused by *Paracoccidioides brasiliensis* and is a chronic granulomatous disease that, after nidation in the lung, disseminates to form ulcerative granulomas of especially the head and gastrointestinal mucosa.[45] Lymph nodes are also often involved. As for *H. capsulatum* var. *capsulatum* and *B. dermatitidis,* the fungus may be isolated from clinical material by inoculation into laboratory animals where, for example, i.test. inoculation of rats, of which the mountain rat (*Proechimys guayanensis*) is particularly susceptible to infection, should be used.[45] Next to mice, hamsters, which are more susceptible than guinea pigs, have been used most extensively in the study of paracoccidioidomycosis.[46,64,65] In mice and other laboratory animals, acute systemic infections are seen after i.v. and i.p. challenge with the yeast form of the fungus. However, as for blastomycosis and coccidioidomycosis, the maturity of the mice is essential when used for experimental infection.[66] Rabbits are relatively resistant to infection.[67]

A chronic progressive model in hamsters inoculated i.test. with yeast cells is somewhat analogous to the human disease.[68,69] However, the pulmonary route of infection with dissemination to other organs, which is the natural route of infection in humans, is established in immunosuppressed mice by inoculation of elements of the saprophytic form of *P. brasiliensis.*[70] Therefore, this model is the most suitable one for the study of paracoccidioidomycosis with respect to, for example, pathogenesis.

ANIMAL MODELS OF MYCOSES DUE TO OPPORTUNISTIC PATHOGENIC FUNGI

Infection due to fungi in this group is normally only established when predisposing factors are present.[71] The list of factors promoting the development of opportunistic mycotic infections is quite large and comprises aspects regarding the fungus (e.g., dose of exposure and virulence of strain), but much more important are predisposing, favoring, or stimulating factors in the host.[72] Among predisposing conditions in humans, the most important ones include diseases such as diabetes mellitus, acute lymphoblastic leukemia, and other hematological neoplasms, and the acquired immunodeficiency syndrome.[72,73] Also, the use of therapeutics that compromise the immunological status of humans and animals or compromise the normal bacterial flora of the outer surfaces and the gastrointestinal tract (e.g., corticosteroids, broad-spectrum antibiotics, and chemotherapeutics) is conductive to opportunistic fungal infections.[73] Some agents directly stimulate the growth of fungal agents, such as deferoxamine (or administration of iron) in aspergillosis, candidosis, and zygomycosis.[72,74,75] In women, pregnancy or the use of high-estrogen-containing oral contraceptives are predisposing factors for developing vaginal candidosis.[76,77]

A number of immunodepressed animal models have been developed to obtain models related to the conditions described in humans and animals. Induced immunosuppression by treatment with, for example, x-irradiation, corticosteroids, cyclophosphamide, mechlorethamine, or splenectomy is frequently used.[72,73,78,79] Spontaneous immunosuppressive animal models such as congenitally athymic nude mice or New Zealand Black (NZB) mice (defective in T lymphocytes) and AKR/J leukemic mice are used not only to mimic the infections in humans under immunocompromised conditions, but also to study of the defense mechanisms involved during different mycoses.[27,73,80] Endocrinological disturbance models such as diabetic models are routinely produced in various animals by administration of alloxan or streptozotocin.[72,73] It should also be noted that sex hormones are also of significant influence on the establishment of some systemic mycoses, such as blastomycosis. Likewise, in the model of vaginal candidosis, it is essential to use oophorectomized animals, usually rats and mice, which are treated with estrogen to bring them into a permanent state of pseudoestrus.[8,18,72,77]

Aspergillosis

Aspergillosis refers to a number of diseases in which *Aspergillus* spp. are involved. Generally, the disease results from toxicity due to contaminated food, allergy mainly due to spore allergens, pulmonary colonization without extension, and invasion with or without subsequent dissemination.[71] *Aspergillus fumigatus* is the most important pathogen, with *A. flavus, A. niger,* and *A. terreus* being less frequent in a decreasing manner.[73] In humans, the lung is the most common site affected, and preexisting or concurrent lung diseases are a major factor predisposing a host to infection.[71] However, most of the predisposing factors mentioned in the introduction to the present section dealing with the opportunistic pathogenic fungi are also responsible for the development of aspergillosis.[71,73] Especially in severely debilitated persons, the course of infection may be dissemination, with localization in a variety of internal organs. In veterinary medicine, avian aspergillosis and bovine proventriculitis and placentitis with subsequent abortion, due especially to *A. fumigatus,* are of great importance.[81–83] Invasive lung aspergillosis may be established in mice, chicks, ducks, rabbits, rats, and other laboratory animals when used as inhalation models (challenged i.n. or i.t.) in which the conidia are given in aerosols in either a dry or wet form.[73,84,85] In these models, the mouse is preferred, and treatment with cortisone is essential for the development of a high incidence of fatal pulmonal

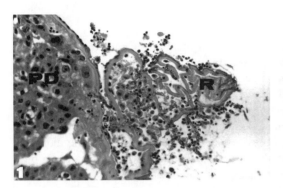 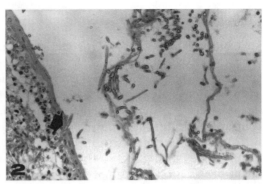

Figure 8.2 Experimental aspergillosis in a pregnant mouse (day 16 of pregnancy) inoculated i.v. with *Aspergillus fumigatus* on day 10 of pregnancy. (1) The growth of hyphae in the periphery of the placental disc (PD) and Reichert's membrane (R) is accompanied by necrosis and polymorphonuclear cell infiltration. (2) Hyphae are seen around amnion and within the fetal skin (arrow). (From Jensen, H.E. and Hau, J., *In Vivo,* 4, 247, 1990. With permission).

aspergillosis as murine alveolar macrophages are capable of preventing germination and can kill spores.[86–88] However, in the cortisone-treated animals, the lysosomal membranes within macrophages are stabilized, making the animals more susceptible to infection.[89,90] An experimental pulmonary aspergilloma model in rabbits is established by artificial bronchostenosis, ligature of pulmonary artery, and injection of *Aspergillus* spores into the distal bronchus. In this model, bronchiectasis, cavity and cyst, and a massive laminated growth of hyphae are found within the bronchial lumen, which is similar to the human aspergilloma.[90] The aerogene route of entry to the body is, compared with i.v. and i.p. inoculations, compatible with the natural entry in humans, in which the lungs are the most frequent portal of entry. By the i.v. route, disseminated forms of aspergillosis are formed regularly, whereas dissemination after i.p. challenge often requires treatment by cortisone or cyclophosphamide.[73] The i.v. model of disseminated aspergillosis, however, has the advantage that a precise dose-related course of infection can be established, which is important in the evaluation of virulence parameters (ID_{50} and LD_{50}) of different fungal strains and of the estimation of therapeutic parameters such as TD_{50}, ED_{50}, and PD_{50}. In the systemic aspergillosis model, the kidneys are the target organs. However, when pregnant animals (cows, sheep, and mice) are inoculated i.v. by spores from *A. fumigatus,* the placenta is also a target organ (Figure 8.2).[92–94]

After the mouse, the rabbit is the dominant animal species used in the study of experimental aspergillosis.[73] By i.v. challenge, the course of disseminated infection may vary from acute to chronic, depending on the size of inoculum. As in mice, administration of immunosuppressive agents will turn the infection into extensive aspergillosis. The rabbit lung has a high susceptibility to aspergillosis. Primary pulmonary aspergillosis in rabbits is established by i.t. inoculation of spores; and as in mice, the use of immunosuppressive drugs is essential for the establishment of fatal infections. In this model, a primary and predominant involvement of the lung tissue is seen with subsequent spread to especially the liver, spleen, and kidneys.[73] Moreover, among laboratory animals, natural occurrence of aspergillosis is especially reported in rabbits.[96]

Localized aspergillosis models of endophthalmitis and endocarditis have also been described. In the latter model, the fungal spores are introduced i.v. into animals that have received an intracardial catheter.[97] From the occlusive vegetations formed on the valves infected, emboli are carried to other organs in which subsequent aspergillosis develops.

Rats have also been extensively used as models for aspergillosis and show no significant differences in the course of infection compared with the other animal species.[73]

A primate model in rhesus monkeys of allergic bronchopulmonary aspergillosis was established by Golbert and Patterson.[98]

Candidosis

Candidosis is an opportunistic infection caused by yeasts of the genus *Candida* and predominantly of the species *Candida albicans*.[71,73] The manifestations of candidosis range from acute and subacute to chronic, and may involve the skin, mucous membranes, or more rarely, become systemic. Here, only experimental infections with *C. albicans* will be considered because it is the dominant cause of human candidosis, and infections by other pathogenic *Candida* spp. show comparable events in laboratory animals. Disseminated infections have been produced in a number of different species (e.g., rats, rabbits, and guinea pigs) by i.v. and i.p. challenge.[73] The mouse is the most-often used model for systemic candidosis. It should be noted, however, that guinea pigs are particularly resistant to i.p. challenge with blastospores of *Candida*, and that rabbits are more susceptible to infection than mice.[73] Among strains of mice, there are prominent differences in the susceptibility to *C. albicans* infections after i.v. challenge, with C57BL/6, C57BL/6J, and Sec/1Rej being most resistant and the C57C57BL/Hej, BALB/c, and CBA/J mice being moderately susceptible. The highest susceptibility is found in AKR/J, CBA/CaJ, DBA/1J, DBA/2J, A/J, and RF/J mice.[73,99] These differences in susceptibility probably reflect different properties in the release of lymphokines, the degrees of natural killer cell activity, and function of the complement system.[99,100]

Systemic candidosis is also seen after i.p. and i.cer. challenge of rabbits and rats with blastospores.[101–103] In systemic infection models, the kidneys are the target organ, which seems to reflect an initial protection from inflammatory cells by intraluminal localization in the tubuli (Figure 8.3).[104] However, recently it was shown that the placenta of pregnant mice showed an even higher susceptibility to infection, which may be a general feature after i.v. challenge of pregnant animals with opportunistic pathogenic fungi (see also Aspergillosis and Zygomycosis; Figure 8.4).[105] In Figure 8.5, the pathogenesis of murine mycotic placentitis is shown. Localized organ manifestations may also be seen after i.v. and i.p. challenge of animals, such as endophthalmitis in rabbits and dermatitis in guinea pigs.[18,73] Localized exogenous candidosis models of endophthalmitis, dermatitis, arthritis, cystitis, and endocarditis (see Aspergillosis) have all been established in rabbits and other animals.[18,72,73,106] Cutaneous candidosis can be produced in a wide range of animals, but the guinea pig is especially susceptible; and when diabetic animals (alloxan treated) are used, the lesions formed are compatible with the human form, and, therefore, the model is commonly used in the screening of new antifungal agents.[9,18,72,73] The model of chronic vaginitis, usually established in rats, is also widely used in the evaluation of new antifungal agents. The infection is established by i. vag. inoculation of blastospores into animals that are oophorectomized and kept in a permanent state of pseudoestrus by weekly injections of estrogen.[9,73,77] Localized oral candidosis (known as thrush) in rats, as well as the crop of several avian species, is produced after p.o. challenge with blastospores. The disease is favored by a carbohydrate-rich diet, antibiotic treatment, and use of germ-free or specific pathogen free (SPF) animals.[73,106,107] Also, localized candidosis in air-filled subcutaneous cysts that imitate thrush is used in the testing of antifungal agents.[108] Intragastric challenge in infant mice results in systemic spread of candidosis, whereas the same course of infection in adult animals requires some compromising treatment with, for example, antibiotic and cytotoxic agents.[73,109,110]

Recently, a murine model of *Candida* mastitis was developed (Figures 8.6 through 8.9).[111] The model, which was found to be discriminative and a model of localized candidosis, was applied to different strains of mice (BALB/c, severely combined immunodeficiency [SCID], and nude BALB/c mice).[112] In several studies, Guhad et al.[113–115] showed that the model was usable to analyze the virulence properties of *C. albicans*, the application of antifungal drugs, and the impact of the immune system on the infection.

In murine models of candidosis, an enhancement of infection is seen after treatment with an overload of iron.[74] Iron also enhances the course of aspergillosis and zygomycosis and seems to be a result of saturation of fungal siderophores, iron-transport cofactors, which bind iron and form

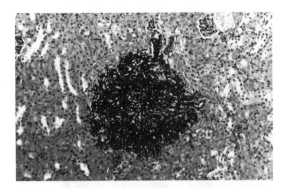

Figure 8.3   Experimental renal candidosis in a mouse after i.v. challenge with *Candida albicans* blastospores.

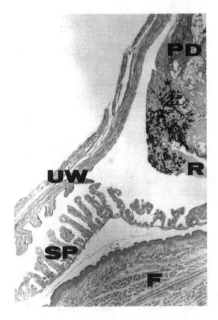

Figure 8.4   Experimental candidosis in a pregnant mouse. The fungi are characteristically restricted to the perifery of the placental disc (PD) and the degenerated Reichert's membrane (R). UW = uterine wall; SP = splanchnopleura; F = fetus. (From Jensen, H.E. et al., *APMIS*, 99, 829, 1991. With permission.)

a chelate that is essential for the growth of the fungi.[72,73,75] Generally, x-irradiated, corticosteroid-treated, and diabetic animals also have a reduced tolerance to challenge with blastospores.[18,72,73]

Finally, it should be mentioned that i.m. injection of *C. albicans* blastospores (viable, heat killed, or lyophilized) is a well-recognized experimental model of murine amyloidosis that may be used in studying pathogenesis and treatment of amyloidosis.[116]

Cryptococcosis

Cryptococcosis is a subacute or chronic, rarely acute, pulmonary, systemic, or meningeal infection caused by the yeast *Cryptococcus neoformans*.[71,73] Classically, two varieties of the fungus are described: *Cryptococcus neoformans* var. *neoformans* and *C. neoformans* var. *gattii*. These two varieties comprise serotypes A, D, and AD and serotypes B and C, respectively. On the basis of

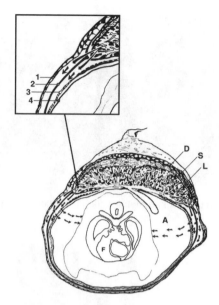

Figure 8.5   The pathogenesis of murine placental candidosis. Arrows indicate the orign and extent of murine candidosis. A = amniotic cavity; D = decidua; F = fetus; L = labyrinth; S = spongiotrophoblasts; 1 = uterine wall; 2 = Reichert's membrane; 3 = splanchnopleura; 4 = amnion. (From Jensen, H.E. et al., *APMIS*, 99, 829, 1991. With permission.)

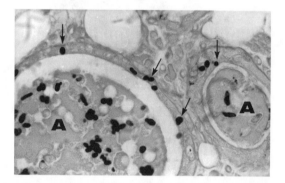

Figure 8.6   Mammary gland from a mouse killed 3 d after intramammary inoculation with 1×10^4 *Candida krusei* cells. Within the lumen and epithelial lining of two alveoli (A), fungal elements (arrows) are seen. (From Guhad, F.A. et al., *J. Comp. Pathol.,* 113, 1995. With permission.)

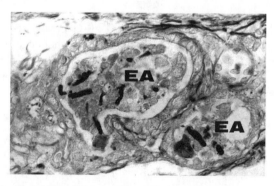

Figure 8.7   Mammary gland from a mouse 2 d after intramammary inoculation of 1×10^5 blastospores of *Candida albicans.* Fungal elements, which are stained black, are present within exudate-filled alveoli (EA). (From Guhad, F.A. et al., *FEMS Microbiol. Lett.*, 166, 1998. With permission.)

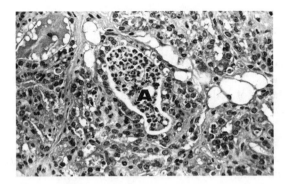

Figure 8.8   Murine mammary gland 4 d after inoculation of 1×10^6 blastospores of *Candida albicans*. Accumulation of heterophils around and within the lumen of an alveolus (A) is present. (From Guhad, F.A. et al., *APMIS*, 106, 1049, 1998. With permission.)

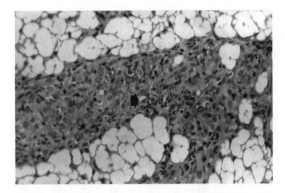

Figure 8.9   Murine mammary gland from a mouse treated with amphotericin B (4 mg/kg intrperitoneally once daily) 6 d after intramammary inoculation of 5×10^7 *Candida albicans* blastospores. In the gland tissue, only a mild infiltration of macrophages and heterophils is seen. Locally, a minor microabscess has formed (arrow). (From Guhad, F.A. et al., *FEMS Microbiol. Lett.*, 26, 125, 1999. With permission.)

phenotypic and genetic differences, serotype A may also be termed *Cryptococcus neoformans* var. *grubii*.

Mice are highly susceptible to cryptococcosis and are frequently used as a model in the study of the disease because it shows a number of similarities to the disease in humans. Dissemination to internal organs is seen after i.v., i.cer., and i.p. challenge of mice with an appropriate amount of *C. neoformans* cells.[73] As for *C. albicans,* variations in susceptibility to infection are seen in mice of different strains. In the disseminated disease models, the histopathological findings are characterized as either granulomatous or cystic, reflecting the presence of macrophages in the different organs.[27,117,118] *C. neoformans* has a propensity for infecting the brain, lungs, and kidneys.[73] Cryptococcal meningitis is so accurately developed in mice after i.v. inoculation of appropriate numbers of cells that this model is used in the differentiation of *C. neoformans* from other *Cryptococcus* species and in the evaluation of antifungal agents.[71] However, when the respiratory system is the portal of entry, dissemination to other organs is delayed, especially to the brain, and allows a more preferable exploration of the course of infection in humans. Mice and rats are the preferred animals, and rabbits and guinea pigs are almost resistant to cryptococcal infections, although chronic cryptococcal meningitis has been developed in cortisone-treated rabbits after i.cer. inoculation.[119–122] In addition to its similarity to the human disease, this rabbit model has the advantage, in comparison with the murine model, that the larger size of the animal allows repeated aspiration of larger volumes of cerebrospinal fluid for analysis.[73]

Localized cryptococcal infection models are produced in other organs after local application, e.g., cutaneous and ocular cryptococcosis.[9,73] After p.o. administration of *C. neoformans* cells to mice, some will have the gastrointestinal tract colonized, and dissemination, however infrequently, to other organs may occur. In that case, the course is not influenced by treatment that compromises the immunological status of the animal.[73,123] Colonization of the nasal mucosa of mice may also be seen after i.n. inoculation of cells of some strains of *C. neoformans*.[124]

Scedosporiosis

Scedosporiosis is caused by *Scedosporium apiospermum (Pseudallescheria boydii)* and *S. inflatum,* and the infection may vary from local infection of, especially, the lung, skin, and cornea to disseminated mycosis.[125] Comparable animal models of local scedosporiosis include granulomas, keratitis, and arthritis in rabbits.[71] Mice are often used in the production of disseminated infections developing subsequent to i.v. inoculation of conidia.[126]

Zygomycosis

Zygomycosis refers to infections caused by fungi of the class Zygomycetes, of which the family Mucoraceae of the order Mucorales are most important in medical and veterinary mycology.[127,128] The course of infection may be acute to long-term chronic. The localization of the infection may be in the cutis or subcutis, lung, or nose, with subsequent spread to the brain (rhinocerebral zygomycosis); or more rarely, the disease may turn out in a disseminated form.[71,127] *Absidia corymbifera, Rhizopus* spp. and *Mucor* spp., are most often found as the causative organism of human and animal zygomycosis.[127,128] Disseminated acute systemic infections by these fungi are easily established in most animals after i.v. challenge (Figure 8.10). Mice, rats, rabbits, and guinea pigs are often used, with guinea pigs being the most appropriate.[19,73] However, these infections are not likely to be used as models because this course of infection is seen only rarely in humans. The i.v. route of challenge is, however, used extensively in studies of etiology, immunology, histopathology, and assessment of new antifungal agents.[19,72,73] Inoculation of spores i.n. and i.t. into cortisone-treated or streptozotocin-diabetic animals results in pulmonary and cerebral zygomycosis with a course of infection and pathology close to that of human cases of zygomycosis.[73,129,130] Also, treatment of mice with deferoxamine and iron (Fe^{3+}) will render them more susceptible to infection, and p.o. challenge of guinea pigs pretreated with aspirin will cause gastric invasion.[72,131,132] Localized chronic pyogranulomatous infections in most animals may also be produced after cutaneous, subcutaneous, or orbital inoculations (Figure 8.10).[73] As for candidosis and aspergillosis, the murine placenta is also highly susceptible to zygomycosis.[133]

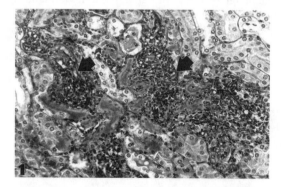 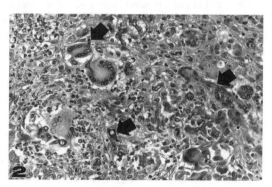

Figure 8.10   Murine zygomycosis due to *Absidia corymbifera*. (1) Acute renal zygomycosis after intravenous challenge. Arrows = hyphae. (2) Chronic subcutaneous granulomatous zygomycosis after subcutaneous challenge. Arrows = hyphae.

Pneumocystosis

Pneumocystis carinii organisms, the cause of pneumocystosis, have been found in a number of domestic (cows, horses, pigs, goats, dogs, and cats) and laboratory animals (mice, rats, and rabbits).[134] In humans and animals, the infection is restricted to the lungs, in which it is the cause of an interstitial pneumonia.[135] *P. carinii* is difficult to culture *in vitro* and is dependent on the presence of feeder cells, such as embryonic chick epithelial lung cells.[136] However, because of the only-moderate replication and the limited number of passages, the basic research on *P. carinii* is mostly based on different kinds of animal models in which immunocompromised host animals harbor the organism.[137] Experimetal animal models are also used as a source of the organism for *in vitro* studies. The immunosuppression required for the development of pneumocysticosis may be achieved pharmacologically (e.g., with cortisone acetate, dexamethasone, and cyclosporin A) or by using genetically altered, immunosuppressed animal strains (e.g., SCID mice).[134]

Animal models of pneumocystosis are primarily used for the study of pathobiology related to the organism and treatment of the disease. Acquired immune deficiency syndrome (AIDS) patients especially will often develop pneumocystosis and, if not treated, die from the disease.[134,135] Therefore, animal models are widely used for the comparative study of pathogenesis, therapy, and especially prophylaxis. Finally, it should be noted that *P. carinii* organisms are not transmissible between different host species.[134]

ANIMAL MODELS OF MISCELLANEOUS MYCOSES AND ALGOSES

Miscellaneous Fungi

Geotrichum spp. may be the cause of mucocutaneous infections. In laboratory animals, it is very difficult to establish infection by the fungi. However, inoculation of mice i.v. and i.p. with clinical isolates of *Geotrichum candidum* may result in systemic infection.[71,138,139]

Penicillium spp. are very common in the environment but are only rarely the cause of infection.[71] However, one exception is *Penicillium marneffei,* which has been recovered from a number of human and animal (especially the bamboo rat *Rhizomys pruinosus*) infections, particularly in Asian countries.[140,141] In humans, infections are often progressive, and disseminated forms similar to those seen in histoplasmosis are formed. A comparable course of disease occurs in mice, rats, and hamsters challenged i.v. or i.p. with the fungus.[140]

Pityrosporum ovale (s. *Malassezia furfur*), a lipophilic fungus, is an etiological agent in the development of pityriasis versicolor, folliculitis, and seborrheic dermatitis in humans.[9] Faergemann[142,143] has successfully infected volunteers by cutaneous infection under occlusive dressing and additional application of olive oil. The positive effect of olive oil was also demonstrated using the insides of ears of rabbits. A number of more low-pathogenic fungi, such as *Rhodotorula rubra, Candida glabrata,* and other *Candida* spp. different from *C. albicans,* produce a moderate skin infection when inoculated onto the backs of diabetic (alloxan-pretreated) guinea pigs.[9]

Adiaspiromycosis, which is seen especially in the lungs of wild rodents, is caused by the inhalation of conidia of the fungal genus *Chrysosporium (Emmonsia).*[71] In humans, adiaspiromycosis is rare, but the knowledge of the infection is important as a differential diagnosis to other fungi in tissues of rodents. Injection of conidia into mice, rabbits, rats, and dogs may result in the development of systemic infection.[71] Localized granulomatous orchitis is produced after i.test. inoculation of the fungi in hamsters (Figure 8.11).

Mycotic keratitis in humans is often caused by members of the genera *Candida* and *Aspergillus*; but in rare situations, infection by more low-pathogenic fungi, such as *Fusarium* spp., may also occur. A variety of rabbit and rat models of mycotic keratitis caused by these fungi are used preferably in the testing of new antifungal agents.[73]

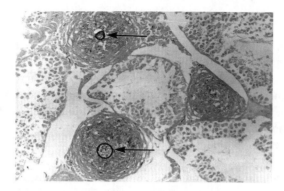

Figure 8.11   Adiaspiromycotic granulomatous orchitis in a hamster after intratesticular inoculation of culture
material. (Arrows = adiaspores.)

Algae

Human and animal infections due to algae are rare. However, infection by *Prototheca* spp.,
especially *Prototheca zopfii* (an achloric alga), may be the cause of superficial or deep cutaneous
infections and bursitis in humans and, more frequently, mastitis in cattle.[144,145] Reports have also
been given on disseminated infections in cows and dogs.[146,147] Some cases of bovine lymphadenitis
caused by infection with green algae of the order *Chlorococcales* are also reported.[148] Mice
inoculated i.v. with *P. zopfii* develop systemic granulomatous infections (Figure 8.12), and skin
infections appear in guinea pigs after i.d. inoculation.[149] In rats, i.p. challenge by green algae results
in the formation of a slowly progressive infection of the serosal peritoneal surface.[148]

APPLICATION OF MODIFIED ANIMAL MODELS IN MYCOLOGY

To obtain more homogeneous infections with pathogenic fungi and to establish an infection
with opportunistic pathogenic or poorly invasive fungi, various methods are used to enhance the
susceptibility of animals to infection. Furthermore, some modified models are also used to mimic
the conditions under which humans are infected, especially with the opportunistic pathogenic fungi.
In the section dealing with these infections, factors were listed that were predisposing, favoring,
and stimulating for the growth of fungi. Here, some other modified models are given that are applied
in the study of transformative fungal changes and defense mechanisms involved in mycoses.

Some fungi adapt themselves by transformation into a parasitic form when growing in tissues,
a phenomenon called *dimorphism*, a unique factor in the pathogenicity of these fungi. To study

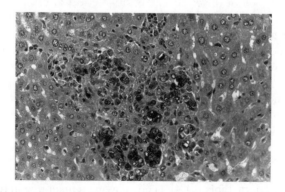

Figure 8.12   Murine hepatic granulomatous protothecosis after intravenous challenge by cells of *Prototheca
zopfii*. In the process, unicellular and multicellular organisms are seen.

this phenomenon, a number of *in vitro* methods have been used. *In vivo* fungal transformation can be followed by consecutive histopathology after challenge (e.g., i.v., s.c., and i.p.). In these models, heavy cell and humoral defense mechanisms will often mask the details of transformation. In the agar implantation model, blocks of agar containing the saprophytic stages of fungi are implanted into the abdominal cavity of mice.[27] From series of mice, the agar blocks are removed after adequate intervals and subjected to histology and electron microscopy. In this model, the development and transformation of fungi are only influenced by humoral defense factors of the host.[27] On the basis of results from the agar implantation model, the study of fungal infections after, for instance, i.v, s.c., and i.p. challenge and natural fungal infections in humans and animals, the pathogenic fungi have been classified into two categories according to their parasitic forms:[27] (1) fungi that are mycelial in their saprophytic stage and spherical in their parasitic stage; the transformation of these fungi is via the stage of arthroconidiae (e.g., *T. rubrum, C. immitis,* and *P. marneffei*), via the stage of chlamydospores (e.g., *B. dermatitidis, P. brasiliensis,* and *Fonsecaea pedrosoi*, a common cause of chromomycosis), or by direct budding from hyphae (*S. schenckii, H. capsulatum* var. *capsulatum,* var. *duboisii,* and var. *farciminosum*; and (2) fungi whose parasitic forms are similar to the saprophytic form, either in the form of mycelia (e.g., *Aspergillus, Absidia, Mucor, Rhizopus, Fusarium,* and *Scedosporium* species), the form of mycelial and yeast forms (e.g., *Candida* spp.), or yeast (e.g., *Cryptococcus neoformans*).

In the study of specific aspects of pathogenicity and defense mechanisms involved in mycotic infections, numerous modified animal models have been used. By these models, important differences of the cell-mediated reactions and the influence of complement in the defense against fungal infections have been elucidated.

Inbred strains of mice that are genetically deficient in the fifth factor of the complement system (C5), that is, DBA/ZN and B.10.D2/oSn mice, and C4D guinea pigs (congenitally deficient in component C4), have been used to study the possible role of the alternative complement pathway in cryptococcosis and candidosis.[27,73]

In the study of the defensive role of T lymphocytes, congenital athymic mice (nu/nu BALB/c mice), New Zealand Black (NZB) mice, which often become defective in their T lymphocytes, and thymectomized mice are used. The number and function of polymorphonuclear (PMN) cells are decreased and suppressed, respectively, by x-irradiation and administration of nitrogen mustard.[27] In these models, the sessile macrophages of the fixed-macrophage system usually remain intact, and the importance of the PMN cells can be analyzed. The defensive role of mononuclear cells in mycoses can be analyzed by challenge of mice treated i.v. with dextran sulfate or silica, which saturate the phagocytic function of monocytes and sessile macrophages.[27] Homozygous severely combined immunodeficiency (SCID/SCID) mice lack both specific humoral and cell-mediated immunity.[112,134] Histopathological examination of tissues from these modified mycotic animal models has contributed greatly to the understanding of which defense mechanisms are involved against different fungi. Table 8.1 is a review of differences in the susceptibility (lethal dose, severity of lesions, and efficacy in killing the fungus) of congenitally athymic nude mice (nu/nu) compared with their heterozygous littermates (nu/+) of BALB/c background to different fungi after i.v. challenge.[27] In the chronic state of deep mycoses in humans and laboratory animals, the formation of granulomas is the main pathological finding. However, in the earlier stages, the inflammatory reaction depends on the fungus involved. Toward some fungi, the cellular reaction is mainly made up by the mononuclear cells, with assistance from only a negligible number of PMN cells. In other mycoses, the cell infiltration is primarily due to PMN cells in the early stages of infection; whereas in the chronic stages, the killing of the fungus is accomplished by the infiltration of macrophages (PMN/mononuclear). Finally, the host defense against aspergillosis and zygomycosis is mainly due to PMN cells, but in the chronic processes of these mycoses, granulomas are also formed. In Table 8.1, the cells playing a main role in the host defense against different fungi are summarized.

Table 8.1 Susceptibility to Mycoses in Congenital Athymic Nude Mice (nu/nu) versus Their Heterozygous Littermates (nu/+) of BALB/c Background after Intravenous Challenge; and the Dominant Type of Cells Involved in the Defense of Infection

Fungal Infection	Susceptibility of Nude Mice	Main Cellular Response
Cryptococcosis		
C. neoformans	Enhanced	Mononuclear
Phaeohyphomycosis		
W. dermatitidis	Enhanced	Mononuclear
Histoplasmosis capsulati		
H. capsulatum var. *capsulatum*	Enhanced	Mononuclear
Histoplasmosis duboisii		
H. capsulatum var. *duboisii*	Enhanced	Mononuclear
Sporotrichosis		
S. schenckii	Enhanced	Mononuclear
Blastomycosis		
B. dermatitidis	Enhanced	Mononuclear/PMN
Paracoccidioidomycosis		
P. brasiliensis	Enhanced	Mononuclear/PMN
Chromomycosis		
F. pedrosoi	Enhanced/lowered[a]	Mononuclear/PMN
Candidosis		
C. albicans	Controversial	PMN/mononuclear
Coccidioidomycosis		
C. immitis	Controversial	PMN/mononuclear
Aspergillosis		
A. fumigatus	None	PMN/mononuclear
Zygomycosis		
A. corymbifera	None	PMN/mononuclear

Note: PMN = polymorphonuclear.

[a] Enhanced at high doses and lowered at low doses.

EVALUATION OF ANTIFUNGAL AGENTS IN ANIMAL MODELS

Therapeutic choices between microbial agents have traditionally been guided by their activity *in vitro*. However, *in vitro* results for antifungal agents are not necessarily indicative of efficacy *in vivo*. In particular, the azole antifungal agents yield inconsistent sensitivity results and tend to produce higher susceptibility endpoints, depending on components and pH of the medium, inoculum size, incubation temperature, and time of reading.[150] Fluconazole reaches an extreme in terms of the disparity between *in vitro* and *in vivo* activity.[151] Moreover, only by use of a wide range of animal models was it possible to select and introduce the first broad-spectrum antifungal drug, ketoconazole.[9] For these reasons and for testing the applicability of different dispensing forms and therapeutic effects, side effects, etc., the use of animal models of mycoses is of significant importance in the screening for new antifungal agents.

When testing new antifungal agents, as many fungal species as possible should be tested. Moreover, because a number of fungi show strain variation in their virulence, expressed by their median infective dose (ID_{50}) and median lethal dose (LD_{50}; the dose, in colony-forming units per kilogram, that will infect and kill, respectively, 50% of the animals), the number of strains tested should also be high.

Models used in the evaluation of efficacy are classified according to the nature of the infection:[152,153]

1. The basic *antimicrobial screening models* are commonly used in early evaluation of antifungal agents, and the animals (usually mice) are challenged with a dose that ensures death of all animals. In this model, the ability of agents to prolong survival of infected animals is determined, and the

estimated median effective dose, ED_{50} (mg/kg), the dose that protects 50% of the animals from death, is calculated. Advantages of these models are as follows: infection and treatment are simple; there are clearly defined endpoints; they are economical; and are of short duration. Disadvantages include: the course of infection is uncharacteristic and fulminant; the antifungal agents are administrated at or close to the infection; the models are highly sensitive to the size of the infective dose; and single or few doses are given, which may result in pharmacokinetic differences that do not allow comparisons between agents.

2. The *ex vivo model* uses a foreign body containing the organism and is implanted (s.c., i.p., etc.) before treatment. During treatment, the bodies are removed and the contents analyzed *in vitro*. The bodies may be fibrin clots or dialysis sacs that permit entry of the agent but restrict entry of the cellular and humoral components of the host defense system. The use of a porous or hollow device permits entry of phagocytes and antibodies, and may be valuable for the determination of these components to penetrate a specific site of infection. This model has thus far not found any practical form in testing antifungal agents, but the agar implantation model is an example of its use in mycopathology.[27]

3. In the *monoparametric model*, a simple indicator of therapeutic effectiveness is measured, as opposed to an ultimative therapeutic cure. In this model, the capacity of agents to sterilize infected tissues (e.g., *C. albicans* in murine kidney infections) and the concentration of the antifungal agent in tissues are evaluated. In the effort to reduce the use of laboratory animals, monoparametric models should be replaced by discriminative models.

4. The *discriminative models* are by far the most technically complicated models and are designed to mimic the initiation and progress of infection in humans and domestic animals. In these models, multiple parameters are measured, and they allow evaluation of drug concentration, adjuvant therapies, etc. In these models, calculated parameters such as the median protective dose (PD_{50}) and median therapeutic dose (TD_{50}; the dose, in milligrams per kilogram, that protects and cures 50% of the animals, respectively) also are determined. In the selection of a discriminative model, the following ideal features should be considered:[153] the technique for infection should be simple; and the fungus, route of entry, spread in the body, and tissues involved should be similar to the situation in humans. The severity, course, and duration of the infection should be predictable, reproductive, and amenable to analysis. Furthermore, susceptibility to therapy must be measurable and reproductive.

Some models seem to satisfy most of these criteria adequately, such as murine pulmonary cryptococcosis, but in most models of mycoses, some compromises have to be offered; for example, in models of dermatophytoses, the fungus is usually a zoophilic dermatophyte, and the prolonged chronic infections as seen in humans are not produced, and relapse of skin infection may be seen from lesions in internal organs when the infection is established through i.v. inoculation.[9] Another example is that to establish and maintain vaginal candidosis in laboratory animals, the animals must be oophorectomized and treated with estrogen during the time of infection.[73,77] In Table 8.2, some common animal models of mycoses used in the testing of antifungal agents are listed.

ANIMAL MODELS AS MYCODIAGNOSTIC TOOLS

A number of fungi are, when only present in a limited amount, grown more regularly *in vivo* than *in vitro*. Therefore, when *in vitro* cultivations of materials under suspicion of content of, for example, *B. dermatitidis, H. capsulatum* var. *capsulatum, P. brasiliensis, S. schenckii,* and *C. neoformans* are negative, animal inoculations (often in mice) are performed with the material.[45] Usually the material is, in combination with antibiotics, given s.c., i.v., i.cer., or i.p.; but for *P. brasiliensis,* the preferred site for inoculation is the testicles of mountain rats.[45] The specimens are usually of environmental or clinical origin, such as soil, pus, granulomas, etc. When growth of the fungus in the animal is suspected at autopsy, its organs are removed and, from these, *in vitro* cultivation is attempted. Experimental inoculations of mice are also used in the differentiation of

Table 8.2   Selected Animal Models Applied in the Evaluation of Antifungal Agents

Fungal Infection	Animal	Predisposing Factors	Inoculation Site	Localization of Infection
Dermatophytosis				
T. mentagrophytes and *M. canis*	Guinea pig	Abraded/none	On skin[a]	Skin
	Guinea pig	None	i.v.	Skin/dissemination
Pityriasis				
P. ovale and *P. orbiculare*	Guinea pig	Clipped	On skin[a]	Skin
Sporotrichosis				
S. schenckii	Guinea pig	None	i.v./i.test.	Dissemination
Penicilliosis				
P. marneffei	Guinea pig	Immunosuppressed/ none	i.v.	Dissemination
Blastomycosis				
B. dermatitidis	Mouse	None	i.n.	Lung/dissemination
	Mouse	None	i.n.	Dissemination
Coccidioidomycosis				
C. immitis	Mouse	None	i.n.	Lung/dissemination
	Mouse	None	i.n.	Dissemination
Histoplasmosis				
H. capsulatum var. *capsulatum*	Mouse	None	i.n.	Lung/dissemination
	Mouse	None	i.v./i.p.	Dissemination
H. capsulatum var. *duboisii*	Guinea pig	None	i.test.	Testicles/dissemination
Paracoccidioidomycosis				
P. brasiliensis	Mouse	None	i.n.	Lung/dissemination
	Mouse	None	i.n.	Dissemination
Aspergillosis				
A. fumigatus	Mouse	Immunosuppressed	i.n.	Lung/dissemination
	Chicken	None	Aerosol	Lung/dissemination
	Rabbit	Immunosuppressed	i.cor.	Cornea
	Rabbit	Intracardial catheter	i.v.	Endocardium/ dissemination
	Guinea pig	Immunosuppressed/ none	i.v.	Dissemination
	Mouse	Immunosuppressed/ none	i.v.	Dissemination
Cryptococcosis				
C. neoformans	Rabbit	Immunosuppressed	Cisterna magnum	Meninges
	Mouse	None	i.cer.	Meninges/dissemination
	Mouse	Immunosuppressed/ none	i.n.	Lung/dissemination
	Mouse	Immunosuppressed/ none	i.v./i.p.	Dissemination
	Guinea pig	Immunosuppressed/ none	i.v.	Dissemination
Candidosis				
C. albicans	Guinea pig	Clipped and diabetic	On skin	Skin
	Mouse	Immunosuppressed	s.c.	Subcutis
	Mouse	Air	s.c.	Subcutis
	Mouse	None	i.mam.	Mammary glands
	Mouse	Immunosuppressed	i.mam.	Mammary glands
	Rat	Pseudoestrus	i.vag.	Vagina
	Rat	Pseudoestrus and diabetic	i.vag.	Vagina
	Guinea pig	Immunosuppressed and antibiotics	p.o.	Gastrointestinal tract

(continued)

Table 8.2 (continued)   Selected Animal Models Applied in the Evaluation of Antifungal Agents

Fungal Infection	Animal	Predisposing Factors	Inoculation Site	Localization of Infection
	Mouse	Immunosuppressed and antibiotics/none	p.o.	Gastrointestinal tract
	Guinea pig	None	i.cor.	Cornea
	Rabbit	Immunosuppressed/ none	i.cor.	Cornea
	Rabbit	None	i.v.	Eye/dissemination
	Rabbit	Intracardial catheter	i.v.	Endocardium/ dissemination
	Guinea pig	Immunosuppressed/ none	i.v.	Dissemination
	Mouse	Immunosuppressed/ none	i.v.	Dissemination
	Rat	Immunosuppressed/ none	i.v.	Dissemination

Note: i.v. = intravenous; i.test. = intratesticular; i.n. = intranasal; i.p. = intraperitoneal; i.cor. = intracorneal; i.cer. = intracerebral; s.c. = subcutaneous; i.mam. = intramammary; i.vag. = intravaginal; p.o. = per oral; diabetic = alloxan- and streptozotocin-treated animals; pseudoestrus = castrated and estrogen-treated animals; immunosuppressed = x-irradiated, mechlorethamine-, prednisolone-, hydrocortisone-, or cyclophospha- mide-treated animals; Antibiotics = streptomycin and chloramphenicol.

[a] Usually performed under occlusive dressing.

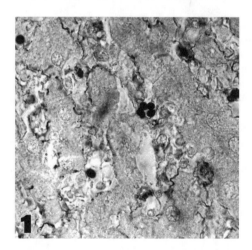 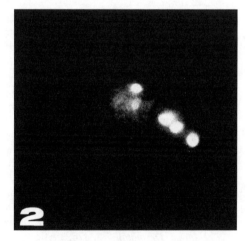

Figure 8.13 Immunohistochemical identification of *Histoplasma capsulatum* var. *capsulatum.* (1) In the Kupffer's cells, yeast-like organisms are located. (2) Staining of the organisms by specific FITC-labeled anti-*H. capsulatum* globulins confirm the diagnosis of hepatic histoplasmosis. (From Jensen, H.E. et al., *APMIS,* 100, 1992. With permission.)

some fungi, such as *C. carrionii* from *C. bantianum,* and the pathogenicity of *C. neoformans* for mice is used in the differentiation of this species from other *Cryptococcus* spp.[26,71] Finally, it should be noted that *in vivo* growth by passage in laboratory animals is presently the only feasible method for the isolation and "cultivation" of *L. loboi.*[26,30]

For the high number of immunological assays used for the diagnosis of different mycoses, the production of specific polyclonal or monoclonal antibodies is essential. Production of polyclonal antibodies is preferably done in rabbits and goats by immunization with different fractions of fungal antigens. Monoclonal antifungal antibodies are produced in mice or rat hybridomas *in vivo* (ascites production) or *in vitro* (cell cultures). In the evaluation of the sensitivity and specificity of antifungal antibodies, controlled experimental infections of laboratory animals are indispensable. For these purposes, animal models have been used extensively in testing, for example, immunohistochemical assays used in the histopathological differentiation of algae and fungi (Figure 8.13)[149,154,155] and in enzyme-linked immunosorbent assays[156,157] and agglutination assays[158] developed for the detection of fungal antigen in serum and urine of infected humans and domestic animals as an aid in the diagnosis of mycoses. Furthermore, well-characterized antifungal antisera also are often included as references in studies of human antibody reactions.[159]

REFERENCES

1. Rippon, J.W., Ed., *Medical Mycology: Dermatophytosis and Dermatomycosis,* 3rd ed.,W.B. Saunders, Philadelphia, 1988, p. 169.
2. Hironaga, M., Okazaki, N., Saito, K., and Watanabe, S., Trichophyton mentagrophytes granulomas, *Arch. Dermatol.,* 119, 482, 1983.
3. Rippon, J.W., Animal models of experimental dermatophyte infections, in *Experimental Models in Antimicrobial Chemotherapy,* Vol. 3, Zak, O. and Sande, M.A., Eds., Academic Press, London, 1986, p. 161.
4. Watanabe, S., Animal models of cutaneous and subcutaneous mycoses, in *Animal Models in Medical Mycology,* Miyaji, M., Ed., CRC Press, Boca Raton, FL, 1987, p. 53.
5. Takahashi, S., Morphological, biological and physiological studies of *Trichophyton rubrum.* I. Morphological studies and experimental inoculation of guinea pigs, *Jpn. J. Dermatol.,* 72, 50, 1962.
6. Reiss, F., Successful inoculation in animals with *Trichophyton parpareum, Arch. Dermatol. Syph.,* 54, 242, 1944.
7. La Touche, C.J., Mouse favus due to *Trichophyton quinckeanum* (zopf) macleod & muende: a reappraisal in the light of recent investigations. I–III. *Mycopathol. Mycopathol. Appl.,* 11, 257, 1959.
8. Calderon, R.A., Immunoregulation of dermatophytosis, *CRC Crit. Rev. Microbiol.,* 16, 339, 1989.
9. Van Cutsem, J., Animal models for dermatomycotic infections, in *Current Topics in Medical Mycology,* Vol. 3, McGinnis, M.R. and Borgers, M., Eds., Springer-Verlag, New York, 1989, p. 1.
10. Hänel, H., Braun, B., and L'schhorn, K., Experimental dermatophytosis in nude guinea pigs compared with infection in Pirbright White animals, *Mycoses,* 33, 179, 1990.
11. Greenberg, J.H., King, R.H., Kerbs, S., and Field, R., A quantitative dermatophyte infection model in the guinea pig — a parallel to the quantitative human infection model, *J. Invest. Dermatol.,* 67, 704, 1976.
12. Kerbs, S. and Allen, A.M., Effect of occlusion on *Trichophyton mentagrophytes* infection in guinea pigs, *J. Invest. Dermatol.,* 71, 301, 1978.
13. Green, F., Lee, K.W., and Balish, E., Chronic *Trichophyton mentagrophytes* dermatophytosis of guinea pig skin grafts on nude mice, *J. Invest. Dermatol.,* 79, 125, 1982.
14. Green, F. and Balish, E., *Trichophyton mentagrophytes* dermatophytosis in germ free guinea pigs, *J. Invest. Dermatol.,* 75, 476, 1980.
15. Van Cutsem, J. and Janssen, P.A.J., Experimental systemic dermatophytosis, *J. Invest. Dermatol.,* 83, 26, 1984.
16. Van Cutsem, J., Van Gerven, F., and Janssen, P.A.J., Activity of orally, topically, and parenterally administrated itraconazole in the treatment of superficial and deep mycoses: animal models, *Rev. Infect. Dis.,* 9, 15, 1987.
17. Van Cutsem, J., Van Gerven, F., and Janssen, P.A.J., Saperconazole, a new potent antifungal triazol: *in vitro* activity spectrum and therapeutic efficacy, *Drugs Fut.,* 14, 1187, 1989.
18. Van Cutsem, J., Van Gerven, F., Fransen, J., and Janssen, P.A.J., Experimental candidosis in animals and chemotherapy, in *Candida and Candidamycosis,* Türnbay, E., Ed., Plenum Press, New York, 1991, p. 107.
19. Van Cutsem, J., Fransen, J., and Janssen, P.A.J., Experimental zygomycosis due to *Rhizopus* spp. infection by various routes in guinea pigs, rats and mice, *Mycoses,* 31, 563, 1988.
20. Eades, S.M. and Corbel, M.J., Metastatic subcutaneous zygomycosis following intravenous and intracerebral inoculation of *Absidia corymbifera* spores, *Sabouraudia,* 13, 200, 1975.
21. Fukushiro, R., Maduromycosis, in *Handbook of Dermatology,* Yamamura, Y., Kukita, A., Sano, S., and Seiji, M., Eds., Nakayama Shoten, Tokyo, 1982, p. 66.
22. Aleksin, R.M., Administration of preparation TF 130, *Veterinariia,* 3, 52, 1974.

23. Dobukovski, E.G., gber methoden der Trichophytie Bekampfung, *Veterinaria,* 39, 32, 1962.

24. Segal, E., Vaccines for the management of dermatophyte and superficial yeast infections, in *Current Topics in Medical Mycology,* McGinnis, M.R. and Borgers, M., Eds., Springer-Verlag, New York, 1989, p. 36.

25. Knight, A.G., A review of experimental human infections, *J. Invest. Dermatol.,* 59, 354, 1972.

26. Rippon, J.W., The subcutaneous mycoses, in *Medical Mycology,* 3rd ed., W.B. Saunders, Philadelphia, 1988, p. 276.

27. Miyaji, M. and Nishimura, K., Experimental fungal infections, in *Animal Models in Medical Mycology,* Miyaji, M., Ed., CRC Press, Boca Raton, FL, 1987, p. 1.

28. Reiss, F., Experimental mycotic infections on laboratory animals, in *Medical Mycology,* Simons, R.D.G., Ed., Elsevier, London, 1954, p. 50.

29. Borelli, D., A method for producing chromomycosis in mice, *Trans. R. Soc. Trop. Med. Hyg.,* 66, 793, 1972.

30. Wiersman, J.P. and Niemel, P.L.A., Lobo's disease in Surinam patients, *Trop. Geogr. Med.,* 17, 89, 1965.

31. Rippon, J.W., Ed., The pathogenic Actinomycetes, in *Medical Mycology,* 3rd ed., W.B. Saunders, Philadelphia, 1988, p. 13.

32. Avram, A., Grains experimentaux maduromycosiques a Cephalosporium falciforme, Monosporium apiospermum, Nadurella mycetomi, et Norcardia asteroides, *Mycopathology,* 32, 319, 1967.

33. Avram, A., Experimental induction of grains with Cephalosporium falciforme, *Sabouraudia,* 5, 89, 1965.

34. Symmers, D., Experimental reproduction of maduromycotic lesions in rabbits, *Arch. Pathol.,* 39, 358, 1945.

35. Fukushiro, R., Kinbara, T., Nagai, T., Ikeda, S., and Kumagai, T., On primary pyoderma-like aspergillosis, *Jpn. J. Med. Mycol.,* 14, 127, 1973.

36. Sternberg, T.H., Tarbet, J.E., Newcomer, V.D., and Winter, L.H., Deep infection of mice with *Trichophyton rubrum, J. Invest. Dermatol.,* 19, 374, 1952.

37. Satterwhite, T.K., Kageler, W.V., Conkoin, R.H., Portnoy, B.L., and Dupont, H.L., Disseminated sporotrichosis, *J. Am. Med. Assoc.,* 240, 771, 1978.

38. Charoenvit, Y. and Taylor, L.R., Experimental sporotrichosis in Syrian hamsters, *Infect. Immunol.,* 23, 366, 1979.

39. Barbee, W.C., Ewert, A., and Davidson, M., Animal model: sporotrichosis in the domestic cat, *Am. J. Pathol.,* 86, 281, 1977.

40. Benham, R.W. and Kesten, B., Sporotrichosis: its transmission to plants and animals, *Infect. Dis.,* 50, 437, 1932.

41. Hopkins, J.G. and Benham, R.W., Sporotrichosis in New York state, *N.Y. State J. Med.,* 32, 595, 1932.

42. Kwon-Chung, K.J., Compararison of isolates of Sporothrix schenckii obtained from fixed cutaneous lesions with isolates from other types of lesions, *J. Infect. Dis.,* 139, 424, 1979.

43. Nakahara, T., Studies on the strains of *Sporotrichum schenckii* isolated from soils, *Jpn. J. Med. Mycol.,* 12, 30, 1971.

44. Mackinnon, J.E. and Conti-Diaz, The effect of temperature on sporotrichosis, *Sabouraudia,* 2, 56, 1962.

45. Rippon, J.W., The systemic mycoses, in *Medical Mycology,* 3rd ed., W.B. Saunders, Philadelphia, 1988, p. 373.

46. Brummer, E. and Clemons, K.V., Animal models of systemic mycoses, in *Animal Models in Medical Mycology,* Miyaji, M., Ed., CRC Press, Boca Raton, FL, 1987, p. 79.

47. Morozumi, P.A., Halpern, J.W., and Stevens, D.A., Susceptibility differences of inbred strains of mice to blastomycosis, *Infect. Immunol.,* 32, 160, 1981.

48. Brass, C. and Stevens, D.A., Maturity as a critical determinant of resistance to fungal infections: studies in murine blastomycosis, *Infect. Immunol.,* 36, 387, 1982.

49. Harvey, R.P., Schmid, E.S., Carrington, C.C., and Stevens, D.A., Mouse model of pulmonary blastomycosis: utility, simplicity, and quantitative parameters., *Am. Rev. Resp. Dis.,* 117, 695, 1978.

50. Sugar, A.M. and Picard, M., Experimental blastomycosis pneumonia in mice by infection with conidia, *J. Med. Vet. Mycol.,* 26, 321, 1988.

51. Landay, M.E., Mitten, J., and Miller, J., Disseminated blastomycosis in hamsters. II. Effect of sex on susceptibility, *Mycopathol. Mycologia,* 42, 73, 1970.
52. Conant, N.F., Smith, D.T., Baker, R.D., Calloway, J.L., and Martin, D.S., Eds., *Manual of Clinical Mycology,* 2nd ed., W.B. Saunders, Philadelphia, 1954.
53. Kirkland, T.N. and Fierer, J., Inbred mouse strains differ in resistance to lethal *Coccidioides immitis* infection, *Infect. Immunol.,* 40, 912, 1983.
54. Clemons, K.V., Leathers, C.R., and Lee, K.W., Systemic Coccidioides immitis infection in nude and beige mice, *Infect. Immunol.,* 47, 814, 1985.
55. Huppert, M., Sun, S.H., Gleason-Jordan, I., and Vokovich, K.P., Lung weight parallels disease severity in experimental coccidioidomycosis, *Infect. Immunol.,* 14, 1356, 1976.
56. Kong, Y.M., Levine, H.B., Madin, S.H., and Smith, C.E., Fungal multiplication and histopathological changes in vaccinated mice infected with *Coccidioides immitis, J. Immunol.,* 92, 779, 1964.
57. Schwarz, J., Ed., *Histoplasmosis,* Praeger Publishers, CBS, New York, 1981.
58. Baughman, R.P., Hendricks, D., and Bullock, W.E., Sequential analysis of cellular immune responses in the lung during *Histoplasma capsulatum* infection, *Clin. Res.,* 33, 425A, 1984.
59. Singh, T., Studies on epizootic lymphangitis. Study of clinical cases and experimental transmission, *Indian J. Vet. Sci.,* 36, 45, 1966.
60. Singh, T. and Varmani, B.M.L., Studies on epizootic lymphangitis. A note on pathogenicity of Histoplasma farciminosum (Rivolta) for laboratory animals, *Ind. J. Vet. Sci.,* 36, 164, 1966.
61. Walker, J. and Spooner, E.T.C., Natural infection of the African baboon *Papio papio* with the large cell form of histoplasma, *J. Pathol. Bacteriol.,* 80, 436, 1960.
62. Butler, T.M., Mystery case no. 16, *Comp. Pathol. Bull.,* 21, 1, 1989.
63. Okudaira, M. and Swartz, J., Infection with *Histoplasma duboisii* in different experimental animals, *Mycology,* 53, 53, 1961.
64. Lutz, A., Uma mucose pseudo-coccidica localisada no boca e observada no Brazil: contirbuiaco ao conhecimento das hypho-blastomycoses americanas, *Bras. Med.,* 22, 121, 1908.
65. Guimeraes, F., Infeccao do hamster (*Cricetus auratus* Waterhouse) pelo agente da micose de Lutz (blastomicose sul-americana), *Hospital (Rio),* 40, 515, 1951.
66. Brummer, E., Restrepo, A., Stevens, D.A., Azzi, R., Gomez, A., Hoyos, G., McEwen, J., Cano, L., and deBedount, C., Murine model of paracoccidioidomycosis. Production of fatal acute pulmonary or chronic pulmonary and disseminated disease: immunological and pathological observations, *J. Exp. Pathol.,* 1, 241, 1984.
67. Pollak, L. and Angulo-Ortega, A., *Pathogenesis of Paracoccidioidomycosis, Proceedings of the 1st Pan American Symposium,* PAHO and World Health Organization Scientific Publication 254, Washington, D.C., 1972, p. 293.
68. DelNegro, G., Lacaz, C., and Fiorillo, A., *Paracoccidioidomycosis: Blastomicose Sub-America,* Sarvier-Edusp., Sao Paulo, Brazil, 1982, p. 78.
69. Iabuki, K. and Montenegro, M.R., Experimental paracoccidioidomycosis in the Syrian hamster: morphology, ultrastructure and correlation of lesions with presence of specific antigen and serum levels of antibodies, *Mycopathology,* 67, 131, 1979.
70. Restrepo, A. and DeGuzman, E.G., Paracoccidioidomycosis experimental del ration inducida por via aerogena, *Sabouraudia,* 14, 299, 1976.
71. Rippon, J.W., Opportunistic infections, in *Medical Mycology,* 3rd ed., W.B. Saunders, Philadelphia, 1988, p. 532.
72. Van Cutsem, J., Fungal models in immunocompromised animals, in *Mycoses in AIDS Patients,* Vanden Bossche, Ed., Plenum Press, New York, 1990, p. 207.
73. Yamaguchi, H., Opportunistic fungal infections, in *Animal Models in Medical Mycology,* Miyaji, M., Ed., CRC Press, Boca Raton, FL, 1987, p. 101.
74. Abe, F., Tateyama, M., Shibuya, H., Azumi, N., and Ommura, Y., Experimental candidiasis in iron overload, *Mycopathology,* 89, 59, 1985.
75. Abe, F., Tateyama, M., Shibuya, H., and Ommura, Y., Experimental candidiasis in iron overload, *Jpn. J. Med. Mycol.,* 25, 290, 1984.
76. Odds, F.C., Candidosis of the genitalia, in *Candida and Candidosis,* 2nd ed., Odds, F.C., Ed., BailliPre Tindall, London, 1988, p. 124.

77. Sobel, J.D., Pathogenesis of *Candida vulvovaginitis,* in *Current Topics in Medical Mycology,* Vol. 3, McGinnis, M.R. and Borgers, M., Eds., Springer-Verlag, Berlin, 1989, p. 86.

78. Mardon, D.N. and Robinnette, E.H., Jr., Organ distribution and viability of *Candida albicans* in noncancerous and tumor-bearing (Lewis lung carcinoma) mice, *Can. J. Microbiol.,* 24, 1515, 1978.

79. Johnson, J.A., Lau, B.H.S., Nuater, R.L., Slatar, J.M., and Winter, C.E., Effect of L1210 leukemia on the susceptibility of mice to *Candida albicans* infections, *Infect. Immunol.,* 19, 146, 1978.

80. Corbel, M.J. and Eades, S.M., The relative susceptibility of New Zealand Black and CBA mice to infection with opportunistic fungal pathogens, *Sabouraudia,* 14, 17, 1976.

81. Jordan, F.T.W., Diseases of poultry, *Br. Vet. J.,* 137, 545, 1981.

82. Jensen, H.E., Basse, A., and Aalbæk, B., Mycosis in the stomach compartments of cattle, *Acta Vet. Scand.,* 30, 409, 1989.

83. Jensen, H.E., Krogh, H.V., and Schønheyder, H., Bovine mycotic abortion — a comparative study of diagnostic methods, *J. Vet. Med., B,* 38, 33, 1991.

84. Van Cutsem, J., Antifungal activity of enilconazole on experimental aspergillosis in chickens, *Avian Dis.,* 27, 36, 1983.

85. Niki, Y., Bernad, E.M., Edwards, F.F., Schmitt, H.J., Yu, B., and Armstrong, D., Model of recurrent pulmonary aspergillosis in rats, *J. Clin. Microbiol.,* 29, 1317, 1991.

86. Bhatia, V.N. and Mohapatra, L.N., Experimental aspergillosis in mice. I. Pathogenic potential of *Aspergillus fumigatus, Aspergillus flavus* and *Aspergillus niger, Mykosen,* 12, 615, 1969.

87. Bhatia, V.N. and Mohapatra, L.N., Experimental aspergillosis in mice. II. Enhanced susceptibility of the cortisone treated mice to infection with *Aspergillus fumigatus, Aspergillus flavus* and *Aspergillus niger, Mykosen,* 13, 105, 1970.

88. Sandhu, D., Sandhu, R.S., Damodaran, V.N., and Randhawa, H.S., Effect of cortisone on broncho-pulmonary aspergillosis in mice exposed to spores of various Aspergillus species, *Sabouraudia,* 8, 32, 1970.

89. Epstein, S.M., Verney, E., Miale, T.D., and Sideransky, H., Studies on the pathogenesis of experimental pulmonary aspergillosis, *Am. J. Pathol.,* 51, 769, 1967.

90. Merkow, L.L., Epstein, S.M., Sideransky, H., Verney, E., and Pardo, M., The pathogenesis of exper-imental pulmonary aspergillosis, *Am. J. Pathol.,* 62, 57, 1970.

91. Sawasaki, H., Horie, K., Naito, Y., Watabe, S., Tajima, G., and Mizutani, Y., Experimental pulmonary aspergilloma, *Mycopathology,* 32, 265, 1967.

92. Hill, M.W.M., Whiteman, C.E., Benjamin, M.M., and Ball, L., Pathogenesis of experimental bovine mycotic placentitis produced by *Aspergillus fumigatus, Vet. Pathol.,* 8, 273, 1971.

93. Cysewski, S.J. and Pier, A.C., Mycotic abortion in ewes produced by *Aspergillus fumigatus,* pathologic changes, *Am. J. Vet. Res.,* 29, 1135, 1968.

94. Jensen, H.E. and Hau, J., A murine model for the study of the impact of *Aspergillus fumigatus* inoculation on the foeto-placental unit, *Mycopathology,* 112, 11, 1990.

95. Jensen, H.E. and Hau, J., Murine mycotic placentitis produced by intravenous inoculation of conidia from *Aspergillus fumigatus, In Vivo,* 4, 247, 1990.

96. Cohrs, P., Jaffe, R., and Meesen, H., Eds., *Pathologie der Laboratoriumstiere,* Vol. 2., Springer-Verlag, Berlin, 1958.

97. Carrizosa, J., Kohn, C., and Levinson, M.E., Experimental aspergillus endocarditis in rabbits, *J. Lab. Clin. Med.,* 86, 746, 1975.

98. Golbert, T.M. and Patterson, R., Pulmonary allergic aspergillosis, *Ann. Intern. Med.,* 72, 395, 1970.

99. Odds, F.C., Pathogenesis of candidosis, in *Candida and Candidosis,* 2nd ed., Odds, F.C., Ed., BailliPre Tindall, London, 1988, p. 252.

100. Cinander, B., Dubiski, S., and Wardlaw, A.C., Distribution, inheritance, and properties of an antigen, MUB1, and its relation to hemolytic complement, *J. Exp. Med.,* 120, 897, 1964.

101. Tarsi, R., Simonetti, N., and Orpianesi, C., Experimental candidiasis in rabbits: protective action of fructose-1,6,-diphosphate, *Mycopathology,* 81, 111, 1983.

102. Parker, J.C., Jr., Cleary, T.J., and Kogure, K., The effects of transient candidemia on the brain: preliminary observations on a rodent model for experimental deep candidosis, *Surg. Neurol.,* 11, 44, 1979.

103. Parker, J.C., Jr., Cleary, T.J., Monji, T., Kogure, K., and Castro, A., Modifying cerebral candidiasis by altering the infectious entry route, *Arch. Pathol. Lab. Med.,* 104, 537, 1980.

104. Louria, D.B., Candida infection in experimental animals, in *Candidiasis,* Bodey, G.P. and Fainstein, V., Eds., Raven Press, New York, 1985, p. 29.

105. Jensen, H.E., Hau, J., Aalbæk, B., and Schønheyder, H., Experimental candidosis in pregnant mice, *APMIS,* 99, 829, 1991.

106. Thienpont, D., Van Cutsem, J., and Borgers, M., Ketoconazole in experimental candidosis, *Rev. Infect. Dis.,* 2, 570, 1967.

107. Balish, E. and Phillips, A.W., Growth, morphogenesis and virulence of *Candida albicans* after oral inoculation in the germ-free and conventional chick, *J. Bacteriol.,* 91, 1736, 1966.

108. Polak, A. and Schaffner, A., A new experimental model of localized candidosis for the study of antifungal chemotherapy, *Mycoses,* 32, 398, 1989.

109. Pope, L.M., Cole, G.T., Guentzel, M.N., and Berry, L.J., Systemic and gastrointestinal candidiasis in infant mice after intragastric challenge, *Infect. Immunol.,* 25, 702, 1979.

110. Cole, G.T., Lynn, K.T., and Seshan, K.R., Evaluation of a murine model of hepatic candidiasis, *J. Clin. Microbiol.,* 28, 1828, 1990.

111. Guhad, F.A., Jensen, H.E., Aalbæk, B., Rycroft, A., and Hau, J., A murine model for the study of mycotic mastitis, *J. Comp. Pathol.,* 113, 315, 1995.

112. Guhad, F.A., Development and Validation of a Localized Murine Candidasis Model, dissertation, Uppsala, Sweden, Reprocentralen, Ekonomikum, 1999, 7.

113. Guhad, F.A., Csank, C., Jensen, H.E., Thomas, D.Y., Whiteway, M., and Hau, J., Reduced pathogenicity of a *Candida albicans* MAP kinase phosphatase (CPP1) mutant in the murine mastitis model, *APMIS,* 106, 1049, 1998.

114. Guhad, F.A., Jensen, H.E., Aalbæk, B., Csank, C., Mohamed, O., Harcus, D., Thomas, D.Y., Whiteway, M., and Hau, J., Mitogen-activated protein kinase-defective *Candida albicans* is avirulent in a novel model of localized murine candidiasis, *FEMS Microbiol. Lett.,* 166, 135, 1998.

115. Guhad, F.A., Jensen, H.E., and Hau, J., Experimental murine mycotic mastitis: a sensitive and lenient model for studies of antifungal chemotherapy, *FEMS Microbiol. Lett.,* 26, 125, 1999.

116. Savage, A. and Tribe, C.R., Experimental murine amyloidosis: experience with *Candida albicans* as an amyloidogenic agent and liver biopsy as a diagnostic tool, *J. Pathol.,* 127, 199, 1979.

117. Miyaji, M. and Nishimura, K., Studies on organ specificity in experimental murine cryptococcosis, *Mycopathology,* 76, 145, 1981.

118. Watanabe, T., Miyaji, M., and Nishimura, K., Studies on relationship between cysts and granulomas in murine cryptococcosis, *Mycopathology,* 86, 113, 1984.

119. Karaoui, R.M., Hall, N.K., and Larsh, H.W., Role of macrophages in immunity and pathogenesis of experimental cryptococcosis induced by the airborne route. I. Pathogenesis and acquired immunity of *Cryptococcus neoformans, Mykosen,* 20, 380, 1977.

120. Ritter, R.C. and Larsh, H.W., The infection of white mice following an intranasal instillation of *Cryptococcus neoformans, Am. J. Hyg.,* 78, 241, 1963.

121. Graybill, J.R., Ahrens, J., Nealon, T., and Raque, R., Pulmonary cryptococcosis in the rat, *Am. Rev. Resp. Dis.,* 127, 636, 1983.

122. Perfect, J.R., Lagn, S.D.R., and Durack, D.T., Chronic cryptococcal meningitis. A new experimental model in rabbits, *Am. J. Pathol.,* 101, 177, 1980.

123. Green, J.R. and Bulmer, G.S., Gastrointestinal inoculation of *Cryptococcus neoformans* in mice, *Sabouraudia,* 17, 233, 1979.

124. Dixon, D.M. and Polak, A., *In vivo* and *in vitro* studies with an atypical rhinotrophic isolate of *Cryptococcus neoformans, Mycopathology,* 96, 33, 1986.

125. Dupont, B., Improvisi, L., and Ronin, O., Aspects epidemiologiques et cliniques des infections a Scedosporium et Pseudallescheria, *J. Mycol. Med.,* 118, 33, 1991.

126. Drouhet, E., Dupont, B., and Ravisse, P., Étude experimentale d'une souche hautement virulente de Scedosporium inflatum isolee d'une arthrite du genou, *J. Mycol. Med.,* 118, 16, 1991.

127. Espinel-Ingroff, A., Oakley, L.A., and Kerkering, T.M., Opportunistic zygomycotic infections — a literature review, *Mycopathology,* 97, 33, 1987.

128. Ainsworth, G.C. and Austwick, P.K.C., Eds., *Fungal Diseases of Animals,* 2nd ed., BPCC Wheatons, Exeter, United Kingdom, 1973, p. 53.

129. Kitz, J.D., Embree, R.W., and Cazin, J., Comparative virulence of *Absidia corymbifera* strains in mice, *Infect. Immunol.,* 33, 395, 1981.

130. Waldorf, A.R., Halde, C., and Vedros, N.A., Murine model of pulmonary mucormycosis in corti-sone-treated mice, *Sabouraudia,* 20, 217, 1982.

131. Van Cutsem, J. and Boelaert, J.R., Effects of deferoxamine, feroxamine and iron on experimental mucormycosis (zygomycosis), *Kidney Int.,* 36, 1061, 1989.

132. Smith, J.M.B., Experimental mycotic ulceration, *Sabouraudia,* 34, 353, 1968.

133. Jensen, H.E., Aalbæk, B., and Hau, J., Induction of systemic zygomycosis in pregnant mice by *Absidia corymbifera, Lab. Anim. Sci.,* 45, 254,1995.

134. Sukura, A., *Pneumocystis carinii* in a Rat Model, dissertation, Helsinki, Finland, Cosmoprint Oy, Helsinki, Finland, 1995, 21.

135. Dei-cas, E., Pneumocystis infection: the iceberg? *Med. Mycol.,* 38(Suppl. 1), 23, 2000.

136. Pifer, L.L., A fifteen-year perspective on the *in vitro* culture of *Pneumocystis carinii, J. Protozool.,* 36, 23, 1989.

137. Smulian, A.G. and Walzer, P.D., The biology of *Pneumocystis carinii, Crit. Rev. Microbiol.,* 18, 191, 1992.

138. Jensen, H.E., Hau, J., Aalbæk, B., and Schønheyder, H., Indirect immunofluorescence staining and crossed immunoelectrophoresis for differentiation of *Candida albicans* and *Geotrichum candidum, Mycoses,* 33, 519, 1990.

139. Spanoghe, L., Devos, A., and Viaene, N., Cutaneous geotrichosis in the red flamingo (*Phoenicopterus ruber), Sabouraudia,* 14, 37, 1976.

140. Segretain, G., *Penicillium marneffei N.* sp., agent d'une mycose du systeme reticulo-endothelial, *Mycopath. Mycopath. Appl.,* 11, 327, 1959.

141. Deng, Z., Yun, M., and Ajello, L., Human penicilliosis marneffei and its relation to the baboo rat (*Rhizomys pruinosus), J. Med. Vet. Mycol.,* 24, 383, 1986.

142. Faergemann, J., Experimental tinea versicolor in rabbits and humans with *Pityrosporum orbiculare, J. Invest. Dermatol.,* 72, 326, 1979.

143. Faergemann, J., Tinea versicolor and *Pityrosporum orbiculare*: mycological investigations, experimental infections and epidemiological surveys, *Acta. Dermatol. Venereol.,* 86, 1, 1979.

144. Connor, D.H. and Neafie, R.C., Prototithecosis, in *Pathology of Tropical and Extraordinary Diseases,* Vol. 2, Bindford, C.H. and Connor, D.H., Eds., Armed Forces Institute of Pathology, Washington, D.C., 1976, p. 684.

145. Frank, N., Ferguson, L.C., Cross, R.F., and Redman, D.R., Prototheca, a cause of bovine mastitis, *Am. J. Vet. Res.,* 30, 1785, 1969.

146. Migaki, G., Garner, F.M., and Imes, G.D., Bovine protothricosis — a report of three cases, *Pathol. Vet.,* 6, 444, 1969.

147. Imes, G.D., Lloyd, J.C., and Brightman, M.P., Disseminated protothecosis in a dog, *Onderstepoort J. Vet. Res.,* 44, 1, 1977.

148. Rogers, R.J., Connole, M.D., Norton, J., Thomas, A., Ladds, P.W., and Dickson, J., Lymphadenitis of cattle due to infection with green algae, *J. Comp. Pathol.,* 90, 1, 1980.

149. Sudman, M.S. and Kaplan, W., Identification of the Prototheca species by immunofluorescence, *Appl. Microbiol.,* 25, 981, 1973.

150. Bennett, G. and Grant, S., Antifungal activity, in *Fluconazole, An Overview,* 3rd ed., Bennett, G. and Grant, S., Eds., Fortune Printing, Hong Kong, 1990, p. 7.

151. Odds, F.C., Cheesman, S.L., and Abbott, A.B., Antifungal effect of fluconazole (UK-49858), a new triazole antifungal, *in vitro, J. Antimicrob. Chemother.,* 18, 473, 1986.

152. Zak, O. and O'Reilly, T., Minireview — animal models in the evaluation of antimicrobial agents, *Antimicrob. Agents Chemother.,* 35, 1527, 1991.

153. Zak, O. and Sande, M.A., Introduction: the role of animal models in the evaluation of new antibiotics, in *Experimental Models in Antimicrobial Chemotherapy,* Vol. 1, Zak, O. and Sande, M.A., Eds., Academic Press, Orlando, FL, 1986, p. 1.

154. Jensen, H.E. and Schønheyder, H., Immunofluorescence staining of hyphae in the histopathological diagnosis of mycoses in cattle, *J. Med. Vet. Mycol.,* 27, 33, 1989.

155. Jensen, H.E., Bloch, B., Henriksen, P., Dietz, H.H., Schønheyder, H., and Kaufman, L., Disseminated histoplasmosis in a badger (*Meles meles*) in Denmark, *APMIS,* 100, 1992.

156. Dupont, B., Huber, M., Kim, S.J., and Bennett, J.E., Galactomannan antigenemia and antigenuria in aspergillosis: studies in patients and experimentally infected rabbits, *J. Infect. Dis.,* 155, 1, 1987.

157. Jensen, H.E., Latge, J.P., Frandsen, P.L., and Schønheyder, H., Application of ELISA and immuno-blotting for the diagnosis of systemic bovine aspergillosis and zygomycosis, in *Proceedings of the VIth International Symposium of the World Association of Veterinary Laboratory Diagnosis,* 1992, p. 39.

158. Van Cutsem, J., Meulemans, L., Van Gerven, F., and Stynen, D., Detection of circulating galactoman-nan by Pastorex Aspergillus in experimental invasive aspergillosis, *Mycoses,* 33, 61, 1990.

159. Latge, J.P., Moutaouakil, M., Debeaupuis, J.P., Bouchara, J.P., Haynes, K., and Prévost, M.C., The 18-kilodalton antigen secreted by *Aspergillus fumigatus, Infect. Immunol.,* 59, 2586, 1991.

CHAPTER 9

Diabetic Animal Models

Karsten Buschard and Rikke Thon

CONTENTS

INTRODUCTION

Diabetes mellitus is an important human disease, divided into two major forms: type 1 diabetes mellitus (T1DM), formerly called insulin-dependent diabetes mellitus (IDDM); and T2DM, earlier called non-insulin-dependent diabetes mellitus (NIDDM). Both diseases are frequent. Among Caucasians, 0.5 to 1% of the population (in a few areas, up to 2%) will be affected by T1DM. T2DM is even more common; and in many Western countries, 5 to 10% of elderly people suffer from the disease. In certain populations, the prevalence of T2DM is even higher; among Pina Indians, it is up to 30%.

Although both T1DM and T2DM are characterized by abnormally high blood glucose levels and glucosuria, the etiologies and pathogeneses are different. Clinically, T1DM has a rather sudden onset, with hypoinsulinemia and ketone molecules in the blood and urine. At onset, maybe only 10% of the β cells of the pancreas (which synthesize and secrete insulin) remain.[1] For survival, the patients are dependent on lifelong exogenous insulin treatment. The goal of T1DM patients is to keep the blood glucose values low without having incidents of hypoglycemia. This is a function of insulin treatment, food intake, and amount of exercise. The better that metabolic control is maintained, the less likely it is that a patient will develop chronic complications, although these nevertheless are seen after some years in most of these diabetic patients. Because of this, diabetes is now the most common course of acquired blindness, the third most common course of renal failure, and about the fifth most common course of death in many countries. In addition, many T2DM patients suffer from complications, which include retinopathy, nephropathy, and neuropathy. T1DM is recognized as an autoimmune disease, and the β-cell destruction is mediated by T cells. Also, autoantibodies can be measured in most patients. In contrast, T2DM has no involvement of the immune system. The disease is characterized by peripheral insulin resistance and relatively insufficient insulin secretion. Lack of first-phase insulin response is seen. Most frequently, patients are overweight, especially because of increased amounts of intraabdominal fat tissue.

Good animal models have been developed for both kinds of diabetes. These models provide an excellent opportunity for studying the multitude of interacting factors that contribute to the syndrome, which is not feasible in afflicted humans. A desirable feature of a model syndrome is, of course, that it approximates the phenotypes of human disease, thereby leading to a more complete understanding of etiology, pathogenesis, and treatment in humans. In particular, the animal models provide material for examining the very early steps in the pathological process because such investigations cannot be conducted in humans because the manifest disease covers up a long preceding process. However, none of the mentioned models are ideal, and none of them resemble human diabetes completely. To establish new findings in the pathogenesis, prevention, or treatment of diabetes, it is therefore highly desirable that a new scientific principle be found in more than one of the animal models. This chapter first describes the following T1DM models: the spontaneously diabetic BB rat, the NOD (non-obese diabetic) mouse, and the induced models of low-dose streptozotocin and virus-induced diabetes in mice. Thereafter, the chapter describes the following T2DM models: *ob/ob* mice, *db/db* mice, and GK rats.

ANIMAL MODELS OF TYPE 1 DIABETES

The BB Rat

The BB-rat syndrome was recognized initially in 1974 by Chappel at the BioBreeding Laboratories, Ottawa, Canada.[2] Overt T1DM, associated with hypoinsulinemia occurred sporadically in this commercial breeding colony of non-inbred Wistar-derived laboratory rats kept under strict gnotobiotic conditions. A breeding program was established, and it was decided that the syndrome would be named "BB" after the initials of the breeding laboratory.

All BB rats are descendants of the original Ottawa litters, but rats in different colonies now vary in frequency of diabetes. To identify the specific strain, all animals are named after the city or institution in which they are bred, for example, BB/W for Worcester.[3]

Clinical Course of the Diabetic Syndrome

Diabetes in the BB rat typically has an abrupt onset, with glucosuria, hyperglycemia, hyperketonemia, ketonuria, and hypoinsulinemia. The age at which diabetes is diagnosed is generally between 60 and 120 d.[4] The mean is about 90 d in most reported data. This age distribution at the diagnosis of T1DM is analogous to that observed in humans; there is a preponderance of cases among the juvenile and adolescent populations. The incidence of diabetes varies in the different rat colonies and is up to 80%. The animals are not obese, and diabetes occurs with almost equal frequency in both sexes.

Acutely diabetic animals die from ketoacidosis within 2 weeks of onset unless insulin is given. Morphological studies show infiltration of mainly mononuclear cells in the islets of Langerhans, a condition called insulitis that is present before the disease is clinically manifest. The pancreas of rats with overt T1DM shows less than 0.1% of normal insulin content.[5,6] The progression from normal to seriously decompensated can be counted in days. The hyperglycemia is associated with hypoinsulinemia and hyperglucagonemia. Until glucosuria begins, absolute values and rates of gain in body weight in the majority of rats are indistinguishable from those of littermates.

Despite hyperphagia and polydipsia, weight loss is rapid and a good indicator of diabetes development. Physical activity is clearly decreased, and tachypnea can be seen. In contrast to humans, the BB rat (diabetic as well as non-diabetic) has an unusual predisposition to lymphopoietic malignancy and to infection, especially with *Mycoplasma pneumoniae,* which is often fatal. The animals exhibit a pronounced decrease in the population of T lymphocytes and thereby a functional deficiency of a variety of lymphocyte-mediated immune reactions — that is, a marked immunoregulatory defect. A line of nonlymphopenic diabetic BB rats has, however, been developed.[7]

Genetics

Human T1DM, as well as the BB-diabetic syndrome, is a heritable disorder. In humans, there is a 30% concordance for T1DM among monozygotic twins; and in the BB-rat model, about 70% of the animals develop diabetes in colonies that have been inbred for many generations, indicating that factors other than genetics must play a role. It is most likely that the mode of inheritance of BB-rat diabetes involves an autosomal-recessive gene or gene cluster with incomplete penetrance (approximately 50%),[8,9] leaving room for environmental factors to influence the expression of the genes or their product. Furthermore, diabetes in the BB rat also shows a major histocompatibility complex association.

Disease Mechanisms

As in humans, diabetes in the BB rat is believed to be an autoimmune disease. Three main causes contribute to this conviction: (1) involvement of the humoral immune system, (2) involvement of the cellular immune system, and as previously discussed, (3) involvement of a genetic factor, that is, the association with the major histocompatibility complex (MHC). The exact series of events that initiates diabetes is still hypothetical.

The Humoral Immune System

A phenotypic feature of diabetic and diabetes-prone (DP) BB rats is the presence of autoantibodies of the IgG class, which bind to smooth muscle, thyroid colloid, and gastric parietal cell antigens.[10,11] Although there is high concordance between the presence of diabetes, thyroiditis, and autoantibodies, 50% of animals without thyroiditis evidence antithyroid colloid antibodies. Perhaps more important is that beta islet cell surface antibodies (ICSA) have been detected as early as 40 d of age. Complement-fixing islet cell antibodies (CF-ICA) have also been detected and may be present 2 weeks before the onset of diabetes. Thus, these two autoantibodies actually antedate the manifest disease. Antilymphocyte antibodies are also prevalent in diabetic animals.[12,13]

The Cellular Immune System

As mentioned, the BB rat is lymphopenic, and this can be recognized before the clinical onset of diabetes.[14] Lymphopenia is characterized by a marked decrease in the number of T lymphocytes in the peripheral blood, lymph nodes, and spleen.[15] Although all T-cell subsets are diminished, the CD8+ T-cell subset (cytotoxic/suppressor) is the most diminished.[16] In addition, the RT6 differentiation alloantigen, which normally is expressed on about half the peripheral T cells (but is absent in bone marrow and thymocytes), is absent in rats with lymphopenia.[17]

Pancreatic lymphocytic insulitis is observed in young asymptomatic BB rats with normal levels of blood glucose and insulin, so insulitis actually precedes overt diabetes. Studies have shown the lymphocytic infiltrate to consist of B cells, CD8, and CD4 T cells, as well as macrophages and natural killer (NK) cells. Macrophages are believed to be the first cells invading the islets, an important cell type both for cytokine production and antigen presentation.[18] Additionally, it has been demonstrated that NK-cell activity is increased in acutely diabetic as well as DP BB rats, and that islet cells can serve as target cells for these large granular lymphocytes *in vitro*, NK cells being capable of lysing islet cells.[19] The exact role of the various cell types is not clarified.

Within a very short time after the detection of hyperglycemia, insulitis rapidly decreases and finally disappears with the appearance of the so-called end-stage islets, consisting almost exclusively of glucagon, somatostatin, and pancreatic polypeptide-synthesizing islet cells.

The presence of lymphocytic thyroiditis in a large proportion of BB rats also suggests that this organ is the target of a cell-mediated autoimmune attack. Lymphocytic thyroiditis occurs in diabetic and normoglycemic BB/W rats but is more frequent among diabetic animals. However, the thyroiditis is not followed by clinical thyroid disease.

Further evidence for the involvement of cellular immunity in the pathogenesis of diabetes in the BB rat is found in the fact that DP rats have been protected from developing diabetes by neonatal thymectomy. Another study has shown incomplete thymectomy to influence the incidence, indicating that the mass of functional thymic tissue is a factor in the pathogenesis.[20] Neonatal bone marrow allografts,[21] sublethal whole-body irradiation,[22] and total lymphoid irradiation[23] have also been shown to protect DP rats from diabetes. Administration of antilymphocyte globulin alone prevents diabetes when given to prediabetic animals, and will cure diabetes in approximately one third of BB rats treated on the day that diabetes is detected. Also, transfusions of whole blood[24] or peripheral T lymphocytes[25] from the diabetes-resistant (DR) subline of BB rats have been reported to prevent the appearance of diabetes in the DP rat. Conversely, Concanavalin A (ConA)-activated splenic lymphocytes have been shown to adoptively transfer insulitis and diabetes upon injection into young DP BB/W-rats[26] or into otherwise DR BB rats[27] and Wistar-Furth rats[28] that have been pretreated with cyclophosphamide. Administration of cyclosporin A will effectively reduce the frequency of diabetes but does not cure the disease.[29,30] Cyclosporin A itself is not cytotoxic but is believed to act by inhibiting T-lymphocyte proliferation in response to antigenic stimulation. Cyclosporin A is able to protect the β cell from injury caused by the cytotoxic effect of interleukin-1 and probably also interleukin-6, which functionally and structurally has been shown to modify beta cells *in vitro*. Cyclosporin A is used to treat prediabetic rats when needed for breeding but cannot be used in humans because the side effects (especially nephrotoxicity) are too serious. On the other hand, Freund's Adjuvant, which causes immunostimulation, lowers the diabetes incidence, maybe because of an influence on the suppressor T cells, in accordance with the fact that elimination of infectious agents from the environment actually increases the frequency and accelerates the tempo of spontaneous diabetes among DP rats.[31]

The Question of Self-Tolerance

As mentioned, diabetes is believed to be an autoimmune disease. Failure to induce islet tolerance may be caused by (1) thymic antigen-presenting cells in DP animals being defective in their ability to present β cells to establish islet tolerance,[32] or (2) the fact that islets from rat neonates, the age at which self-tolerance is normally induced, lack certain antigenic determinants that develop later, leaving them susceptible to destruction by their own immune system. A study has shown that diabetes in BB rats can be prevented by neonatal stimulation of β cells, a procedure that is thought to induce or enhance antigen expression on the β cells, which facilitates the ability of the immune system to develop self-tolerance.[33,34] The neonates were stimulated for the first 6 d after birth by glucose accompanied by glucagon or arginin, the immature β cells producing only a basal amount of insulin and being unresponsive to glucose alone in order to accelerate β-cell maturation and possibly to induce antigen expression and tolerance. Over the first 200 d of life, only about 40% of the treated rats developed diabetes, compared with 65% of untreated controls. This may explain the observation that children of mothers who have T1DM are three times less likely to develop the disease than are children of fathers with T1DM. Earlier maturation of the β cells during the diabetic pregnancy may thus protect against diabetes in later life.

Intrathymic injections also have been carried out.[35] This was done on the assumption that the introduction of islet cells into the thymus might directly induce islet tolerance — a mechanism for the establishment of self-tolerance might then be an enhancement of the activity of the above-mentioned antigen-presenting cells. The islets needed for injection were isolated from DR rats. In fact, only 35% of the rats that had an intrathymic injection of islets developed diabetes, compared with 88% of the control sham-operated rats. Thus, it seems that exposing the cells of the thymus directly to islet antigen can prevent an autoimmune attack, induce tolerance, and significantly reduce the incidence of the disease.

Environmental Factors

The concordance of only about 30 to 50% in human monozygotic twins and the fact that the incidence of diabetes varies from 50 to 80% in highly inbred BB rat colonies can be considered very strong arguments for the involvement of environmental factors. They may either trigger the autoimmune process or modify its course.

An environmental influence operating on a basis of genetic susceptibility may be the diet.[36] Diet has clearly been shown to modify the frequency of diabetes among BB rats; substitution of a defined diet for rat chow lowers the frequency of disease to about half of that seen for rats fed normal rat chow, and feeding a diet containing only a casein hydrolysate further decreases the frequency of disease. It is unknown whether the lower incidence is secondary to removal of a specific dietary protein or whether it is caused by the removal of many components (e.g., fibers, lectins, viral and bacterial toxins) that may be present in chow and thus affect the gut of the young weanlings.

Other environmental factors have been evaluated. Castration, vagotomy, hypophysectomy, and stress produced by ultrasound, for example, could not prevent diabetes.[37]

Administration of nicotinamide,[38,39] a precursor for the synthesis of nicotinamide adenine dinucleotide (NAD), has proven to be able to delay the onset of diabetes. Histological examinations of pancreata collected from treated animals showed a reduction of insulitis and preservation of the number of β cells and the overall islet architecture. Moreover, treatment with large doses of nicotinamide from the first day of glucosuria precipitated the disappearance of glucosuria and an improvement of glucose tolerance during the treatment period.

Exogenous insulin treatment is another way of trying to influence the incidence through environmental factors: reduction of diabetes incidence of BB rats has been seen with early prophylactic insulin treatment of DP animals. In a specific study, BB rats were given insulin from day 50 to day 142 of age.[40] At withdrawal, this group was compared with a control group of rats given insulin only from the first day of glucosuria. The incidence in the prophylactically treated group was 22%, compared with 44% among the controls. The findings of this study suggest that administration of exogenous insulin to BB rats during the prediabetic period could render the β cells, characterized by a low rate of insulin synthesis, less vulnerable to immune aggression. Specifically, a reduction of endogenous insulin secretion might reduce the amount of antigens on the β-cell surface that is recognized by the immune system to such a level that the autoimmune cascade is either not initiated or is alleviated.[41] In another study, when insulin treatment was started earlier in life (day 35), the diabetes incidence was reduced from 56 to 2%.[42]

Another study concerning prophylactic insulin treatment has been carried out using the DR BB rat, in which diabetes and thyroiditis occur in less than 1% of the animals and the RT6 alloantigen is present on about 60% of the T cells. Thirty-day-old DR rats were treated with anti RT6 monoclonal antibody, exogenous insulin, or both, until the age of 60 d.[43] *In vivo* depletion of RT6 T cells by giving cytotoxic monoclonal antibodies induced diabetes and thyroiditis in more than 50% of treated animals by 60 d of age. Coadministration of insulin during this prediabetic period prevented nearly all cases of diabetes, but not thyroiditis. Spleen cells from these insulin-treated and RT6-depleted nondiabetic DR rats were still capable of adoptive transfer of diabetes.

The precise mechanism of insulin action is unproven, but the possibility exists that the action could take place either at the β-cell level or at the T-cell level (*vaccination*). On the other hand, as is obvious from, for example, the case of prophylactic insulin treatment not being able to prevent thyroiditis, a great deal of evidence exists that insulin treatment acts on the β-cell level, where it suppresses insulin secretion: prolonged insulin treatment means prolonged hypoglycemia, which again causes reduced β-cell mitotic activity and suppressed endogenous insulin production, secretion, and stores. Such depression of β-cell metabolic activity might very well render the β cells resistant to the cytotoxic effect of cytokines such as interleukin-1 released in the course of the autoimmune process. Interestingly, prophylactic insulin treatment does show effect in the BB rat only when given in metabolic doses.

As already partly discussed, alteration of antigens that are targets of the autoimmune process could also occur in response to exogenous insulin keeping the blood glucose low. Studies have been carried out that demonstrate that islet cells incubated at different glucose concentrations showed different labeling with specific autoantibodies.[41] Labeling was found to be more frequent and more pronounced in islet cells incubated at high glucose concentrations. The labeling was of cell surface antigens, which were detected by the β-cell-specific monoclonal antibody IC2, and A2B5, the latter directed against a ganglioside. Thus, β-cell antigen expression very likely depends on the functional state of the cells.

The Non-Obese Diabetic Mouse

Like the BB-rat model, the non-obese diabetic (NOD) mouse model is a genetically determined model and the NOD mouse is in many ways the mouse equivalent to the BB rat. The ultimate effector mechanisms, however, are different.

The pedigree of the NOD mouse is as follows. In 1966, a cataract-prone mouse arose from outbred ICR mice and gave rise to the CTS strain. Because cataract is frequent in diabetic patients, the suspicion of a pathogenetic relationship to diabetes arose. Selective breeding was carried out and two sister strains, one euglycemic and the other slightly hyperglycemic, arose after 13 generations of breeding. The mouse that developed non-obese diabetic symptoms was obtained in the 20th generation and ironically in the euglycemic sister strain. The mouse was female and exhibited polyuria, severe glycosuria, and weight loss. The strain was established in 1974 by Makino et al. in Osaka, Japan. Breeding was continued using offspring selected for both spontaneous diabetes and reproductive ability, leading after the 6th generation to the NOD mouse, which is not cataract-prone.[44,45]

In 1980, the original NOD strain had a cumulative diabetes incidence by 30 weeks of age of 60 to 80% in females versus only about 10% in males.[45] The main period of diabetes manifestation was between 80 and 200 d.[46] A corresponding nondiabetic substrain was also maintained, to serve as a control strain and termed non-obese normal (NON).

Clinical Course of the NOD Diabetic Syndrome

Many NOD lines have been established around the world and they differ significantly in diabetes incidence, time of onset, and degree of female preponderance. Apart from a higher frequency, NOD females also exhibit permanent hyperglycemia at an earlier age than males: peak onset between 16 and 20 weeks as compared with between 21 and 28 weeks in males.[47] Gonadal sex steroids are important modulators of pathogenesis: castrated males show a higher incidence of diabetes and oophorectomized females a lower incidence.[48] Castration of mice up to the age of 7 weeks results in an increase in males and a decrease in females.[49]

The clinical features of the diabetes syndrome in NOD mice are quite similar to human T1DM and characterized by hypoinsulinemia, hyperglycemia, glycosuria, hypercholesterolemia, ketonuria, polydipsia, polyuria, and polyphagia. The blood glucose rises from a normal level of approximately 7 to 9 mM to permanent hyperglycemia, that is, a blood glucose level greater than 25 mM over a period of 3 to 4 weeks, and in contrast to the BB rat, the NOD mouse can survive quite a long time without insulin treatment (i.e., 1 to 12 weeks).[47,48]

Histopathology

Despite the sex difference in incidence, almost all animals (>95%) display mononuclear cellular infiltration insulitis.[50,51] In fact, 80% of males and 30% of females show insulitis without developing diabetes up to the 30th week of age. So somehow a much higher frequency of male NOD mice avoid pancreatic lesions severe enough to cause overt glycosuria.

The pathological features of lymphocytic infiltration become evident at about 4 to 5 weeks of age;[51,52] by week 6, initial insulitis is seen in greater than 50% of NOD mice; at 8 weeks, the lymphocytes begin to invade the islets,[53] and the insulitis process is virtually completed as the animals approach 12 weeks of age. Overt glycosuria (i.e., manifest disease) appears several weeks after the completion of insulitis.

The earliest change is periinsulitis adjacent to the pancreatic ducts, followed by invasion of the islet capsule by small lymphocytes that penetrate the islets. The final stage is characterized by small islets from which β cells have disappeared, with resolution of insulitis.[50] The different stages of the process can, however, be found within the same pancreas at any time, so intact islets may be seen not far from severely affected ones. Phenotyping of lymphocyte subsets involved in insulitis has produced conflicting results.[54-57] Monocytes, NK cells, and B lymphocytes, as well as CD4 and CD8 T-cells, are the predominant cell populations.

The NOD mice lymphocytic infiltration is not restricted to islets but also occurs in the submandibular glands, as well as in the lacrimal, thyroid, and adrenal glands, suggesting a wider disturbance of immune tolerance in this animal. Human T1DM has also been associated with other endocrine abnormalities; however, infiltration of salivary glands has not been described.

Genetics

Basically, the genes involved are recessive because animals of the F1 generation from mating between the NOD and a non-diabetic strain do not develop diabetes or insulitis. From backcross experiments with, for instance, C57BL mice and the NON strain, a minimum of three recessive genes have been suggested.[58,59] One is MHC (H-2)-linked and is not needed for insulitis to evolve but is necessary for the development of diabetes. The dominant H-2 types are $H-2K^d$ and $H-2D^b$.[60] A second recessive gene controls the development of severe insulitis and the third gene is involved in the progression to diabetes, perhaps via a lack of specific regulator cells.

Because NOD mice can be considered genetically identical, but not all develop diabetes, it is susceptibility to diabetes that is inherited rather than the expressed disease, as is also the case in humans (identical twins) and the BB rat.

Disease Mechanisms

There is every indication that the spontaneous diabetic syndrome of the NOD mouse is an autoimmune disorder because there is (1) involvement of the humoral immune system, (2) involvement of the cellular immune system, and (3) involvement of a genetic factor.

Humorally Mediated Immunity

One of the immunological observations in the NOD mouse is the occurrence of autoantibodies. Islet cell antibodies (ICA) have been described in about 50% of NOD mice up to the 21st week of age. Islet cell surface antibodies (ICSA) appear at 3 to 6 weeks and reach peak incidence and titer at 12 to 18 weeks. The ICA as well as the ICSA tend to respectively disappear or decline later on.[61,62] The question is whether these autoantibodies are primarily involved in β-cell destruction or are secondary to islet cell destruction/damage and massive leakage or expression of antigens. The last suggestion could be correlated with the time course of insulitis.

The presence of insulin autoantibodies (IAA) before development of diabetes has been reported.[63] A study showed that IAA were only found in sera from NOD mice with insulitis and not from those without insulitis. This study showed that the prevalence of IAA was 0% before the appearance of insulitis, 80% at 12 to 14 weeks of age, and 30% after 20 weeks of age in females. In males, IAA were found in 45% at 12 to 14 weeks of age and 20% after 20 weeks. The IAA were detected by the polyethylene glycol method.[64] Two different studies, however, report that IAA could be detected by an ELISA assay before insulitis developed.[62,63] Antilymphocyte antibodies also appear, most frequently at 3 weeks of age, and decrease thereafter.[58]

Cell-Mediated Immunity

Strong evidence for the involvement of the cellular immune system is found in the fact that neonatally thymectomized and nude NOD mice do not develop diabetes.[65] This means that T lymphocytes are required for diabetes pathogenesis, but the T-lymphopenia characteristic of the BB rat is not found in the NOD mouse, or for that matter in human diabetics. On the contrary, a markedly increased concentration of T lymphocytes in the spleen and peripheral blood is found in NOD, but not in NON mice.[66] This is reflected in an enlargement of thymic cortex and lymph nodes. The increase in T-cell number appears to include both Lyt1[+] and Lyt2[+] phenotypes. This lymphoproliferation is very likely the result of an underlying immunoregulatory defect.

If the insulitis and overt diabetes observed in the NOD mouse are based on cellular mechanisms, the disease should be transferable with lymphocytes. Direct demonstration of the involvement of the cellular immune system was actually made in a study concerning transfer of splenocytes from overtly diabetic NOD to non-diabetic NOD mice:[55]

Splenocytes from overtly diabetic NOD mice were unable to transfer diabetes to very young (<7 weeks) irradiated NOD mice, but effectively transferred the disease to irradiated mice more than 6 weeks of age; overt diabetes was induced within 12 to 22 d in greater than 95% of the recipients. This transfer to young mice induces them to become diabetic at a higher frequency and at a younger age than their untreated littermates. An explanation of the failure to induce diabetes in the very young mice could be that the immune or hormonal system of the recipient must reach a certain degree of maturation before the transfer can be accomplished. Another very likely possibility is that the beta cells of the very young mice may not express the critical antigenic determinants for which the transferred splenocytes are specific until about 6 to 7 weeks after birth.[54]

Not only the age of the recipient seems important, because spleen cells obtained from 7-week-old non-diabetic mice were unable to transfer diabetes, presumably reflecting that an insufficient number of effector cells are present in the spleen at this age. On the other hand, non-diabetic mice donors more than 15 weeks of age have high levels of intraislet insulitis but their ability to transfer diabetes is variable, suggesting that in at least some older non-diabetic NOD mice, either an insufficient number of effectors are present in the spleen or suppressor cells can interrupt effector cell function. NOD mice that have been insulin dependent for 2 months presumably lack β cells and fail to express the antigenic stimulus for the autoimmune response. A splenic transfusion from these animals, however, showed retained ability to transfer diabetes, indicating that long-lived memory cells are present for at least several months after the destruction of β cells.

It is noteworthy that transfer of diabetes, as mentioned above, was not limited to female donors and recipients; splenocytes from diabetic males consistently induced diabetes in non-diabetic NOD males. This is of interest as male mice display a lower spontaneous incidence of diabetes than females, as already mentioned. All the transfers were carried out with as few as 5×10^6 spleen cells, which did not have to be stimulated by ConA in advance, as is necessary in similar spleen transfusion experiments performed in BB rats.

Notable also is the fact that treatment with anti-Thy 1.2 mAb (T cells) prevents diabetes but does not influence the progression of insulitis.[67] Prevention of diabetes as well as insulitis is obtained by administration of L3T4 (CD4) mAb. The necessity of the presense of CD8 cells and macrophages for the development of insulitis was proved by admission of anti-Lyt2 antibodies and silica particles, thereby preventing β-cell destruction.[68]

Immunotherapy and Other Environmental Factors

Cyclosporin A can prevent the onset of diabetes and reduce insulitis in the NOD mouse.[69,70] By contrast, cyclophosphamide strikingly enhances diabetes development, especially in males, perhaps via depression effects on regulator cells.[71] The effect of cyclophosphamide can be prevented by admission of nicotinamide.[72] Nicotinamide and cyclosporin A are discussed further in the BB-rat section. Nicotinamide itself reduces the incidence of insulitis and diabetes in NOD mice and the blocking of the cyclophosphamide effect is probably brought about by inhibition of ADCC.[76]

As was the case with the BB rat, prophylactic insulin treatment of NOD mice during the prediabetic phase has been shown to prevent and/or delay the clinical onset of the disease.[73] Insulin therapy has also proven to be able to protect non-diabetic NOD mice from the effects of transferred splenocytes.[74] In this last study, the maximum tolerable dosage of fast-acting insulin was given until 30 d after the cell transfer. The diabetes incidence of the insulin-treated group was about 27%, compared with 83% in a control group.

Diet can also influence the incidence; the amount of fat especially seems to be important for the development of the syndrome in the male NOD mouse, that is, a diet reduced in fat can strongly increase incidence.[76] In contrast, administration of gluten-free diet dramatically reduces the diabetes incidence.[76a] The admission of γ-interferon to NOD mice did not alter diabetes development and treatment with interleukin-2 could only reduce blood glucose values slightly.[75] A preparation of group A streptococcus pyogenes, however, protects mice from diabetes and insulitis.[76] Generally, it is a problem for the NOD mouse that prevention of diabetes in this model is may be too easy to obtain and is seen after treatment with many different compounds.

Low-Dose, Streptozotocin-Induced Diabetes

Streptozotocin (SZ) is a naturally occurring broad-spectrum antibiotic produced by *Streptomyces acromogenes.*[77] The drug possesses oncolytic, oncogenic, as well as diabetogenic properties, diabetogenesis being mediated by pancreatic β-cell destruction, and is widely used as a method for induction of diabetes in experimental animals.

SZ consists of a nitrosamine group linked to a glucose molecule. The glucose moiety is apparently the essential component that specifically leads SZ into the β cell. SZ is rapidly cleared from the bloodstream with a serum half-life of 15 min.

In 1963, SZ was conventionally administered as a single dose (200 mg/kg body weight), causing complete β-cell necrosis and diabetes within 24 h.[78] The islets, however, were virtually inflammation-free. In 1976, Like and Rossini presented a new model where multiple subdiabetogenic doses to mice were applied.[79] The result was a delayed onset of hyperglycemia, which for reasons of kinetics could not be due to the direct and rapid toxic activity of the drug. Fortunately, this new model also showed islets with insulitis; and until the discovery of the two spontaneously occurring models (the BB rat and the NOD mouse), this model provided one of the few experimental ways to study insulitis.

The mouse strain used by Like and Rossini was outbred CD-1 mice. The dosage used was 40 mg per kilogram body weight and was administered for five consecutive days, that is, a total dose equal to the single dosage used previously. Seven days after the completion of injections, the animal evidenced mild hyperglycemia, and plasma glucose elevation became progressively more pronounced 10 to 25 d after the last injection, that is, long after SZ was cleared from the bloodstream and the short-lived SZ β-cytotoxic activity was completed. Severe insulitis and disruption of islet cytoarchitecture was noted by experimental day 11. Light microscope examination revealed large numbers of lymphocytes, moderate numbers of macrophages, and few neutrophils surrounding and permeating the islets of Langerhans. Ultrastructural studies unexpectedly showed the presence of large numbers of type C virus particles within the many partially degranulated β cells, a discovery that was not made in usually well-granulated β cells, nor in α, δ, or inflammatory cells. Obviously, SZ was somehow responsible for the activation of virus replication.

Gender seemed to be an important modifier of the diabetogenic action of SZ because only males were susceptible. Later investigations confirmed this by showing that orchiectomy of CD-1 males depressed the level of hyperglycemia induced by SZ, whereas testosterone treatment restored full sensitivity. Testosterone treatment of both ovariectomized and normal CD-1 females also increased hyperglycemic responsiveness to levels comparable with those observed in intact males.[80]

Mechanisms of Action

There appear to be two ways by which the low-dose streptozotocin model can produce diabetes; one does not exclude the other: (1) by direct cytotoxic effect of SZ and (2) by immune mechanisms (possibly autoimmune).

Direct Cytotoxic Action of Streptozotocin

The very specific toxicity of SZ within islets for β cells is linked to the capacity of the drug to accumulate rapidly in these cells. It seems probable, although not proved *in vitro,* that SZ binds with a glucose recognition site on β cells, because 3-O-methylglucose and at a higher dose D-glucose (partially) protect against streptozotocin.[81] Once inside the cell, SZ decomposes to other components, one of which is a highly reactive carbonium ion that is able to alkylate various cellular components such as DNA or protein. Lesions in DNA of this type are removed by excision repair. Part of this excision repair process is the activation of the enzyme poly(ADP-ribose) synthetase to form poly(ADP-ribose) using nicotinamide adenine dinucleotide (NAD) as a substrate. It is probable that the enzyme becomes activated to such an extent in the beta cells that NAD becomes critically depleted, resulting in a cessation of cellular function and ultimately cell death.[82] Perhaps SZ, on entering the cell, alkylates not only DNA but also important components necessary for the generation of ATP (e.g., glycolytic and mitochondrial enzymes). A drop in ATP generation would further impair the resynthesis of NAD, causing this key component to drop below critical levels.[83]

Immune Mechanisms

There is also the possibility of SZ causing point mutation. This type of lesion could cause the expression of a repressed gene that codes for a protein or other hapten not normally recognized by the immune system, for example, a fetal protein or a retrovirus.[91] In support of the latter is the finding of the low-dose SZ model inducing the expression of type C retrovirus (or type A in the C57BL/KsJ strain). Although there seems to be little cytotoxic activity of these vira, they may increase islet cell antigenicity. Alkylation of DNA bases or the phosphate backbone could, if not repaired, cause conformational changes in DNA. These conformational lesions could alter the binding of a repressor protein and lead to the expression of a normally silent gene, which could elicit an immune reaction. SZ could also cause the expression of neoantigens by simply altering surface proteins on the β cell surface directly. These altered surface proteins are very likely to be immunogenic.

The involvement of the immune system is supported by the fact that (1) T-cell-deficient mice do not develop hyperglycemia[84–87] and that (2) conventional immunosuppression protects from diabetes: irradiation, prednisolone, cyclophosphamide, anti-lymphocyte serum and antibodies to T-cells.[88–94] Cyclosporin A, however, is not able to inhibit diabetes development, probably because it is also β-cytotoxic in mice and might thereby amplify the effects of streptozotocin.[95]

Involvement of immune processes normally leads to an immunological "memory," that is, transfer of diabetes from diabetic SZ-treated mice to normal mice should be possible. However, permanent hyperglycemia has not been convincingly transferred into normal mice receiving splenocytes from SZ-treated donors.[91] This is explainable if one considers that the memory cells are specific for β cells only when the β cells have been modified by streptozotocin. This is not an autoimmune mechanism in the classical sense because the organism has not lost tolerance to normal cells, but immune mechanisms have been induced by altered cells. A normal mouse not treated with SZ does not, of course, possess these altered cells.

Several investigations have examined susceptibility to SZ in different mice strains. Studies have shown "BALB/cBOM-nu/+" males to be susceptible and nu/nu males to be resistant unless reconstituted with T-lymphocyte-enriched splenocytes from euthymic donors,[92–94] clear demonstrations of the diabetogenic potential of T lymphocytes. On the other hand, studies have also shown BALB/cBOM-nu/nu males to be as sensitive to SZ as euthymic littermates, using 60 mg/kg for 5 consecutive days.[96] Yet another study of low-dose streptozotocin showed nude mice of the C57BL/KsJ background to develop blood glucose levels not significantly lower than their thymus-intact littermates.[97] Possible explanations for this variety include different dosage regimes (as already mentioned); different contents of the α and β isomers of SZ, α having the highest β-cell cytotoxicity; and (genetically) different sensitivity among different mouse strains.

Virus-Induced Diabetes: The EMC Virus

A viral agent has been suggested as a trigger of diabetes. This is based on the seasonal trend, the presence of viral antibodies with rising titers in paired sera from newly diagnosed T1DM patients,[98] the presence of inflammatory cells in the islets of Langerhans, the decrease in the number of β cells, and the concordance of only about 30% between monozygotic twins, which speaks in favor of an ethiological importance of the environment — this might very well be viral.

Evidence that viruses may be involved in β-cell destruction comes from experiments in animals. The experimental model most extensively studied has been the diabetogenic encephalomyocarditis (EMC) virus introduced by Craighead and McLane in 1968.[99] The EMC virus is a small RNA virus belonging to the picornavirus family and is categorized as an enterovirus. It is a pantropic virus, which can attack all organs, but only the laboratory-selected M-variant of the virus has a specific tropism for β cells. When inoculated into mice, the virus attacks and destroys the β cells, and a diabetes-like syndrome evolves. However, the development of diabetes by EMC-M virus varied with different virus pools and passage history of the virus: plaque purification of the EMC-M virus resulted in the isolation of two stable variants, the highly diabetogenic EMC-D and the non-diabetogenic EMC-B.[100,101] A new variant, EMC-DV$_1$, which is non-diabetogenic, was, however, recently obtained by plaque purification of the EMC-D variant stock pool and comparison between nucleotide sequence and biological characteristics of the three variants made it likely that only two amino acids (one on the leader peptide, the other on the capsid protein) are responsible for the diabetogenicity of the EMC virus.[102]

Tissue culture experiments showed that EMC-D induced little, if any, interferon, whereas substantial amounts of interferon were produced by EMC-B.[103,113] These results suggested that the interferon system might be one of the factors limiting the number of β cells that become infected and thereby might inhibit the induction of diabetes. In support of this, studies have shown that repeated administration of interferon or an interferon inducer reduces the development of diabetes in mice infected with the D variant.[104] Mice treated with the interferon inducer had less virus, fewer pathological changes, and higher concentrations of immunoreactive insulin in the islets of Langerhans in comparison with untreated mice. In this study the normally non-diabetogenic EMC-B variant was also inoculated into mice given antibody to interferon. The result was an increased content of EMC-B virus in islets and other tissues, which resulted in diabetes in about 40% of the surviving animals. This result demonstrates that EMC-B is, in fact, able to infect islet cells, which therefore probably have receptors for both the EMC-B and EMC-D variants.

Although interferon clearly influences diabetes incidence, the importance of the cytokine has been seriously questioned by the fact that the EMC-DV$_1$ variant is neither diabetogenic nor interferon inducing.[115] Actually, it has been proposed that the protection against diabetes by interferon is merely strain dependent and not the cause of the different diabetogenicity of the B and D variants. The difference in diabetogenic properties of the D and B variants might, however, be related to the affinity of the vira for β-cell receptors. Thus, a study has shown that up to six times more EMC-D than EMC-B virus attaches to primary β cells extracted from male ICR-Swiss mice.[105] As mentioned, two amino acid changements between the B and D variants might be responsible for the diabetogenicity and one of the changements, a change from Thr (EMC-B) to Ala (EMC-D), has been shown to reduce the hydrophilicity of the region by 37%. Thus, this change unique to EMC-D may be responsible for the diabetogenicity of the EMC-D virus by increasing the efficiency of viral attachment to the β cells of mice. The resistance of certain mouse strains to the diabetogenic effects of the EMC-D virus could be due to genetically determined modifications in virus receptors on the surface of β cells.

Clinical Course of the Diabetes-Like Syndrome

After subcutaneous inoculation, the virus multiplies under the skin and disseminates in the blood, but viremia is transient (48 to 72 h). The infected mice develop necrotizing lesions of the β cells and immunofluorescence studies have demonstrated viral antigens exclusively in the islets of Langerhans. During the acute stages of infection, virus multiplication is associated with degranulation of the β cells and the release of insulin into the circulation. Promptly thereafter, blood levels of insulin fall and hyperglycemia develops.

A variable number of animals survive the infection, and mortality during the acute stages varies with animal age, dosage, and strain.[106] Surviving animals either recover, exhibit abnormal glucose tolerance, or develop chronic hyperglycemia and a frank diabetes-like syndrome.[107] Metabolically, many appear normal although they were hyperglycemic at some time during the first 2 weeks after virus inoculation.

Histological changes of the pancreatic islets become evident after about 4 d. At this time disruption of the overall architecture of the islets can be found. Mononuclear cells appear around the islets; in particular, macrophages are present in the tissue early in the course of infection. The inflammatory response varies from islet to islet and is relatively transient because foreign mononuclear cells are rarely found after the second week of infection.[119] Other things being equal, the insulitis in the EMC virus model is more moderate than described in the other animal models of diabetes.

Genetic Susceptibility and Environmental Factors

When mice are infected with EMC virus (D or M variants), only certain inbred strains such as C3H/J, SJL/J, SWR/J, DBA/1J, and DBA/2J are susceptible and develop diabetes, while other strains such as C57BL/6J, CBA/J, and AKR/J remain unaffected.[108] As mentioned previously, there seem to be considerable genetic variations among certain well-characterized BALB/c substrains: the BALB/c/BOM mouse is susceptible to EMC-virus infection[109] while the BALB/cJ mouse is resistant.[110] Backcross studies have indicated that susceptibility is inherited as an autosomal recessive trait.

It appears that although mice seem uniformly susceptible to EMC regarding diabetes development, the insular tissue of some strains is more readily damaged by the virus. The course of the infection in two susceptible strains, DBA/2J and C3H/J, has been compared; it was found that the amounts of virus in the pancreas of the two strains were similar, but the morphological changes in the islets of Langerhans differed because the β cells of the DBA/2J animals were strikingly degranulated and exhibited evidence of necrosis, whereas the insular cells of C3H mice were less severely affected.[119]

As it is only the susceptibility to EMC-induced diabetes that is inherited, it is not surprising that environmental factors also influence the expression of diabetes. Metabolic stress, for instance, has been shown to influence the severity of the disease; by inducing hyperphagia and thus obesity in mice by administration of gold-thio-glucose, which has a damaging effect on the satiation center of the hypothalamus, hyperglycemia occurred more often and was of greater severity than in infected non-obese controls. Corticosteroid hormones are able to increase the severity of the pancreatic lesions of the EMC virus; the islets often exhibit frank necrosis and significantly greater amounts of insulin are found in the blood than in controls.[119]

Immune Mechanisms

The importance of the immune system in this animal model is a highly interesting question. Does the diabetic state occur predominantly on the basis of direct islet-cell destruction by the beta tropic virus, or are immune mechanisms, especially T cells, involved in the pathogenesis? Using the M-strain of the EMC virus (originating from Craighead), Buschard et al. in 1976 demonstrated the absence of a diabetogenic effect of EMC virus in nude mice of the C57/B16 strain.[111] These mice did not, like heterozygotic littermates and homozygotic mice, develop diabetes as shown by abnormal glucose tolerance. Diabetes in the latter developed 2 to 3 weeks after administration of the virus, at a time when the virus could no longer be isolated from the mice. Similar investigations in support of the role of an immune mechanism have been carried out using other strains.[112,113] Thymectomy[114] and irradiation[115] have also been shown to prevent the development of diabetes in DBA/2 mice after EMC-virus inoculation, whereas treatment of the same mice with antilymphocyte serum reduced both the degree and duration of hyperglycemia.[116] Thymectomized and irradiated BALB/cBy mice also fail to develop diabetes when infected.[117,118] Interestingly enough, Buschard et al.[126] observed that the thymus-intact BALB/c mice developed not only diabetes, but also paresis (like in the Guillain–Barré syndrome) after administration of EMC-M virus, suggesting that neural and islet tissue have antigenic components in common. Another study, in which mice (BALB/cByJ) were treated with the anti-T-lymphocyte monoclonal anti-L3T4 and anti-Lyt 2.2 antibodies before virus inoculation, showed that mice depleted of L3T4+ cells exhibited a reduced incidence and severity of diabetes compared with both untreated and anti-Lyt 2.2-treated animals. All mice sustained pancreatic infection, but islet lesion with β-cell degranulation only occurred in immune intact and anti-Lyt 2.2-treated animals.[119] These data clearly support the involvement of the immune system, especially suggesting a pivotal role for helper T lymphocytes in the pathogenesis of the disease.

On the basis of studies showing that depletion of lymphocytes failed to alter the incidence of diabetes,[120] and that athymic nude mice infected with EMC-D virus showed a response nearly identical to the diabetogenic response of heterozygous littermates,[121] Yoon et al. did not find a primary role for the T cells in pathogenesis using their strain of virus. What seems important in this connection is that the passage histories of the virus used by Buschard and Yoon are different; the virus used by Yoon is passaged in β-cell cultures, a process known to increase direct β-cell toxicity, whereas the virus used by Buschard is passaged in mouse fibroblast cultures. Using very β-cell toxic vira, the direct action of the vira on the beta cells overrules a role of the T-immune system, which is obvious when less β-cell toxic vira are used. The model using the very toxic EMC virus makes an interesting experimental model, but the T-cell-dependent model is probably more relevant to human T1DM because the human disease very seldom has an acute onset, as would be expected from the actions of a toxic virus.

However, even Yoon demonstrated immune mechanisms to be involved in his experimental model.[134] It was determined by various MAbs against mouse immunocytes that Mac-2-positive macrophages were predominant at an early stage of viral infection, whereas helper/inducer T cells and cytotoxic/suppressor T cells were present at intermediate and late stages of viral infection. Because it has been reported that Mac-2 expression is induced only by strong inflammation stimuli and appears to be specific for mononuclear phagocyte subpopulations, it was examined whether macrophages truly play a role in destruction of β cells. This was done by depleting mice of macrophages by administration of silica, and long-term (but not short-term) treatment with silica resulted in complete prevention of diabetes in animals given a low dose of the virus.

ANIMAL MODELS OF TYPE 2 DIABETES

Type 2 diabetes (or T2DM) is responsible for 75 to 90% of the cases of diabetes seen and a growing problem in the Western world today. The disease was formerly predominantly seen in persons above the age of 45 years but today an increasing number of young people, including children, are diagnosed.

It seems to be caused by a reduced sensitivity to insulin rather than a reduced production of insulin. Some of the animal models show an increased production of insulin in the early stages that develops into a significantly decreased production of insulin in the late stages. In some models, the disease is connected with obesity.

The clinical signs of type 2 diabetes can be significantly altered by environmental factors. Infections, nutritional content of the diet, and chemical factors are known to be able to influence the development of the disease.

No sharp division between type 1 and type 2 diabetes can be made in animal models. However, most models resemble one type more than the other.

Type 2 diabetes is an inherited condition in several strains but it can also be induced in rats by different methods: neonatal injection of streptozotocin, partial pancreas ectomy, and chronic infusion of glucose. The plasma insulin levels differ in the three models. The streptozotocin-induced model is hypoinsulinemic, the pancreas ectomized model is normoinsulinemic, and the glucose-infused model is hyperinsulinemic.

Diabetes mellitus has been described in several species but the following will concentrate on rodents commercially available.

The Obese Diabetic Mice (ob/ob)

The obese diabetic mouse is characterized by marked obesity, hyperphagia, transient hyperglycemia and markedly elevated plasma insulin concentration associated with an increase in the number and size of the β cells in the islets of Langerhans.

The obesity is linked to an autosomal recessive mutation on chromosome 6 (ob), which occurred in the Jackson Laboratories as early as 1949. The mutation was propagated in C57BL/6J, but also in C57BLKS.[122] Homozygous obese (ob/ob) animals developed hyperglycemia, hyperinsulinemia, and obesity. From about 26 d of age, ob/ob animals can be phenotypically distinguished from littermates on the basis of body weight, while heterozygous ob/+ or homozygous +/+ are lean animals and phenotypically normal.

Obese mice reach a maximum body weight of 60 to 70 g at an age of 7 to 8 months, while lean littermates reach their maximal weight of 30 to 40 g in 3 to 4 months.[123,124] A decrease in thermogenesis can be recognized by 10 to 18 d of age.[125,126]

Genetic Background — The mutation was spread before the backcrossing was completed, and several colonies with obese mice carrying the mutation on different genetic backgrounds are maintained.

Obese mice are kept both on an inbred and non-inbred background, for example, the Bom:Umeå-ob is maintained as a non-inbred strain. The more common C57BL/6JBom-ob is congenic with the C57BL/6J strain and maintained by inbreeding.

The diabetes-like syndrome seems to be more severe in some non-inbred stocks of obese mice than in the more common inbred C57BL/6J obese mouse. Because the metabolic abnormalities are dependent on the interaction between the mutation itself and the genetic background,[127] it is necessary for the interpretation of experimental data to mention the source and genetic background of the obese mouse studied.

Phenotypically, the obese mouse (C57BL/6J *ob/ob*) is identical with the diabetic mouse (C57BLKS *db/db)*; however, the syndrome in C57BLKS *db/db* is far more severe than in the C57BL/6J *ob/ob* mouse. The clinical picture is dependent on the background strain in which the gene is expressed. If the *ob* gene is transferred to C57BLKS, this strain will develop a more severe form of diabetes than that observed in the C57BL/6J strain, indicating that these two strains differ in their capacity to adapt to diabetogenic stimuli.[128] This indicates that the clinical expression of the mutant gene is a result of the interaction between the gene (*ob* or *db*) and the genetic background.[129,130]

Metabolism — Serum insulin level is increased by day 17 to 21 and hypoglycemia develops. However, by the rapid increase in serum insulin level, hyperglycemia soon becomes a prominent feature of the obese mouse (350 to 450 mg%, 19 to 22 mmol/l). Marked insulin resistance associated with loss of insulin receptors in several tissues follows hyperinsulinemia. Decreased glucose tolerance also precedes the appearance of obesity.[131–133] Serum insulin level reaches a peak by 6 to 8 months (200 to 400 microU/ml, 25 to 30 ng/ml), and the blood glucose level seems to normalize.[134]

Food intake is greatly increased; however, this might first be evident 2 to 3 weeks after weaning. Hyperphagia is accompanied by an increased efficiency of energy utilization. The rate of lipogenesis in the liver and adipose tissue is more than doubled, and both intraperitoneal and subcutaneous deposit of fat is increased.[135] The fat deposit continues despite food restriction and exercise in young *ob/ob* mice,[136] indicating a more efficient absorption from the intestine and a higher metabolic utilization of the nutrient.[137]

Gluconeogenesis is enhanced despite the hyperinsulinemic state in obese mice.[138] The adrenal glands of obese mice are enlarged compared with controls; the enlargement is related to the cortical part; and there is an increased synthesis of corticosterone. Caloric deprivation leads to regression of the adrenal cortex assuming that the hypercorticism is a secondary phenomenon in this syndrome.[139]

The secretion of glucagon is also elevated and it has been suggested that the hyperfunction of the α- cells in the pancreas of obese mice is involved in the pathogenesis of the obese-hyperglycemic syndrome. The morphological appearance of the pancreas in the obese mice is characterized by a marked hypertrophy and hyperplasia of the islets of Langerhans. Both β and α cells are increased in number and size; however, up to 90% of the cells in the islets are β cells. The size of the islets is related to body weight, and the islets will decrease in size after caloric deprivation.[140]

The lack of thyroid-dependent Na^+-K^+-ATPase in the tissue of *ob/ob* mice has been suggested to explain the observed abnormalities in this mutant, including the failure to thermoregulate, the increased metabolic efficiency, the hypothalamic defects that contribute to hyperphagia, the hypogonadism, and the hypothyroidism.[141]

Breeding of ob/ob *Mice* — Infertility is characteristic of the *ob/ob* females, the ovaries and uterus being atrophic.[142] The *ob/ob* male will occasionally breed. The level of LH and FSH in serum is lower in obese mice compared with their lean littermates. It has been suggested that there is a persistent immaturity of the hypothalamic–pituitary axis in obese mice.[143]

Therefore, the breeding is performed by mating heterozygous (*ob/+)* animals. As there is no phenotypical difference between the lean *ob/+* and *+/+*, the PCR (polymerase chain reaction) is used to identify the presence of the *ob* gene when selecting breeders.

The Diabetic Mouse (db/db)

The diabetic mouse C57BLKS (*db/db*) is an inbred strain that, despite the name, is also obese and phenotypically very close to the *ob/ob* mouse.

The condition is linked to an autosomal recessive mutation on chromosome 4 and is characterized by obesity, hyperphagia, temporary increased plasma insulin level, degeneration of the β cells, and hyperglycemia. Several alleles of independent origin, db^{ad}, db,[2J] db^{3J} and db^{Pas}, are known and described. The alleles are probably similar,[144–147] and no differences in clinical manifestations have been observed when the different alleles are transferred to the same genetic background.

The clinical features of the *db* mouse can be divided into two phases: a hyperinsulinemic phase (phase I), is followed by a hypoinsulinemic phase at age 2 to 3 months (phase II).

An increased food consumption (hyperphagia) leads to an increase in body weight and obesitas can be recognized as early as the age of 4 weeks. The body weight increases quickly during the next 5 weeks to 40 to 60 g, but does not increase any further. Increased plasma insulin level is seen at an age of 10 d and increases until the age of 2 to 3 months (phase I), at which time it decreases abruptly to normal levels. The blood glucose content is close to normal in phase I (7.7 to 8.8 mmol/l [140 to 160 mg%]) or slightly elevated (8.8 to 16 mmol/l [160 to 300 mg%]). However, at the age of 2 to 3 months (phase II), the blood glucose level shows a marked increase. The blood glucose is maintained at a high level until death at age 5 to 8 months.

Genetic Background — The syndrome in C57BLKS *db/db* is far more severe than in the C57BL/6J *ob/ob* mouse. The clinical picture is dependent on the background strain in which the gene is expressed. For further details, see "Genetic Background" of the obese diabetic mice.

Metabolism — The increase in body weight is a result of not only hyperphagia, but also an increase in the efficiency of food utilization and reduced physical activity.[148] The mutant also exhibits intestinal hypertrophy, abnormalities in the nutrient absorption, and changes in the regulatory neuronal peptides of the intestine.[149]

The severity of clinical signs can be modified by food restriction and alterations in the composition of the diet. Food restriction and a diet with a low content of carbohydrate might prolong the life span of the *db/db* mouse.[150,151]

Gluconeogenesis is increased as the enzyme activity of glucose-6-phosphatase, fructose-1,6-diphosphatase, pyruvatecarboxylase, and phosphenol pyruvatecarboxykinase is elevated both in old and young animals compared with controls.[152] Hyperfunction of the pancreatic α cells (glucagon) is also evident in the *db* mouse.[153]

The clinical symptoms are far more severe in male mice than in female mice, suggesting an effect of sex steroids.[154,155] Some substrain variation in this respect has been reported. In the initial phase (phase I), the size and number of β cells are markedly increased, probably as a compensatory reaction to a decreased sensitivity toward insulin in the peripheral tissue. The decrease in plasma insulin level is correlated with a degeneration of the pancreatic islets and destruction of the islet β cells. The clinical symptoms and course of the disease are more severe than in the *ob/ob* mouse, which explains the shorter life span of the *db/db* mouse.

Immune System — Abnormalities in the immune system are seen in the *db/db* mouse, supporting the theory that the immune system might be involved in the pathogenesis of the clinical symptoms observed in the *db/db* mouse. The *db/db* mouse has a diminished ability to reject skin grafts and to generate cytotoxic T lymphocytes. The lymphokine production is reduced and a depressed delayed hypersensitivity reaction is seen. An increased plaque-forming β-cell response is observed in the *db/db* mouse. Thymus involution is accelerated and there is T-cell lymphopenia. Cytotoxic antibodies against β cells and T cells isolated from the spleen inhibit insulin release from β cells *in vitro*.[156]

Class II MHC autoreactive T cells found in the spleen and lymph nodes indicate the presence of ongoing autoreactivity in *db/db* mice, and treatment with anti-I-A^d monoclonal antibodies can prolong the life span compared with untreated controls. However, insulitis is not found, suggesting that the autoreactivity is not directed toward islet cells but may be a consequence of the disease.[157] Moreover, diabetes does develop in the absence of T and B lymphocytes, as revealed by transfer of genes causing an immune deficiency in *db/db* mice.[158,159] The organ reactive autoantibody production may be modified by sex-linked factors.[160]

Diabetic neuropathy is observed in the C57BLKS *db/db* mouse.[161,162] Lesions are also seen in the kidneys,[163] and the kidney function is impaired compared with controls.[164] Myocardial disease has also been described.[165]

Breeding of db/db *Mice* — The diabetic mouse is an inbred strain maintained by brother × sister mating of heterozygous *(db/+)* animals because the homozygous animals are infertile.

A mutant coatcolor gene closely linked to the *db* gene has been incorporated into the C57BLKS *(db)* strain to facilitate the identification of heterozygotes for breeding. The recessive mutant gene misty *(m)* is linked to the wild (not diabetic) type of the *db* gene. This way, wild-type animals *(+/+)* will become lean and grey *(m/m)*; *(db/+)* will become lean and black; and *(db/db)* will become fat and black. The presence of the *(db)* gene can also be identified using PCR.

The New Zealand Obese Mouse

The New Zealand obese (NZO) mouse is an inbred strain that was developed by Bielschowsky at the Otago University Medical School, New Zealand.[166] It was bred for the purpose of developing a mouse strain for cancer research, and by chance it was found that a substrain became obese and diabetic.

The NZO strain is a model of type 2 diabetes and can be used for the study of obesity and islet dysfunction.

The median life span is about 460 d in males and 530 d in females.[167] The coat color is agouti.

Genetic Background and Metabolism — The precise mode of inheritance is not understood; it is thought to be of a polygenic nature. Lesions are seen within the islets of Langerhans.[168] The NZO mouse accumulates fat mainly within the abdomen, in contrast to the generalized fat distribution observed in other obese diabetic models *(ob* and *db).*[169] Depositing fat starts at about 4 weeks of age, although divergence of growth curves between NZOs and controls is not detectable before about 2 to 4 months. At 5 to 6 months of age, the body weight is approximately 50 g.

Blood glucose varies with age and sex but rarely exceeds 300 mg/100 ml, corresponding to 16 mmol/l. A moderate hyperinsulinemia develops, and the plasma insulin level increases with age to reach levels up to 200 μU/ml before declining. The hypersecretion is associated with a marked hypertrophy of the islet tissue and an increase in pancreatic insulin content. The hyperinsulinemia and obesity are accompanied by an increasing insulin resistance. This is demonstrated by the loss of sensitivity of adipose tissue and muscle glucose metabolism to insulin stimulation and by the drop in insulin-receptor numbers on liver cell plasma membranes.[170]

Other Features of the NZO Mouse — Other features of the NZO mouse include intermediate incidence of ovarian granulosa cell tumors, a high incidence of malignant lymphomas of Peyer's Patches, and a high incidence of duodenal and lung tumors.[171–174]

The Goto Kakizaki Rat

The GK (Goto Kakizaki) rat is a model of non-insulin-dependent diabetes mellitus (T2DM), type 2 diabetes. The model shows a mild diabetes with several type 2-related characteristics, including fasting hyperglycemia, impaired secretion of insulin in response to glucose both *in vivo* and in isolated pancreatic cells, and hepatic and periferal insulin resistance.

Late complications such as retinopathy, microangiopathy, neuropathy, and nephropathy have been described in the literature.[175–177]

Characteristics of the Strain

Contrary to other rodent models of type 2 diabetes, the GK rat is nonobese. Body weight is slightly lower than that of the Wistar rat. There is no difference in the weights of the pancreas and the liver, but that of the kidney is greater and that of the fat pad is lower than in the Wistar rat.

In the GK rat, changes are seen in the pancreas islets. The shape of these is oval or round at the age of 2 months; but at 3 months, the islets lose the smooth round or oval shape and become irregular with a starfish-like shape.

The mean islet area is not different from the Wistar rat but the number of endocrine cells per islet is significantly lower. Instead, it contains mostly fibrous tissue.

The number of β cells decreases with age, and the insulin and glucagon contents of the pancreas are lower in the GK rat than in the Wistar.[178]

Development of the Strain

The GK rat strain has been developed from normal outbred Wistar rats by repeated selective breeding using glucose intolerance as a selection index. This work was started in 1973 by Goto and Kakizaki at the Tohoku University, Sendai, Japan. The animals were exposed to an oral glucose tolerance test (OGTT) and the grade of glucose tolerance was expressed as the sum of blood glucose values at five time points. This resulted in all offspring having a diabetic OGTT after the 10th generation. The strain had some difficulties in keeping a stable glucose tolerance level for some generations, probably due to disease outbrakes in the breeding units; but after moving the strain to new, clean falilities in 1983, the diabetic state became stable and the litter size stabilized.[179]

A Heritable Condition

The genetics and physiology of T2DM is still poorly understood but it clearly has a heritable component and is believed to be of a polygenic nature.[180]

Galli et al.[181] found three independent loci involved in the disease. These loci were located on the chromosomes 1, 2, and 10. The locus on chromosome 1 showed the largest effect on postprandial hyperglycemia but no effect on the fasting level. This locus seems to affect early-stage insulin secretion. The loci on chromosome 2 and 10 affect both fasting and postprandial hyperglycemia.

The T2DM of the GK rat is reported to exhibit an excess of maternal inheritance.

Characteristics of the Disease

A wide range of parameters have been studied in the GK rat to explain the physiological background of the disease. Nagamatsu et al.[182] tested the expression of the target receptor proteins (t-SNAREs) and found that a decreased expression of the t-SNAREs in isolated GK rat islets is, in part, the defect responsible for the characteristic impared insulin secretion.

The exact mechanism of the progressive reduction of pancreatic islet β cells in the GK rat is not clear but it can be inhibited by treatment with Voglibose, an alpha-glucosidase inhibitor. GK rats treated with Voglibose show progressive loss of cells but it is mitigated by the treatment. Voglibose does not seem to stimulate β-cell proliferation but has an effect via a reduction of the hyperglycemia.[183]

Chronic hyperglycemia results in oxidative stress which damages the pancreatic β cells. Administration of the antioxidant α-tocopherol (vitamin E) has resulted in a significant increment of insulin secretion and a significant decrement of blood glucose levels.[184]

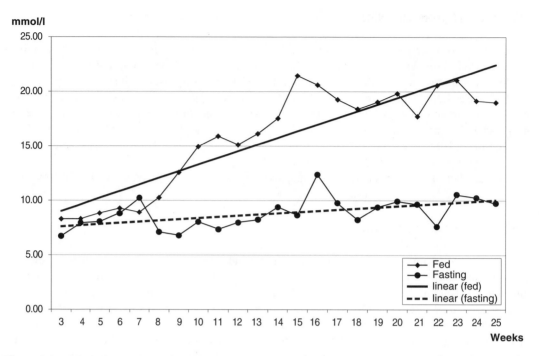

Figure 9.1 Blood glucose levels (mmol/l) in GK fasting and fed male rats from the age of 3 to 25 weeks.

Development of the Disease

In this strain, 100% of the animals develop diabetes at an early stage; and at the age of 2 months, the postprandial blood glucose level is often greater than 10 mmol/l.

The blood glucose level in fasting GK rats is relatively stable but the level of fed animals is constantly rising during the first 6 months of their lives, indicating the impared insulin secretion/insulin resistance typical of type 2 diabetes (Figure 9.1).

Polydipsia and polyuria are seen but the general health of the GK rat is good, and it is able to breed without any treatment although the number of pups per female is smaller than that of the normal Wistar rat.

Substrains of the GK rat have been developed and differences in the diabetic symptoms are seen.

Oral Glucose Tolerance Test

The GK rat has developed on the basis of selective breeding of animals with a positive oral glucose tolerance test (OGTT). Fasting animals are treated orally with a glucose solution at a dose of 2 g/kg and the blood glucose level is measured at 0, 30, 60, and 120 min after the application. The results can be seen in Figure 9.2. Among other characteristics, the GK rat has a slower metabolic decomposition rate of glucose than the normal Wistar rat.

Late Complications

Retinopathy — The GK rat is a model of the retinopathy seen in T2DM. Several authors have described retinal proliferative changes and many parameters were evaluated to explain this. Some of these are the glutathione level, ocular vascular endothelial growth factor, endothelial/perisyte ratio, and retinal microcirculatory alterations.[185–187]

Miyamoto et al.[188] evaluated the microcirculatory conditions of the GK rat compared with age-matched controls. This was tested over an extended period of 5 months.

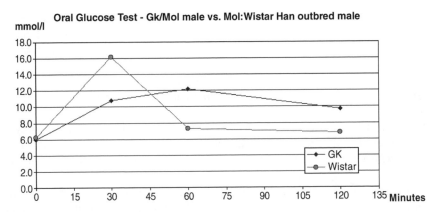

Figure 9.2 Oral glucose tolerance test in 20 GK/Mol fasting males vs. 20 Mol:Wistar fasting males, both born in week 33, 1999.

The eye dilution technique with scanning laser ophthalmoscope-based fluorescein angiography was used to evaluate the circulation in GK rats. Retinal mean circulation times (MCTs), retinal segmental blood flows (SBFs), and vessel diameters were determined by computer-assisted image analysis on a frame-by-frame basis.

Miyamoto et al.[188] found that the MTCs were significantly prolonged and the SBFs significantly reduced in the GK group. No significant differences were observed in the retinal arterial and venous diameters between the two groups.

However, the GK rat did not exhibit dense cataract, and morphological changes of diabetic retinopathy did not develop during the 5-month period, indicating that retinal circulatory abnormalities are found before observable retinopathy development in GK rats.

This pathological picture makes the GK rat a useful model of T2DM for the evaluation of retinal circulation over an extended time period.[188]

Neuropathy — The GK rat also serves as a model of neuropathy seen as a chronic complication of T2DM. Nerve conduction velocity of the nerves of the GK rat is significantly slower than that of age-matched normal Wistar rats and morphological abnormalities are described.[189]

Wada et al.[190] investigated the peripheral nerve function and structures of the GK rat. The chronic hyperglycemia in T2DM is implicated in the pathogenesis of the late complications seen but it is not well known how and to what extent the development of neuropathy is inhibited by blood glucose control. To address this, Wada et al.[190] investigated the effects of an α-glucosidase inhibitor (Voglibose; Vg) on neuropathic changes in the GK rat.

Motor nerve conduction velocity (MNCV) and the structure of the peripheral nerves were examined and compared with Wistar controls. The treatment significantly lowered the blood glucose levels. The MNCV in the GK rat was 80% of the normal controls and Vg treatment inhibited this delay by 24% at 24 weeks and 57% at 36 weeks of age. The Vg treatment also reduced the development of demyelinative nerve fiber abnormalities.[190]

Nephropathy — Diabetic nephropathy is one of the most common causes of end-stage renal failure in the Western world, and the mechanisms underlying its development seem very complex and unfortunately still incompletely understood.

The GK rat shows several pathological changes resembling nephropathy in human type 2 diabetes.

Phillips et al.[191] showed definitive renal structural changes. Thickening of the glomerular and tubular membrane was seen, as was glomerular hypertrophy. There was evidence of immunohistochemical podocyte injury and an increase of interstitial monocyte/macrophage influx. Macrophage infiltration was also seen in the glomeruli.

There is some dispute as to whether or not the GK rat is a model of progressive kidney disease. Riley et al.[192] describe the GK rat as a model in which progressive kidney disease does not develop spontaneously, whereas Marcelo et al.[193] consider it a model of progressive renal disease.

Influence of Environment — The severity of the T2DM of the GK rat can be influenced by external factors. As seen in other diabetes models, the nutritional contents of the feed can change the course of the disease.

A high-fat diet is known to increase hyperglycemia in the GK rat. In F2 progeny of an intercrossing between the GK and the F344 rat, the incidence of diabetes increased 3.7 times after 4 weeks of treatment with a high-fat diet. Four loci on different chromosomes have been found responsible for this effect.[194]

Early dietary restriction has been found to lower the weight gain but not aggravate basal hyperglycemia or glucose intolerance, despite a decrease in basal plasma insulin level. Also, glucose uptake mediated by insulin in the peripheral tissues was clearly improved.[195]

REFERENCES

1. Colle, E., Genetic susceptibility to the development of spontaneous insulin-dependent diabetes mellitus in the rat, *Clin. Immunol. Immunopathol.,* 57, 1, 1990.
2. Chappel, C.I. and Chappel, W.R., The discovery and development of the BB-rat colony: an animal model of spontaneous diabetes mellitus, *Metabolism,* 32, 7, 8, 1983.
3. Marliss, E.B., Recommended nomenclature for the spontaneously diabetic syndrome in the BB-rat, *Metabolism,* 32, 7, 6, 1983.
4. Mordes, J.P., Desemone, J., and Rossini, A.A., The BB-rat, *Diabetes Metab. Rev.,* 3, 725, 1987.
5. Nakhooda, A.F., Like, A.A., and Chappel, C.I., The spontaneously diabetic Wistar rat, *Diabetes,* 26, 100, 1977.
6. Marliss, E.B., Nakhooda, A.F., and Poussier, P., Clinical forms and natural history of the diabetic syndrome and insulin and glucagon secretion in the BB-rat, *Metabolism,* 32, 7, 11, 1983.
7. Like, A.A., Guberski, D.L., and Butler, L., Diabetic BioBreeding/Worcester (BB/Wor) rats need not be lymphopenic, *J. Immunol.,* 136, 3254, 1986.
8. Butler, L., Guberski, D.L., and Like, A.A., Genetic analysis of the BB/W diabetic rat, *Can. J. Genet. Cytol.,* 25, 7, 1983.
9. Like, A.A. and Rossini, A.A., Spontaneous autoimmune diabetes mellitus in the BioBreeding/Worcester rat, *Surv. Synth. Pathol. Res.,* 3, 131, 1984.
10. Elder, M., Macloren, N., Riley, W., and McConnell, T., Gastric parietal and other antibodies in the BB-rat, *Diabetes,* 31, 816, 1982.
11. Like, A.A., Appel, M.C., and Rossini, A.A., Autoantibodies in the BB/W rat, *Diabetes,* 31, 816, 1982.
12. Rossini, A.A., Mordes, J.P., and Like, A.A., Immunology of insulin-dependent diabetes mellitus, *Annu. Rev. Immunol.,* 3, 291, 1985.
13. Dyrberg, T., Poussier, P., Nakhooda, A.F., Bokkeskov, S., Marliss, E.B., and Lernmark, A., Islet cell surface and lymphocyte antibodies often precede the spontaneous diabetes in the BB-rat, *Diabetologia,* 26, 159, 1984.
14. Poussier, P., Nakhooda, A.F., Falk, J.F., Lee, C., and Marliss, E.B., Lymphopenia and abnormal lymphocyte subsets in the "B" rat: relationship to the diabetic syndrome, *Endocrinology,* 110, 1825, 1983.
15. Elder, M.E. and Maclaren, N.K., Identification of profound peripheral T lymphocyte immunodeficiencies in the spontaneously diabetic BB-rat, *J. Immunol.,* 130, 1723, 1983.
16. Nakamura, N., Woda, B.A., Tafuri, A., Greiner, D.L., Reynolds, C.W., Ortaldo, J., Chick, W., Handler, E., Mordes, J.P., and Rossini, A.A., Intrinsic cytotoxicity of natural killer cells to pancreatic islets *in vitro, Diabetes,* 39, 836, 1990.
17. Greiner, D.L., Handler, E.S., Nakano, K., Mordes, J.P., and Rossini, A.A., Absence of the RT-6 cell subset in diabetes prone BB/W-rats, *Am. Assays Immunol.,* 136, 1, 148, 1986.

18. Appel, S.B., Burkart, V., Kantwerk-Funke, G., Funda, J., Kolb-Bachaofen, V., and Kolb, H., Spontaneous cytotoxicity of macrophages against pancreatic islet cells, *J. Immunol.*, 142, 3803, 1989.

19. Mackay, P., Jacobsen, J., and Rabinovitch, A., Spontaneous diabetes mellitus in the BioBreeding/Worcester rat: evidence *in vitro* for NK cell lysis of islet cells, *J. Clin. Invest.*, 77, 916, 1986.

20. Like, A.A., Kislauskis, E., Williams, R.M., and Rossini, A.A., Neonatal thymectomy prevents spontaneous diabetes mellitus in the BB/W rat, *Science,* 216, 644, 1982.

21. Naji, A., Silvers, W.K., Belgrau, D., Anderson, A.O., Plotkin, S., and Barker, C.F., Prevention of diabetes in rats by bone marrow transplantation, *Ann. Surg.*, 194, 328, 1981.

22. Like, A.A., Rossini, A.A., Appel, M.C., Guberski, I., and Williams, R.M., Spontaneous diabetes mellitus: reversal and prevention in the BB/W rat with antiserum to rat lymphocytes, *Science,* 206, 1421, 1983.

23. Rossini, A.A., Slavin, S., Woda, B.A., Geisberg, M., Like, A.A., and Mordes, J.P., Total lymphoid irradiation prevents diabetes in the Bio-Breeding/Worcester (BB/W) rat, *Diabetes,* 33, 543, 1984.

24. Rossini, A.A., Mordes, J.P., Pelletier, A.M., and Like, A.A., Transfusions of whole blood prevents spontaneous diabetes mellitus in the BB/W rat, *Science,* 210, 975, 1983.

25. Rossini, A.A., Faustman, D., Woda, A., Like, A.A., Szymanski, and Mordes, J.P., Lymphocyte transfusions prevent diabetes in the Bio-Breeding/Worcester rat, *J. Clin. Invest.*, 74, 39, 1984.

26. Koevary, S., Rossini, A.A., Stoller, W., Chick, W., and Williams, R.M., Passive transfer of diabetes in BB/W rats, *Science,* 2, 220, 727, 1983.

27. Like, A.A., Weringer, E.J., Holdash, A., McGill, P., and Rossini, A.A., Adoptive transfer of autoimmune diabetes in BioBreeding Worcester (BB/W) inbred and hybrid rats, *J. Immunol.*, 134, 1583, 1985.

28. Koevary, S.B., Williams, D.E., Williams, R.M., and Chick, W., Passive transfer of diabetes from BB/W to Wistar-Furth rats, *J. Clin. Invest.*, 75, 1904, 1985.

29. Like, A.A., Anthony, M., Guberski, D.I., and Rossini, A.A., Spontaneous diabetes mellitus in the BB/W rat. Effects of glucocorticoids, cyclosporin-A, and antiserum to rat lymphocytes, *Diabetes,* 32, 326, 1983.

30. Laupacis, A., Stiller, C.R., Gardell, C., Keown, P., Dupre, J., Wallace, A.C., and Thibert, P., Cyclosporin prevents diabetes in BB Wistar rats, *Lancet,* 1, 10, 1983.

31. Like, A.A., Guberski, D.L., and Butler, L., Influence of environmental viral agents on frequency and tempo of diabetes mellitus in BB/Wor rats, *Diabetes,* 40(2): 259, 1991.

32. Georgiou, H.M., Lagarde, A.C., and Bellgrau, D., T cell dysfunction in the diabetes-prone BB-rat: a role of thymic migrants that are not T cell precursors, *J. Exp. Med.*, 167, 132, 1988.

33. Buschard, K., Jörgensen, M., Aaen, K., Bock, T., and Josefsen, K., Prevention of diabetes mellitus in the BB rats by neonatal stimulation of B cells, *Lancet,* 335, 134, 1990.

34. Ihm, S.H., Lee, K.H., and Yoon, J.W., Studies on autoimmunity for initiation of beta cell destruction, VII, evidence for antigenic changes on beta cells leading to autoimmune destruction of beta cells in BB rats, *Diabetes,* 40, 269, 1991.

35. Koevary, S.B. and Blomberg, M., Prevention of diabetes in the BB/W rat by intrathymic islet injection, *J. Clin. Invest.*, 89, 512, 1992.

36. Scott, F.W., Dietary initiators and modifiers of BB-rat diabetes, in *Lessons from Animal Diabetes II*, Shafrir, E. and Remold, A.E., Eds., Libbey, London, 1988.

37. Rossini, A.A., Mordes, J.P., Gallina, D.L., and Like, A.A., Hormonal and environmental factors in the pathogenesis of BB rat diabetes, *Metabolism,* 32, 1, 33, 1983.

38. Yamada, N., Nonaka, K., Hanafusa, T., Miyazaki, A., Toyoshima, H., and Tarui, S., Preventive and therapeutic effects of large-dose nicotinamide injections on diabetes associated with insulitis, *Diabetes,* 31, 749, 1982.

39. Boitard, C., Timsit, J., Sempe, P., and Bach, J.F., Experimental immunoprevention of type I diabetes mellitus, *Diabetes Metab. Rev.*, 7, 1, 15, 1991.

40. Gotfredsen, C.F., Buschard, K., and Frandsen, E.K., Reduction of diabetes incidence of BB Wistar rats by early prophylactic insulin treatment of diabetes-prone animals, *Diabetologia,* 28, 933, 1985.

41. Buschard, K., Brogren, C.H., Ropke, C., and Rygaard, J., Antigen expression of the pancreatic beta-cells is dependent on their functional state, as shown by a specific, BB rat monoclonal autoantibody IC2, *APMIS J.*, 96, 342, 1988.

42. Like, A.A., Insulin injections prevent diabetes (DB) in BioBreeding/Worcester (BB/Wor) rats, *Diabetes,* 35, 1, 74A, 1986.

43. Gottlieb, P.A., Handler, E.S., Appel, M.C., Greiner, D.L., Mordes, J.P., and Rossini, A.A., Insulin treatment prevents diabetes mellitus but not thyroiditis in RT6-depleted diabetes resistant BB/Wor rats, *Diabetologia,* 34, 296, 1991.

44. Makino, S., Kunimoto, K., Muraoka, Y., Mizushima, Y., Katagiri, K., and Tochino, Y., Breeding of a non-obese, diabetic strain of mice, *Exp. Anim.,* 29, 1, 1980.

45. Makino, S., Hayashi, Y., Muraoka, Y., and Tochino, Y., Establishment of the nonobese-diabetic (NOD) mouse, *Curr. Top. Clin. Exp. Asp. Diabetes Mellitus,* 25, 1985.

46. Kolb, H., Mouse models of insulin dependent diabetes: low-dose streptozotocin-induced diabetes and nonobese diabetic (NOD) mice, *Diabetes Metab. Rev.,* 3, 3, 751, 1987.

47. Leiter, E.H., Prochazka, M., and Coleman, D.L., Animal models of human disease: the non-obese diabetic (NOD) mouse, *Am. J. Pathol.,* 128, 2, 380, 1987.

48. Makino, S., Kunimoto, K., Muraoka, Y., and Katagiri, K., Effect of castration on the appearance of diabetes in NOD mouse, *Exp. Anim.,* 30, 137, 1981.

49. Lampeter, E.F., Signore, A., Gale, E.A.M., and Pozzilli, P., Lessons from the NOD mouse for the pathogenesis and immunotherapy of human type I (insulin-dependent) diabetes mellitus, *Diabetologia,* 32, 703, 1989.

50. Fujita, T., Yui, R., Kusumoto, Y., Serizawa, Y., Makino, S., and Tochino, Y., Lymphocyte insulitis in a non-obese diabetic (NOD) strain of mice: an immunohistochemical and electron microscope investigation, *Biochem. Res.,* 3, 429, 1982.

51. Tochino, T., The NOD mouse as a model of type I diabetes, *Crit. Rev. Immunol.,* 8, 49, 1987.

52. Kataoka, S., Satoh, J., Fujiya, H., Toyota, T., Suzuki, R., Itoh, K., and Kumagai, K., Immunologic aspects of the nonobese diabetic (NOD) mouse: abnormalities of cellular immunity, *Diabetes,* 32, 247, 1983.

53. Wicker, L.S., Miller, B.J., and Mullen, Y., Transfer of autoimmune diabetes mellitus with splenocytes from nonobese (NOD) mice, *Diabetes,* 35, 855, 1986.

54. Signore, A., Cooke, A., Pozzilli, P., Butcher, G., Simpson, E., and Beverley, P.C.L., Class II and IL2 receptor positive cells in the pancreas of NOD mice, *Diabetologia,* 30, 902, 1987.

55. Miyazaki, A., Hanafusa, T., Yamada, K., Miyagawa, J., Fujino-Kurihara, H., Nakajima, H., Nonaka, K., and Tarui, S., Predominance of T lymphocytes in pancreatic islets and spleen of prediabetic non obese diabetic (NOD) mice: a longitudinal study, *Clin. Exp. Immunol.,* 60, 622, 1985.

56. Signore, A., Gale, E.A.M., Adreani, D., Beverley, P.C.L., and Pozzilli, P., The natural history of lymphocyte subsets infiltrating the pancreas of NOD mice, *Diabetologia,* 32, 282, 1989.

57. Kanazawa, Y., Komeda, K., Sato, S., Mori, S., Akanuma, K., and Takuku, F., Non-obese-diabetic mice: immune mechanisms of pancreatic B-cell destruction, *Diabetologia,* 27, 113, 1984.

58. Wicker, L.S., Miller, B.J., Coker, L.Z., McNally, S.E., Scott, S., Mullen, Y., and Appel, M.C., Genetic control of diabetes and insulitis in the nonobese diabetic (NOD) mouse, *J. Exp. Med.,* 165, 1639, 1987.

59. Prochazka, M., Leiter, E.H., Serreze, D.V., and Coleman, D.L., Three recessive loci required for insulin-dependent diabetes in nonobese diabetic mice, *Science,* 237, 286, 1987.

60. Komeda, K. and Goto, N., Genetic monitoring of the NOD mice, in *Insulitis and type I diabetes — Lessons from the NOD Mouse,* Tarui, S., Tochino, Y., and Nonaka, K., Eds., Academic Press, New York, 1986, p. 11.

61. Reddy, S., Bibby, N.J., and Elliot, R.B., Ontogeny of islet cell antibodies, insulin autoantibodies and insulitis in the non-obese diabetic mouse, *Diabetologia,* 31, 322, 1988.

62. Pontesilli, O., Carotenuto, P., Gazda, L.S., Pratt, P.F., and Prowse, S.J., Circulating lymphocyte populations and autoantibodies in non-obese diabetic (NOD) mice: a longitudinal study, *Clin. Exp. Immunol.,* 70, 84, 1987.

63. Maruyama, T., Takei, I., Asba, Y., Yanagawa, T., Takahashi, T., Katoka, K., and Ishii, T., Insulin autoantibodies in non-obese diabetic mice and low-dose streptozotocin-induced diabetes in mice, *Diabetes Res.,* 7, 93, 1988.

64. Maruyama, T., Takei, I., Asaba, Y., Tatsuo, Y., Takahashi, T., Itoh, H., Suzuki, Y., Kataoka, K., Saruta, T., and Ishii, T., Insulin autoantibodies in mouse models of insulin-dependent diabetes, *Diabetes Res.,* 11, 61, 1989.

65. Ogawa, M., Maruyama, T., Hasegawa, T., Kanaya, T., Kobayashi, F., Tochino, Y., and Uda, H., The inhibitory effect of neonatal thymectomy on the incidence of insulitis in non-obese diabetic (NOD) mice, *Biomed. Res.,* 6, 103, 1985.

66. Leiter, E.H., Serreze, D.V., Le, P.H., Coleman, D.L., and Shultz, L.D., Autoimmunity in non-obese diabetic (NOD) mice, *J. Cell Biochem.*, 108, S10A, 1986.

67. Harada, M. and Makino, S., Immunological manipulation of diabetes production in NOD mice, in *Insulitis and type I diabetes — Lessons from the NOD Mouse*, Tarui, S., Tochino, Y., and Nonaka, K., Eds., Academic Press, New York, 1986, p. 143.

68. Charlton, B., Bacelj, A., and Mandel, T.E., Administration of silica particles or anti-Lyt2 antibody prevents beta-cell destruction in NOD mice given cyclophosphamide, *Diabetes*, 37, 930, 1988.

69. Mori, Y., Suko, M., Okudaira, H., Matsuba, I., Tsuruoka, A., Sasaki, A., Yokoyama, H., Tanase, T., Shida, T., Nishimura, M., Terada, E., and Ikeda, Y., Preventive effects of cyclosporin on diabetes in NOD mice, *Diabetologia*, 29, 244, 1986.

70. Formby, B., Miller, N., Garret, R., and Peterson, C.M., Effects of low-dose cyclosporin prophylaxis in nonobese diabetic mice, *J. Pharm. Exp. Ther.*, 241, 1106, 1987.

71. Harada, M. and Makino, S., Promotion of spontaneous diabetes in non-obese diabetic prone mice by cyclophosphamide, *Diabetologia*, 27, 604, 1984.

72. Nakajima, H., Yamada, K., Hanafusa, T., Fujino-Kurihara, H., Miyagawa, J., Miyazaki, A., Siatoh, R., Minami, Y., Kono, N., Nonaka, K., Tochino, Y., and Tarui. S., Elevated antibody-dependent T cell-mediated cytotoxicity and its inhibition by nicotinamide in diabetic NOD mice, *Immunol. Lett.*, 12, 83, 1987.

73. Atkinson, M.A., MacLaren, N.K., and Luchetta, R., Insulitis and diabetes in NOD mice reduced by prophylactic insulin therapy, *Diabetes*, 39, 933, 1990.

74. Thivolet, C.H., Goillot, E., Bedossa, P., Durand, A., Bonnard, M., and Orgiazzi, J., Insulin prevents adoptive transfer of diabetes in autoimmune non-obese diabetic mouse, *Diabetologia*, 34, 314, 1991.

75. Toyota, T., Kataoka, S., Oya, K., Shintani, S., Sato, J., Okano, K., Suzuki, S., and Goto, Y., Characterization of abnormalities of immune response in NOD mice as type I diabetes animal model, *Diabetes Res. Clin. Pract.*, Suppl. 1, S564, 1985.

76. Toyota, T., Satoh, J., Oya, K., Shintani, S., and Okano, T., Streptococcal preparation (OK-432) inhibits development of type I diabetes in NOD mice, *Diabetes*, 35, 496, 1986.

76a. Funda, D.P., Kaas, A., Bock, T., Tlaskalová-Hogenová, H., and Buschard, K., Gluten-free diet prevents diabetes in NOD mice, *Diab. Metab. Res. Rev.*, 15, 323–327, 1999.

77. Herr, R.R., Eble, T.E., Bergy, M.E., and Jahnke, H.K., Isolation and characterization of streptozotocin, *Antibiot. Annu.*, 236, 1959.

78. Rakieten, N., Rakieten, M.L., and Nadkarni, M.V., Studies on the diabetogenic action of streptozotocin, *Cancer Chemother. Rep.*, 29, 91, 1963.

79. Like, A.A. and Rossini, A.A., Streptozotocin-induced pancreatic insulitis: new model of diabetes mellitus, *Science*, 193, 415, 1976.

80. Rossini, A.A., Williams, R.M., Appel, M.C., and Like, A.A., Sex differences in the multi-dose streptozotocin model of diabetes, *Endocrinology*, 103, 1518, 1978.

81. Rossini, A.A., Like, A.A., Dulin, W.E., and Cahill, G.F., Pancreatic beta cell toxicity by streptozotocin anomers, *Diabetes*, 26, 1120, 1977.

82. Yamamoto, H., Uchigata, Y., and Okamoto, H., Streptozotocin and alloxan induce DNA strand breaks and poly (ADP-ribose) synthetase in pancreatic islets, *Nature*, 294, 284, 1981.

83. Wilson, G.L. and Leiter, E.H., Streptozotocin interactions with pancreatic beta cells and the induction of insulin-dependent diabetes, *Curr. Top. Microbiol. Immunol.*, 156, 29, 1990.

84. Kim, Y.T., and Steinberg, C., Immunologic studies on the induction of diabetes in experimental animals: cellular basis for the induction of diabetes by streptozotocin, *Diabetes*, 33, 771, 1984.

85. Paik, S., Fleischer, N., and Shin, S., Insulin-dependent diabetes mellitus induced by subdiabetogenic doses of streptozocin: obligatory role of cell-mediated autoimmune processes, *Proc. Natl. Acad. Sci. U.S.A.*, 77, 6129, 1980.

86. Nakamura, M., Nagafuchi, S., Yamaguchi, K., and Takaki, R., The role of thymic immunity and insulitis in the development of streptozotocin-induced diabetes in mice, *Diabetes*, 33, 894, 1984.

87. Buschard, K. and Rygaard, J., Is the diabetogenic effect of streptozotocin in part thymus dependent? *Acta Pathol. Microbiol. Scand.*, 86, 23, 1978.

88. Rossini, A.A., Like, A.A., Chick,W.L., Appel, M.C., and Cahill, G.F., Studies of streptozotocin-induced insulitis and diabetes, *Proc. Natl. Acad. Sci. U.S.A.*, 74, 2485, 1977.

89. Paik, S., Blue, M.L., Fleischer, N., and Shin, S., Diabetes susceptibility of BALB/c BOM mice treated with streptozotocin: inhibition by lethal irradiation and restoration by splenic lymphocytes, *Diabetes,* 31, 808, 1982.

90. Nedergaard, M., Egeberg, J., and Kromann, H., Irradiation protects against pancreatic islet degeneration and hyperglycemia following streptozotocin treatment of mice, *Diabetologia,* 24, 382, 1983.

91. Rossini, A.A., Williams, R.M., Appel, M.C., and Like, A.A., Complete protection from low-dose streptozotocin-induced diabetes in mice, *Diabetologia,* 24, 382, 1983.

92. Hahn, H.J., Barnstorff, K., Nadrowitz, R., and Schmidt, W., The effect of irradiation on the development of low-dose streptozotocin diabetes in mice, *Diabetes Metab.,* 9, 42, 1983.

93. Oschilewski, M., Schwab, E., Kiesel, U., Opitz, U., Stonkel, K., Kolb-Bachofen, V., and Kolb, H., Administration of silica or monoclonal antibody to Thy-1 prevents low-dose streptozotocin induced diabetes in mice, *Immunol. Lett.,* 12, 289, 1986.

94. Kolb, H., Oschilewski, M., Oschilewski, U., Schwab, E., Moume, C.M., Greulich, B., Burkart, V., Zielasek, J., and Kiesel, U., Analysis of 22 immunomodulatory substances for efficacy in low-dose streptozotocin-induced diabetes, *Diabetes Res.,* 6, 21, 1987.

95. Andersson, A., Borg, H., Hallberg, A., Hellerstrom, C., Sandler, S., and Schnell, A., Long-term effects of cyclosporin A on cultured mouse pancreatic islets, *Diabetologia,* 27, 66, 1984.

96. Beattie, G., Lonnom, R., Lipsick, J., Kaplan, N.O., and Osler, A.G., Streptozotocin-induced diabetes in athymic and conventional BALB/c mice, *Diabetes,* 29, 146, 1980.

97. Leiter, E.H., Multiple low-dose streptozotocin-induced hyperglycemia and insulitis in C57BL mice: influence of inbred background, sex and thymus, *Proc. Natl. Acad. Sci. U.S.A.,* 79, 630, 1982.

98. Yoon, J.W., Austin, M., Onodera, T., and Notkins, A.L., Virus-induced diabetes mellitus isolation of a virus from the pancreas of a child with diabetic ketoacidosis, *N. Engl. J. Med.,* 300, 1173, 1979.

99. Craighead, J.E. and McLance, M.F., Diabetes mellitus: induction in mice by encephalomyocarditis virus, *Science,* 162, 913, 1968.

100. Yoon, J.W., McClintock, P.R., Onodera, T., and Notkins, A.L., Virus-induced diabetes mellitus. (XVII). Inhibition by a non-diabetogenic variant of encephalomyocarditis virus, *J. Exp. Med.,* 152, 878, 1980.

101. Yoon, J.W. and Notkins, A.L., Virus-induced diabetes in mice, *Metabolism,* 32, 37, 1982.

102. Bae, Y.S., Eun, H.M., Pon, R.T., Giron, D., and Yoon, J.W., Two amino acids, Phe 16 and Ala 776, on the polyprotein are most likely to be responsible for the diabetogenicity of encephalomyocarditis virus, *J. Gen. Virol.,* 71, 639, 1990.

103. Cohen, S.H., Bolton, V., and Jordan, G.W., Relationship of interferon-inducing particle phenotype to encephalomyocarditis virus-induced diabetes mellitus, *Infect. Immunol.,* 42, 605, 1983.

104. Yoon, J.W., Cha, C.Y., and Jordan, G.W., The role of interferon in virus-induced diabetes, *J. Infect. Dis.,* 147, 155, 1983.

105. Kaptur, P.E., Thomas, D.C., and Giron, D.J., Differing attachment of diabetogenic and nondiabetogenic variants of encephalomyocarditis virus to cells, *Diabetes,* 38, 1103, 1989.

106. Craighead, J.E., The role of viruses in the pathogeneis of pancreatic disease and diabetes mellitus, *Prog. Med. Virol.,* 19, 161, 1975.

107. Craighead, J.E. and Steinke, J., Diabetes mellitus-like syndrome in mice infected with encephalomyocarditis virus, *Am. J. Pathol.,* 63, 119, 1971.

108. Notkins, A.L., Yoon, J.W., Onodera, T., and Jenson, A.B., Virus-induced diabetes, *Perspect. Virol.,* XI, 141, 1981.

109. Buschard, K., Hastrup, N., and Rygaard, J., Virus-induced diabetes in mice and thymus-dependent immune system, *Diabetologia,* 24, 42, 1983.

110. Yoon, J.W., The role of viruses and environmental factors in the induction of diabetes, *Curr. Top. Microbiol. Immunol.,* 164, 95, 1990.

111. Buschard, K., Rygaard, J., and Lund, E., The inability of a diabetogenic virus to induce diabetes mellitus in athymic (nude) mice, *Acta. Pathol. Microbiol. Scand. Sect. C,* 84, 299, 1976.

112. Jansen, F.K., Thyrneyssen, O., and Montefering, H., Virus induced diabetes and the immune system II — Evidence for an immune pathogenesis of the acute phase of diabetes, *Biomedicine,* 31, 1, 1979.

113. Buschard, K., Hastrup, N., and Rygaard, J., Virus-induced diabetes in mice and thymus-dependent immune system, *Diabetologia,* 24, 42, 1983.

114. Petersen, K.G., Schloter, K., Kasimir, H., Treiber, A., Montefering, K., and Kerp, L., Prevention of EMC-virus-induced diabetes by neonatal thymectomized mice, *Excerpta Med. Int. Congr. Ser.,* 481, 184, 1979.

115. Jansen, F.K., Montefering, H., and Schmidt, W.A.K., Virus induced diabetes and the immune system. I. Suggestion that appearance of diabetes depends on immune reactions, *Diabetologia,* 13, 545, 1977.

116. Dafoe, D.C., Naji, A., Kirby, W., and Barker, C.F., Role in immunity in induction of and recovery from viral immune diabetes, *Surg. Forum,* 31, 51, 1980.

117. Babu, P.G.,Huber, S., Sriram, S., and Craighead, J.E., Genetic control of multisystem autoimmune disease in encephalomyocarditis virus infected BALB/cCum and BALB/cBYJ mice, *Curr. Top. Microbiol. Immunol.,* 154, 1985.

118. Babu, P.G., Huber, S.A., and Craighead, J.E., Contrasting features of T lymphocyte mediated diabetes in encephalomyocarditis virus-infected BALB/cBy and BALB/cCum mice, *Am. J. Pathol.,* 124, 193, 1986.

119. Haynes, M.K., Huber, S.A., and Craighead, J.E., Helper-inducer T-lymphocytes mediate diabetes in EMC-infected BALB/cBYJ mice, *Diabetes,* 36, 877, 1987.

120. Yoon, J.W., McClintock, P.R., Bachurski, C.J., Longstreth, J.D., and Notkins, A.L., Virus-induced diabetes mellitus. No evidence for immune mechanisms in the destruction of ?-cells by the D-variant of encephalomyocarditis virus, *Diabetes,* 34, 922, 1985.

121. Baek, H.S. and Yoon, J.W., Role of macrophages in the pathogenesis of encephalomyocarditis virus-induced diabetes in mice, *J. Virol.,* 64, 5708, 1990.

122. Coleman, D.L., Obese and diabetes: two mutant genes causing diabetes-obesity syndromes in mice, *Diabetologia,* 14, 141, 1978.

123. Westman, S., Development of the obese-hyperglycaemic syndrome in mice, *Diabetologia,* 4, 141, 1968.

124. Bray, G.A. and York, D.A., Genetically transmitted obesity in rodents, *Phys. Rev.* 51, 3, 598–634, 1971.

125. Herberg, L. and Coleman, D.L., Laboratory animals exhibiting obesity and diabetes syndromes, *Metabolism,* 26, 59–99, 1977.

126. Bray, G.A. and York, D.A., Hypothalamic and genetic obesity in experimental animals: an autonomic and endocrine hypothesis, *Phys. Rev.,* 59, 3, 719–785, 1979.

127. Bailey, C.J., Flatt, P.R., and Atkins, T.W., Influence of genetic background and age on the expresssion of the obese hyperglycaemic syndrome in Aston ob/ob mice. *Int. J. Obesity,* 6, 11–21, 1982.

128. Cohn, J.A. and Cerami, A., The influence of genetic background on the susceptibility of mice to diabetes induced by alloxan and on recovery from alloxan diabetes, *Diabetologia,* 17, 187–191, 1979.

129. Coleman, D.L. and Brodoff, B.N., Spontaneous diabetes and obesity in rodents, in *Diabetes Mellitus and Obesitas,* Brodoff, B.N. and Bleicher, S., Eds., Baltimore, 1982, 283–293.

130. Berelowitz, M., Coleman, D.L., and Frohman, L.A., Temporal relationship of tissue somatostatin-like immunoreactivity to metabloic changes in genetically obese and diabetic mice, *Diabetes,* 29, 717–723, 1980.

131. Coleman, D.L., Obese and diabetes: Two mutant genes causing diabetes-obesity syndromes in mice, *Diabetologia,* 14, 141–148, 1978.

132. Coleman, D.L., Diabetes-obesity syndrome, in *The Mouse in Biomedical Research.* Vol. IV, Foster, H.L. et al., Eds., Academic Press, New York, 1983, 125–132.

133. Danielsson, Å., Hellman, B., and Täljedal, I., Glucose tolerance in the period preceding the appearance of the manifest obese-hyperglycemic syndrome in mice, *Acta Physiol.Scand.,* 72, 81–84, 1968.

134. Herberg, L. and Coleman, D.L., Laboratory animals exhibiting obesity and diabetes syndromes. *Metabolism,* 26, 5999, 1977.

135. Bray, G.A. and York, D.A., Hypothalamic and genetic obesity in experimental animals: an autonomic and endocrine hypothesis, *Phys. Rev.,* 59, 3, 719–785, 1979.

136. Dubuc, P.U., Cahn, J., and Willis, P., The effects of exercise and food restriction on obesity and diabetes in young ob/ob mice, *Int. J. Obesity,* 8, 271–278, 1984.

137. Bihler, I. and Freund, N., Sugar transport in the small intestine of obese hyperglycaemic, fed and fasted mice, *Diabetologia,* 11, 387–393, 1975.

138. Herberg, L. and Coleman, D.L., Laboratory animals exhibiting obesity and diabetes syndromes. *Metabolism,* 26, 59–99, 1977.

139. Hellerström, C., Hellman, B., and Larsson, S., Some aspects of the structure and histochemistry of the adrenals in obese-hyperglycemic mice. *Acta Pathol.Microbiol.Scand.*, 54, 365–372, 1962.

140. Hellman, B., Brolin, S., Hellerström, C., and Hellman, K., The distribution pattern of the pancreatic islet volume in normal and hyperglycaemic mice, *Acta Endocrinol.*, 36, 609–616. 1961.

141. York, D.A. et al., An enzymatic defect in the obese (ob/ob) mouse: loss of thyroid-induced soidum- and potassium-dependent adenosinetriphosphatase, *Proc. Natl. Acad. Sci.*, 75, 477–481, 1978.

142. Batt, R.A. and Harrison, G.A., The reproductive system of the adipose mouse, *J. Hered.*, 54, 135–138, 1963.

143. Swerdloff, R.S., Peterson, M., Vera, A., Batt, R.A.L., Heber, D., and Bray, G.A., The hypothalamic-pituitary axis in gentically obese (ob/ob) mice: response to luteinizing hormone-releasing hormone. *Endocrinology*, 98, 1359–1364, 1977.

144. Herberg, L. and Coleman, D.L., Laboratory animals exhibiting obesity and diabetes syndromes, *Metabolism*, 26, 59–99, 1977.

145. Leiter, E.H., Coleman, D.C., and Hummel, K.P., The influence of genetic background on the expression of mutations at the diabetes locus in the mouse, *Diabetes*, 30, 1029–1034, 1981.

146. Guenet, J.L., Avner, P., Babinet, C., Bishop, C., and Renard, J.P., The "obese-like" mutation reported is allelic with diabetes (db chromosome 4), *MNL*, 70, 95, 1984.

147. Guenet, J.L. and Babinet, C., A mutation in the DW inbred line producting an obese phenotype, *MNL*, 67, 30, 1982.

148. Bray, G.A. and York, D.A., Hypothalamic and genetic obesity in experimental animals: an autonomic and endocrine hypothesis, *Phys. Rev.*, 59, 3, 719–785, 1979.

149. Bailey, C.J., Wilkes, L.C., Flatt, P.R., Conlon, J.M., and Buchanan, K.K., Effects of growth hormone-releasing hormone on the secretion of islet hormones and on glucose homeastasis in lean and genetically obese-diabetic (ob/ob) mice and normal rats, *J. Endocrin.*, 123, 19–24, 1989.

150. Bray, G.A. and York, D.A., Genetically transmitted obesity in rodents, *Phys. Rev.*, 51, 3, 598–634, 1971.

151. Leiter, E.H., Coleman, D.L., Eisenstein, A.B., and Strack, I., Dietary control of pathogenesis in C57BL/Ks db/db diabetes mice, *Metabolism*, 30, 554–562, 1981.

152. Herberg, L. and Coleman, D.L., Laboratory animals exhibiting obesity and diabetes syndromes, *Metabolism*, 26, 59–99, 1977.

153. Bray, G.A. and York, D.A., Hypothalamic and genetic obesity in experimental animals: an autonomic and endocrine hypothesis, *Phys. Rev.*, 59, 3, 719–785, 1979.

154. Coleman, L.L., Schwizer, R.W., and Leiter, E.H., Effect of genetic background on the therapeutic effects of Dehydroepiandrosteron (DHEA) in diabetes-0besity mutants and in aged normal mice, *Diabetes*, 33, 26–32, 1984.

155. Leiter, E.H., Coleman, D.C., and Hummel, K.P., The influence of genetic background on the expression of mutations at the diabetes locus in the mouse, *Diabetes*, 30, 1029–1034, 1981.

156. Leiter, E.H., Prozhazka, M., and Serreze, D.V., B-cell pathogenesis in absence of T- and B-lymphocyte function in genetically diabetic mice, *MNL*, 75, 33, 1986.

157. Singh, B. and Cliffe, W.J., Treatment of diabetic (db/db) mice with anti-class-II MHC monoclonal antibodies, *Ann. N.Y. Acad. Sci.*, 475, 353–355, 1986.

158. Leiter, E.H., Prozhazka, M., and Serreze, D.V., B-cell pathogenesis in absence of T- and B-lymphocyte function in genetically diabetic mice, *MNL*, 75, 33, 1986.

159. Leiter, E.H., Prozhazka, M., and Schultz, L.D., Effect of immunodeficiency on diabetogenesis in genetically diabetic (db/db) mice, *J. Immunol.*, 138, 3224–3239, 1987.

160. Yoon, J.-W., Leiter, E.H., Coleman, D.L., Kim, M.K., Pak, C.Y., McArthur, R.G., and Roncari, D.A.K., Genetic control of organ-reactive autoantibody production in mice by obesity (ob) diabetes (db) genes, *Diabetes*, 37, 1287–1293, 1988.

161. Sima, A.A.F. and Robertson, D.M., Peripheral neuropathy in diabetic mutant mice. An ultrastructural study, *Lab.Invest.*, 40, 627–632, 1979.

162. Sima, A.A.F. and Robertson, D.M., Peripheral neuropathy in mutant diabetic mice (C57BL/Ks (db/db)), *Acta Neuropathol.*, 41, 85–89, 1978.

163. Like, A.A., Lavine, R.L., Peffenberger, P.L., and Chick, W.L., Studies in the diabetic mutant mouse VI. Evaluation of glomerula lesions and associated proteinuria, *Am. J. Pathol.*, 66, 193–224, 1972.

164. Bray, G.A. and York, D.A., Hypothalamic and genetic obesity in experimental animals: an autonomic and endocrine hypothesis, *Phys. Rev.,* 59, 3, 719–785, 1979.

165. Giacomelli, F. and Wiener, J., Primary myocardial disease in the diabetic mouse, *Lab. Invest.,* 40, 460–473, 1979.

166. Bielschowsky, M. and Bielschowsky, F., A new strain of mice with hereditary obesity, *Proc. Univ. Otago Med. School,* 31, 29–31, 1953.

167. Goodall, C.M., Bielschowsky, M., Forster, D.R., and D'Ath, E.F., Incidence and metastatic pattern of lymphoreticular neoplasms in untreated NZO/Bl inbred mice, *Lab. Anim.,* 6, 85, 1972.

168. Gates, R.J., Hunt, M.I., Smith, R., and Lazarus, N.R., Return to normal of blood-glucose, plasma-insulin and weight gain in New Zealand Obese mice after implantation of islets of Langerhans, *Lancet,* 2, 507–570, 1972.

169. Bielschowsky, M. and Bielschowsky, F., A new strain of mice with hereditary obesity, *Proc. Univ. Otago Med. School,* 31, 29–31, 1953.

170. Bray, G. A. and York, D.A., Genetically transmitted obesity in rodents, *Phys. Rev.,* 51(3), 598–634, 1971.

171. Bielschowsky, M. and D'Ath, E.F., Spontaneous granulosa cell tumors in mice of strains NZC/bl, NZO/Bl, NZY/Bl and NZB/Bl, *Pathology,* 5, 303–308, 1973.

172. Rappaport, H., Bielschowsky, M., D'Ath, E.F., and Goodall, C.M., Malignant lymphomas arising in Peyer's patches and other organs of untreated NZO/Bl mice, *Cancer Res.,* 31, 2047–2052, 1971.

173. Goodall, C.M., Bielschowsky, M., Forster, D.R., and D'Ath, E.F., Incidence and metastatic pattern of lymphoreticular neoplasms in untreated NZO/Bl inbred mice, *Lab. Anim.,* 6, 85, 1972.

174. Goodall, C.M., Bielschowsky, M., Forster, D.R., and D'Ath, E.F., Oncological and survival references data for NZO/Bl inbred mice, *Lab. Anim.,* 7, 65, 1973.

175. Suzuki, K.-I., Goto, Y., and Toyota, T., Spontaneously diabetic GK (Goto-Kakizaki) rats, in *Lessons from Animal Diabetes,* Shafrir E., Ed., Smith–Gordon, London. 1992, 107–116.

176. Hughes, S.J., Suzuki, K., and Goto, Y., The role of islet secretory function in the development of diabetes in the GK Wistar rat, *Diabetologia,* 37, 863–870, 1994.

177. Villar-Palasi, C. and Farese, R.V., Impaired skeletal muscle glycogen synthase activation by insulin in the Goto-Kakizaki (GK) rat, *Diabetologia,* 37, 885–888, 1994.

178. Goto, Y., Suzuki, K.-I., Sasaki, M., Ono, T., and Abe, S., GK rat as a model of nonobese, noninsulin-dependent diabetes. Selective breeding over 35 generations, in *Frontiers in Diabetes Reasearch. Lessons from Animal Diabetes II,* Shafrir, E. and Renold, A.E., Eds., Smith–Gordon, London, 1988, 301–303.

179. Goto, Y., Kakizaki, M., and Masaki, N., Spontaneous diabetes produced by selective breeding of normal Wistar rats, *Proc. Jap. Acad. Sci.,* 51, 80–85, 1975.

180. Nobrega, M.A., Roman, R.J., and Jacob, H.J., Genetics of progressive renal disease in the GK rat, a model for spontaneous non-insulin dependent diabetes mellitus (NIDDM), *Abstracts of 13th Workshop on Genetic Systems in the Rat,* 2000, 52.

181. Galli, J. et al., Genetic analysis of non-insulin dependent diabetes mellitus in the GK rat, *Nature,* 12, 1996.

182. Nagamatsu, S. et al. Decreased expression of t-SNARE, syntaxin 1, and SNAP-25 in pancreatic beta-cells is involved in impared insulin secretion from diabetic GK rat islets: restoration of decreased t-SNARE proteins improves impared insulin secretion, *Diabetes,* 48(12): 2367–2373, 1999.

183. Koyama, M., Wada, R., Mizukami, H., Sakuraba, H., Odaka, H., Ikeda, H., and Yagihashi, S., Inhibition of progressive reduction of islet beta-cell mass in spontaneously diabetic Goto-Kakizaki rats by alpha-glucosidase inhibitor, *Metabolism,* 49(3), 347–352, 2000.

184. Ihara, Y., Yamada, Y., Toyokuni, S., Miyawaki, K., Ban, N., Adachi, T., Kuroe, A., Iwakura, T., Kubota, A., Hiai, H., and Seino, Y., Antioxidant alpha-tocopherol ameliorates glucemic control of GK rats, a model of type 2 diabetes, *FEBS Lett.,* 4. 473(1), 24–26, 2000.

185. Agardh, C.D., Agardh, E., Hultberg, B., Qian, Y., and Ostenson, C.G., The glutatione levels are reduced in Goto-Kakizaki rat retina, but are not influenced by amino guanidine treatment, *Curr. Eye Res.,* 17(3), 251, 1998.

186. Sone, H., Kawakami, Y., Okuda, Y., Sekine, Y., Honmura, S., Matsuo, K., Segawa, T., Suzuki, H., and Yamashita, K., Ocular vascular endothelial growth factor levels in diabetic rats are elevated in observable retinal proliferative changes, *Diabetogogica,* 40(6), 726, 1997.

187. Agardh, C.D., Agardh, E., Zhang, H., and Ostenson, C.G., Altered endothelial/pericyte ratio in Goto-Kakizaki rat retina, *J. Diab. Complications,* 11(3), 158, 1997.
188. Miyamoto, K., Ogura, Y., Nishiwaki, H., Matsuda, N., Honda, Y., Kato, S., Ishida, H., and Seino, Y., Evaluation of retinal microcirculatory alterations in the Goto-Kakizaki rat, a spontaneous model of non-insulin-dependent diabetes, *Invest. Ophthalmol. Vis. Sci.,* 37(5), 898, 1996.
189. Goto, Y., Suzuki, K.-I., Sasaki, M., Ono, T., and Abe, S., GK rat as a model of nonobese, noninsulin-dependent diabetes. Selective breeding over 35 generations, in *Frontiers in Diabetes Reasearch. Lessons from Animal Diabetes II,* Shafrir E. and Renold. A.E., Eds., 1988, 301–303.
190. Wada, R., Koyama, M., Mizukami, H., Odaka, H., Ikeda, H., and Yagihashi, S., Effects of long-term treatment with alpha-glucosidase inhibitor on the peripheral nerve function and structure in Goto-Kakizaki rats: a genetic model for type 2 diabetes, *Diabetes Metab. Res. Rev.,* 15(5), 332, 1999.
191. Phillips, A.O., Baboolal, K., Grone, H.J., Janssen, U., Davies, M., Steadman, R., Williams, J.D., and Floege, J., Metabolic and renal structural changes in a nonobese, normotensive rat model of type II diabetes, *J. Am. Soc Nephr.,* 9, 639, 1998.
192. Riley, S.G., Steadman, R., Williams, J.D., Floege, J., and Phillips, A.O., Augmentation of kidney injury by basic fibroblast growth factor or platelet-derived growth factor does not induce progressive diabetic nephropathy in the Goto Kakizaki model of non-insulin-dependent diabetes, *J. Lab. Clin. Med.,* 134(3), 304, 1999.
193. Nobrega, M.A., Roman, R.J., and Jacob, H.J., Genetics of progressive renal disease in the GK rat, a model for spontaneous non-insulin dependent diabetes mellitus (NIDDM), *Abstracts of 13th Workshop on Genetic Systems in the Rat,* 2000, 53.
194. Li, L., Jiao, H., Olsson, M., Luthman, J., Eriksson, C., and Luthman, H., Genome-wide linkage analysis for high-fat-induced hyperglycemia in the GK rat, *Abstracts of 13th Workshop on Genetic Systems in the Rat,* 2000, 52.
195. Alvarez, C., Bailbe, D., Picarel-Blanchot, F., Bertin, E., Pascual-Leone, A.M., and Portha, B., Effect of early dietary restriction on insulin action and secretion in the GK rat, a spontaneous model of NIDDM, *Am. J. Physiol. Endocrinol. Metab.,* 278(6), 1097, 2000.

CHAPTER **10**

Animal Models of Skeletal Disease

Kurt D. Hankenson, Christi M. Cavaliere, and Ryan P. Frank

CONTENTS

INTRODUCTION

The current decade, 2000 to 2010, has been designated the "Bone and Joint Decade" by the World Health Organization. One of the four goals of this initiative is "advancing understanding of musculoskeletal disorders through research to improve prevention and treatment."[1] Two chronic, age-associated conditions, osteoporosis and osteoarthritis, are particularly problematic because

(1) the natural history of the diseases is extremely complex and poorly understood, and (2) no treatments have been devised to reliably restore complete function once the diseases have clinically progressed. Because musculoskeletal conditions are often age associated, it is anticipated that the prevalence of skeletal-related diseases across the entire population will reach epidemic proportions as the average life expectancy of the population climbs. However, musculoskeletal conditions are not only age-related, chronic disorders. Acute bone and joint trauma, as well as developmental and heritable conditions of bone and cartilage, represent significant causes of pain and disability across all of society.

Animal models have contributed significantly to our understanding of skeletal development, function, pathology, and healing. Specifically, genetically engineered murine (GEM) models and spontaneous mutations in rats and mice have provided insight into molecular mechanisms that regulate skeletal development, homeostasis, and disease. As well, induced skeletal pathology in various laboratory animals, from birds to non-human primates, can be used to successfully mimic human disease. This chapter reviews common animal models of bone and cartilage disorders, focusing specifically on GEM models and on inducible systems that can be adapted for studies using rodents. Obviously, it is not possible to include all skeletal models nor all pertinent GEM models, but we will highlight representative models in Tables 10.1 through 10.14 and make reference to review articles throughout the text. As well, a comprehensive volume, *Animal Models in Ortho-paedic Research*, covers the topic of animal models of skeletal disease in much greater detail and highlights topics that are not within the scope of this chapter.[2]

When choosing a skeletal animal model, it is essential that a number of points be considered. First, how well the animal model mimics the disease condition in humans must be addressed. For instance, although the induction of bone resorption after estrogen removal may mimic postmeno-pausal bone loss, whether the model adequately mimics other causes of osteopenia must be considered. As well, although mice and rats are ideal models for studying molecular mechanisms and gene expression, depending on the goals of the study, higher mammals more accurately mimic human skeletal disease at the organ level and may be a better choice. Second, whether the animal model can be exploited to understand events at the molecular level irrespective of the events at the whole organ must be considered. For example, although the disease state between humans and mice may differ significantly, using GEM models to study molecular mechanisms may still be the best option. Third, skeletal studies, whenever possible, should be conducted with the contralateral limb acting as a negative control. This not only improves statistical power but also reduces the number of animals. The limb chosen should be selected randomly.[3] Finally, because skeletal tissues are slowly remodeled organs, the time course of experiments and sampling must be considered.

BONE

Overview

Bone is a mineralized collagenous tissue. It functions to support and protect the soft tissues of the body, enables ambulation by functioning as the lever to the action of skeletal muscle, acts as a calcium store, and is the primary site for adult hematopoeisis. Bone develops via two develop-mental processes: intramembranous bone formation and endochondral bone formation. The appen-dicular skeleton is composed primarily of endochondral bone, whereas craniofacial bones are primarily intramembranous in origin. Endochondral bone growth occurs secondary to vascular invasion into a cartilage anlage.[4,5] Chondroclastic cell activity occurs coincident with vascular invasion, and bone is formed on the remnants of the cartilage template by osteoblasts (OBs). This primary bone is then modeled throughout development and growth to achieve a functional homeo-stasis. In general, modeling of long bones results in resorption at the endosteal surface and formation at the periosteal surface. This leads to a mechanically superior bone. Trabecular modeling results in bony trabeculae that are aligned along the axis of maximum load.

In response to a variety of normal and pathological processes, properly modeled bone is continuously remodeled throughout an animal's life. Bone is removed by monocytic-lineage osteo-clasts (OCLs), followed by bone deposition by OBs on the resorptive surface.[6,7] Remodeling is a dynamic process that, under normal circumstances, results in the replacement of older bone with new bone. In adult humans, 10% of bone is resorbed and replaced every year; thus, it is estimated that complete skeletal turnover occurs every 10 years.[8] Bone metabolic units (BMUs) are the hallmark of remodeling in humans and most other species. However, rodents lack traditional BMUs; therefore, it is debatable whether the coupled processes of formation and resorption that occur in mice and rats represent true remodeling.[9] As well, rodents lack osteons, which are the cortical manifestations of BMUs. Defects in bone modeling or remodeling that result in either greater bone production or reduced bone resorption lead to increases in bone content (osteosclerosis), whereas modeling or remodeling defects that result in reduced bone production or increased resorption result in decreased bone mass (osteopenia).

OBs and OCLs are under the influence of mechanical load and a variety of humoral and local factors that affect cell maturation, cell proliferation, protein synthesis, or degradation. These two counteracting cell types can control the development, function, and apoptosis of one another. Increases in mechanical load result in a net increase in bone deposition.[10] Systemic factors, such as parathyroid hormone (PTH), estrogen, vitamin D, and growth hormone (GH), regulate both bone resorption and formation. As well, a wide variety of growth factors, such as the bone morphogenetic protein (BMP) family, fibroblast growth factors (FGF), and insulin-like growth factors (IGF), and inflammatory mediators, such as prostaglandin E2 and interleukin 1 (IL-1), influence bone remod-eling.[11,12] Components of the extracellular matrix (ECM) also control bone matrix production.

OBs are derived from undifferentiated mesenchymal progenitors.[13,14] At the periosteal bone surface, the OB progenitors are associated with the fibrous periosteum, whereas in the endosteal compartment, OB progenitors are mesenchymal cells located throughout the marrow cavity. Func-tional OBs have three fates. They can become quiescent bone-lining cells, they can become osteocytes surrounded by bone matrix, or they can undergo apoptosis.[15]

OCLs are derived from common macrophage progenitors in the marrow cavity.[16] The develop-ment of these cells is dependent on a variety of cytokines, including the common cytokines, granulocyte-macrophage colony-stimulating factor (GM-CSF), and macrophage colony-stimulating factor (mCSF), but also on more specific cytokines such as tumor necrosis factor (TNF) and IL-6. Recently, a TNF-related molecule that binds the RANK receptor, RANK ligand (RANKL), was identified that is absolutely required for OCL formation. A soluble, RANK-like protein, osteopro-tegerin (OPG), can bind to RANKL and limit its activity. OCLs are characterized as multinucleated, tartrate-resistant acid phosphatase (TRAP)-positive cells that express the calcitonin receptor and the proteolytic enzyme, cathepsin K.

Models of Increased Bone Mass

A number of heritable disease conditions in humans are associated with increased bone mass, including sclerosteosis, osteopetrosis, and Paget's disease. In sclerosteosis, there is an increase in the amount of bone that forms, such that the marrow cavity of long bones can become ablated. Osteopetrosis, on the other hand, is characterized by retention of primary trabecular bone and cartilage because of a failure to remodel through OCL activity. Paget's disease is an acquired bone abnormality that is likely multietiologic and includes a heritable component associated with viral infection. Disease progression results in proliferative osteogenic lesions characterized by both increased bone formation and resorption.

The gene associated with sclerosteosis in humans was recently identified, SOST,[17] and neither knockout nor transgenic-overexpressing mice of this gene have been reported. SOST appears to function in a normal state as an inhibitor of BMP activity; thus, it is assumed that the defect in SOST is a loss-of-function mutation. The knockout of the gene should provide key data regarding the natural history of this disease in humans and may represent a model that can be used to test treatment options for sclerosteosis. In addition, humans with a gain-of-function mutation in the LRP5 gene have high bone mass and resistance to fracture, although not clinical sclerosteosis.[18] Mice with this gene knocked out show a decrease in bone mass, similar to the human disease osteoporosis pseudoglioma, which occurs in patients with a loss-of-function mutation in LRP5.[19] On the basis of these findings, we speculate that mice overexpressing LRP5 will have enhanced bone mass and mimic the human disease.

Several GEMs show increased bone mass due to enhanced bone formation (Table 10.1; reviewed by Boyce et al.[20] and McCauley[21]). These include knockouts for the ECM proteins osteocalcin[22] and thrombospondin-2.[23] Mice overexpressing an inhibitor of G-coupled protein desensitizer, GRK, from an OB-specific promoter have enhanced bone mass, presumably because of the maintenance of PTH-related protein receptor (PTHRP) signaling in OBs. As well, mice with gene defects that are associated with lipid metabolism, including leptin- and leptin receptor-null mice, and mice lacking white fat, A-ZIP/F1 transgenic, all show increases in bone mass relative to WT controls.[24]

Table 10.1   Murine Models with Increased Bone Mass

Model	Origin	Pathology Description	Ref.
Osteocalcin-null	Targeted disruption	Defect in mineralization results in enhanced BFR	22
Thrombospondin-2 null	Targeted disruption	Increased cortical bone, osteoprogenitor number, and BFR; OCL activity normal	23
Osteopontin-null	Targeted disruption	Mice maintain bone mass in response to OVX, unloading, and PTH	143, 144
ob/ob — leptin deficient	Spontaneous mutation	In the absence of leptin, increased trabecular bone mass and BFR, but OB number is normal	24
db/db — leptin receptor deficient	Spontaneous mutation	Similar to ob/ob	24
High-bone mass mice	Spontaneous — inbred line C3H/HeJ	C3H mice show a higher bone mass due to an increase in systemic IGF-1	56
A-ZIP/F1 mice	Transgenic overexpression of c-fos and c-jun transcription factor dominant negative in adipoyctes	Low leptin levels that are present in these fat-deficient mice result in enhanced bone mass	24
GRK inhibitor overexpression — osteocalcin promoter	Transgenic overexpression in OBs of an inhibitor of G-coupled protein receptor desensitization	Increased bone density and trabecular bone volume; associated increases in OCL activity	145
DeltaFosB	Transgenic — tetracycline-regulated promoter	Bone formed at the expense of adipocytes in the endocortical compartment; increased OB differentiation	146
Fra-1	Transgenic overexpression	Progressive osteosclerosis due to increased endocortical BFR and MAR; OB proliferation unchanged, differentiation increased	147
IGF-1 — osteocalcin promoter	Transgenic overexpression in OB	Increased trabecular bone formation due to enhanced OB life span, but not an increase in OB proliferation	148
Vitamin D receptor — osteocalcin promoter	Transgenic overexpression in OB	Increased periosteal MAR; increased bone strength; endocortical resorption inhibited	149

Note: BFR, bone formation rate; IGF, insulin-like growth factor; MAR, mineral apposition rate; OB, osteoblasts; OCL, osteoclast; OVX, ovariectomy; PTH, parathyroid hormone.

The importance of IGF-1 has also been revealed because mice overexpressing IGF-1 using the osteocalcin promoter have enhanced trabecular bone due to enhanced OB activity.

Models of osteopetrosis in small-animal species are plentiful; have been reviewed by Boyce et al.,[20] de Vernejoul and Benichou,[25] and McCauley;[21] and are outlined in Table 10.2. In these animal models, like in human osteopetrosis, bone is not properly resorbed, resulting in retention of cartilage and an inability to remodel bone. An absence of tooth eruption is a common abnormality that is associated with faulty resorption. Thus, these lines of mice are difficult to maintain because of malnutrition. In general, these models fall into one of three categories: (1) an absence of OCL precursor cells, (2) failure of precursors to develop into mature OCLs, or (3) a failure of mature OCLs to function. Defects at any point do not necessarily indicate an endogenous cellular defect and may rather be related to a loss of or inappropriate function of a supportive marrow stromal cell (MSC). A defect that is not correctable by marrow transplantation suggests that the abnormality is due to an MSC alteration. MSCs regulate OCL differentiation and are not transferred in marrow transplant. For instance, op/op mice do not produce m-CSF, thus marrow transplantation is ineffective at compensating for the abnormality.[26] As well, marrow transplant would not be expected to correct the defect in OPG-overexpressing mice.[27]

Four spontaneous murine lines have been used as models of osteopetrosis. The mutated gene has been identified in three of the models. The op/op mouse lacks mCSF, and virtually no OCLs form.[26] The oc/oc mouse lacks a vacuolar adenosine triphosphatase, and although OCLs form, they do not function normally.[28] Mice with microphthalmia (mi/mi) also develop OCLs, but the OCLs are immature. The mi locus codes for bHLH-zip transcription factor, mitf, which is required for OCL maturation.[29] There are four recognized rat osteopetrosis models but the defective genes have not been identified in three of the models. The mutation in the tl/tl rat is a defect in mCSF. Spontaneous osteopetrotic rabbits have an unknown defect in OCL function and display the characteristics of normal osteoporosis; however, bone marrow transplantation is not effective at correcting the problem, thus mimicking the models of null mutations in mCSF. However, one difference from mCSF-deficient models is that in the os/os rabbit, OCLs form but are incapable of bone resorption.[30] In animal studies of osteopetrosis, selection of the appropriate model is essential. For instance, if the goal of the study is to test a compound that may promote OCL number in osteopetrosis, then it would be shortsighted to select a model in which OCL function is abnormal.

To date, there are no reported animal models of Paget's disease. It has been difficult to reproduce in animals because of the failure to isolate a linked gene and the likely contribution of secondary infectious disease.[31] An elegant murine model that begins to mimic the OCL abnormality observed in Paget's disease overexpresses the measles virus receptor (hCD46) in OCL, but a likely defect in OB function has not been identified.[32]

Models of Decreased Bone Mass

A decrease in bone mass (osteopenia) occurs when bone resorption outpaces bone formation during remodeling. This may result from a down-regulation in OB activity or an increase in OCL activity relative to OB. The most widely recognized bone-loss condition in humans is postmenopausal osteoporosis. *Osteoporosis* is a clinical designation that is used when a patient has a decrease in bone mass of 2.5 standard deviations below the mean peak bone mass for the population. Osteoporotic patients have a significantly enhanced risk of fracture. For the sake of this discussion, we refer to all conditions of decreased bone mass, including osteoporosis, as osteopenia. It should be noted that the term *osteoporosis* has not been used as a clinical term to describe osteopenia in any animal because of the failure to recognize an increased risk of fracture clinically.

Osteopenia is a complex, multifactorial disease.[33,34] Loss of bone is age associated, increased in cases of sex steroid deficiency (loss of estrogen or testosterone), secondary to unloading, and also occurs as a result of corticosteroid treatment. As well, decreases in bone mass have been documented after chronic alcohol and nicotine exposure. There is a heritable component to

Table 10.2   Common Models of Osteopetrosis

Model	Mutated Gene and Common Name	Pathology Description	Corrected by BMT	Ref.
Murine, spontaneous	Osteosclerosis (oc/oc)	Vacuolar ATPase; no ruffled borders on OCLs	Yes	28
Murine, spontaneous	Microphthalmia (mi/mi)	Mutation in bHLH transcription factor	Yes	29
Murine, spontaneous	Grey-lethal (gl/gl)	Defect in formation of OCLs; unknown mutation	Yes	150
Murine, spontaneous	Osteopetrotic (op/op); mCSF null mutation	Equivalent to mCSF knockout; no OCL	No	26
Murine, targeted disruption	src-null	Can not resorb bone due to the failure to form ruffled borders	Yes	151
Murine, targeted disruption	c-fos	No OCL development	Yes	152
Murine, targeted disruption	Cathepsin-null	Can not resorb bone due to the absence of this key enzyme	Yes	153
Murine, targeted disruption	RANKL-null	No OCL development due to the lack of production of a OCL inducing factor by MSC	No	154
Murine, targeted disruption	RANK-null	No OCL development; OCL precursors lack required receptor	Yes	155
Murine, targeted disruption	TRAP-null	Reduced bone resorption; OCL number increases, but cells are dysfunctional	Yes	156
Murine, targeted disruption	TRAF6-null	No OCL development; gene product is an intermediate signaling molecule	Yes	157
Murine, targeted disruption	Beta3-null	OCLs unable to attach to bone due to dysfunctional integrin complexes	Yes	158
Murine, targeted disruption	mCSF receptor-null	OCL precursors lack required cellular receptor, no OCLs form	Yes	159
Murine, transgenic	OPG overexpressor	Reduced OCL development OPG inhibits RANKL activity	No	27
Murine, transgenic	RANK-Fc soluble overexpressor	Decreased OCL development	No	160
Rat, spontaneous	Toothless (tl/tl)	Apparent alteration in CSF1; no OCL formation	No	161
Rat, spontaneous	Incisor absent rat (ia/ia)	Reduction in the number of formed OCLs	Yes	162
Rat, spontaneous	Osteopetrotic rat (op/op)	Defect localizes to chromosome 10; OCLs form ruffled borders, but they are ineffective at resorbing bone	Yes	163
Rat, spontaneous	Microphthalmia bland (mib/mib)	Mild osteoporosis that recovers with maturity	Yes	164
Rabbit, spontaneous	Osteosclerotic (os/os)	No ruffled borders on OCLs; no bone resorption	No	30

Note: ATP, adenosine triphosphate; BMT, bone marrow transplant; mCSF, macrophage colony-stimulating factor; MSC, marrow stromal cell; OCL, osteoclasts; OI, osteogenesis imperfecta; OPG, osteoprotegerin; RANKL, RANK ligand.

osteopenia, and mutations in a number of known genes are associated with osteopenia, including collagen type I, vitamin D receptor, and estrogen receptor genes. Animal models of decreased bone mass can be used to better understand the complex molecular mechanisms regulating bone remodeling and represent a practical model for testing antiresorptive and anabolic therapeutics. The U.S. Food and Drug Administration requires that all antiosteoporosis therapeutics be tested in both small-animal and large-animal models. The large-animal model requirement is a function of the difference in remodeling between rodents and larger mammals.

Given the intense interest in developing new treatment modalities for osteopenia, a large body of literature has been generated on the use of various animal models. For a more in-depth discussion of these models, the reader is referred to excellent reviews by R.T.F. Turner et al.,[35] Jerome and Peterson,[36] Miller et al.,[37] Thompson et al.,[38] and Mosekilde.[39] As well, the reader is referred to papers presented at the International Conference on Animal Models in the Prevention and Treatment of Osteopenia, held in 1995 in Cairns, Australia, and presented as a supplement to the journal *Bone* (*Bone*, Vol. 17 Suppl., 1995). The most common and reliable model for the induction of osteopenia is gonadectomy. This has been used as a model of osteopenia in the mouse,[40] rat,[41,42] rabbit, dog,[43] sheep,[44] and non-human primate.[36] Typically, females undergo ovariectomy (OVX) in an attempt to mimic postmenopausal osteoporosis; however, orchidectomy in males also effectively induces bone loss. In most mammals examined, this results in a decrease in bone mass characterized by an overresorption of bone. In general, an increase in OCL activity is accompanied by an increase in OB activity that does not keep pace with the resorption. OVX has been used to test the efficacy of antiresorptive agents, such as bisphosphonates in these varying models. As well, OVX has been used to induce remodeling changes as a test of phenotype in a variety of GEM that did not otherwise show bone phenotypes. For instance, osteopontin-null mice do not have a bone defect unless challenged by OVX.[45]

OVX has varying bone effects that are dependent on the species selected and time points examined; thus, validation of bone loss in any chosen model, relative to established parameters of bone loss, is an essential consideration. Rats most frequently have been used as a small-animal model of osteoporosis, and the response of growing rats to osteoporosis has been extremely well characterized.[41] In the rat model, an increase in serum markers of resorption is evident within the first week after OVX, and bone loss is evident within 2 weeks. It is interesting to note that OVX in the dog is not a particularly reliable inducer of bone loss but has been used with success in the primate.[36] Although previous investigators have expressed concern over the reliability of primate OVX as an inducer of bone loss, changes in bone mass density, bone strength, and dynamic parameters have been demonstrated in a large number of published and unpublished studies. As well, a recent study by Stroup et al.[46] showed that inhibition of gonadotropin-releasing hormone could mimic postestrogen bone loss in non-human primates.

There are several other models of induced bone loss in addition to gonadectomy. Bone loss can be induced by mechanical unloading (which is covered in the next section of this chapter, "Models of Mechanical Loading and Unloading") or can be secondary to the systemic administration of a number of compounds. Long-term administration of PTH leads to a loss of bone in the rat.[47] Interestingly, this contrasts with the case of intermittent PTH administration, which has been shown to increase endosteal bone mass.[48] The administration of RANKL systemically enhances OCL formation and bone loss.[49] Corticosteroid, cyclosporin-A, and calcium-restricted diets lead to bone loss in the rat.[50,51,52,53]

A surprising number of GEM show decreased bone mass, and representative models are outlined in Table 10.3. As well, the reader is referred to reviews that highlight transgenic and knockout mice that are shown to have osteopenic bone phenotypes.[21,35,54] It is interesting to note that the affected genes cannot be classified into a single functional family. For instance, mice deficient in osteonectin (an ECM protein), FGF2 (a growth factor), and LRP5 (a lipoprotein cell receptor) all have a reduction in bone mass secondary to a decrease in the number of osteoprogenitors. Interestingly, most of the other GEM models have decreased bone mass, not because of OB insufficiency but because of greater OCL activity.

A special comment should be made regarding both the SAMP6 mouse model and low bone mass inbred strains of mice. SAMP6 is a spontaneous mutation that results in an age-associated decrease in bone.[55] Low bone mass, C57/BL6, as opposed to high bone mass, C3H/HeJ, mice have been studied in an attempt to determine genetic factors that are involved in regulating bone mass.[56]

Table 10.3   Murine Osteopenia Models

Model Type	Origin	Pathology Description	Ref.
SAMP6	Spontaneous	Low-turnover osteopenia; both decreased OB and OCLs with age	55
LRP5	Targeted disruption	Decreased OB proliferation in this knockout for a putative wnt cofactor	19
Aromatase	Targeted disruption	Enzyme required for estrogen production; decreased bone in females	165
Estrogen receptor alpha and beta (double knockout)	Targeted disruption	Low turnover osteopenia; gender-specific effects; decreased OB function	166
Osteoprotegerin	Targeted disruption	Greater OCL formation in these mice lacking a soluble inhibitor of RANKL binding	167
c-Abl	Targeted disruption	Defect in OB maturity; reduced mineral apposition; OCL normal	168
IRS-1	Targeted disruption	Impaired OB proliferation, differentiation, and OCL support; IRS-1 mediates IGF-1 signaling	169
Biglycan	Targeted disruption	Decreased bone formation due to decreased OB precursors; ECM protein	170
Osteonectin	Targeted disruption	Decreased OB precursors; ECM protein	171
Klotho	Targeted disruption	Low turnover; decreased OB and OCL	172
MT-MMP	Targeted disruption	Multiple connective tissue phenotypes in mice deficient in a required collagenolytic protein	173
eNOS	Targeted disruption	Decreased bone formation; no anabolic response to OVX	174
FGF2	Targeted disruption	Decrease in osteoprogenitor number leads to a decrease in bone mass	175
IGF-1	Targeted disruption	Reduced mouse size and decreased cortical thickness, but increased trabecular bone volume	176
Beta1 integrin dominant negative	Transgene driven by osteocalcin promoter	Impaired adhesion of OBs to bone	177
Cbfa1	Transgene driven by collagen I promoter	Thinned cortical bone with increased endosteal compartment size; decreased trabecular bone volume; both OB and OCL defects present	178
HSV-thymidine kinase	Transgene driven by osteocalcin promoter	Gancyclovir administration ablates OBs in osteocalcin-TK expressing mice; OCLs are maintained	179
TRAP	Transgene	Decreased trabecular bone	180
TGF-beta2	Transgene driven by osteocalcin promoter	Progressive bone turnover	181

OI (Osteogenesis Imperfecta) Models

Model Type	Origin	Pathology Description	Ref.
Mov13	Retroviral insertion in col1a1 first intron	Mimics human type I OI; decreased collagen transcription from mutated allele	182
oim/oim	Spontaneous	No alpha2 chain of type I collagen; collagen forms as homotrimers	183
fro/fro	Spontaneous	90% perinatal lethality similar to human OI type II subgroup A; 10% survive and are similar to human OI type III	184
Gly to Cys mutation in Col1A1 transgene	Transgene	Similar to OI type II	185
Col1A1 minitransgene	Transgene	Disrupts trimer formation at the level of procollagen association; procollagen suicide; severe, lethal OI in high-expressing lines	186
Brtl1V	Cre/*lox* targeted substitution	Gly(349) → Cys mutation mimicking human type IV OI	59

Note: ECM, extracellular matrix; MSC, marrow stromal cell; OB, osteoblasts; OCL, osteoclast; IGF, insulin-like growth factor, RANKL, RANK ligand; TRAP, tartrate-resistant acid phosphatase.

These low bone mass inbred strains show a reduction in circulating levels of IGF-1 and a decrease in OB progenitors.[57] Any of the murine models would allow an investigator to study a variety of bone mass effectors, rather than the traditional OVX model, which mimics estrogen deficiency. This is an important distinction because the etiology of osteoporosis is multifactorial and not due to androgen loss exclusively.

A final consideration in discussing osteopenia is the human disease condition, osteogenesis imperfecta (OI). OI is an autosomal-dominant disorder characterized by a decreased bone mass resulting in fracture with minimal trauma due to a decrease in matrix quantity, quality, or both. Affected patients often have blue sclera, hearing loss, and associated dental abnormalities. OI typically results from a single base mutation in the α1 chain of type I collagen that results in a glycine amino acid substitution. The abnormally produced protein results in dominant-negative inhibition of the normal gene product produced from the other allele. Less severe cases of OI actually result from a stop codon in the procollagen alpha 1 gene and are the result of haploinsufficiency. Several murine models of OI have been identified and are listed in Table 10.3 (reviewed by Kuivaniemi et al.[58]) Definitively, Forlino et al.[59] introduced a germ-line mutation that specifically mimics a human mutation (BrtlIV). The targeted mutation was generated using Cre/*LoxP*. However, this is a fairly new model, and the other models of OI have been more extensively characterized. In fact, the oim/oim mouse and the mouse developed by Khillan et al.[186] have been used in studies of OI treatment using cell replacement[60] and gene therapy.[61]

Models of Mechanical Unloading and Loading

Force plays a crucial role in normal bone metabolism. Alterations in both formation and resorption occur in response to applied loads and are dependent upon the magnitude, type, and location of the load. *In vitro* systems with bone cells stretched or subjected to fluid flow have provided valuable information regarding the mechanical-cellular response at the molecular level. However, whole-animal studies are necessary for investigating the complex interplay between mechanical force, endocrine function, age, gender, body weight, diet, baseline activity level, and possible pharmacological treatments. Experimental changes in force can be characterized as mechanical unloading or loading of the skeleton.

Unloading Models

Skeletal unloading occurs as a result of microgravity during space flight or as a result of immobilization, suspension, or paralysis. Models of microgravity include experimental rats that have been on numerous space missions for later study of bone structure and architecture (Table 10.4). Efforts to develop a ground-based model of microgravity led to the development of the rat hind-limb suspension (HLS) models (Table 10.4). In the HLS models, the back or tail is suspended from a pulley, leaving the animal's head in a 30° downward tilt with the hind limbs mobile but bearing no weight.[62,63] Studies reviewing HLS models using back suspension or tail suspension showed that the back suspension model was more stressful to the animal and resulted in poor weight gain and changes in bone mass that were unrelated to limb suspension.[64] Tail suspension models are therefore more widely used and have been adapted for use in mice.

Animal models of immobilization have been studied to determine the effects of disuse on bone metabolism (Table 10.4). Methods of partial body immobilization include confinement in a small cage, casting or limb taping, bed rest, lower-body positive pressure, and water immersion (for review, see Morey-Holton and Wronski[65]). Paralysis through nerve or spinal cord transection leads to denervation and total immobility. The effects of denervation are not completely understood, and a denervated limb may differ from a limb that has been mechanically immobilized. This factor must be taken into account when comparing study results. Total-body immobilization has been described using a body cast, body mold, or water immersion.

Table 10.4   Limb Immobilization Models

Model	Age	Experimental System	Time Span	Ref.
		Space Flight		
Rat, Sprague-Dawley (male)	6–7 weeks	Vivarium: sham vs. adrenalectomy (ADX) Flight chamber/normal gravity: sham vs. ADX Flight: sham vs. ADX	17-d space flight	187
Rat	2–3 mo	Control Flight	18.5–19.5 d space flight	188
		Nerve Transection		
Rat, Sprague-Dawley (male)	200 g	Sham-operated control Unilateral tenotomy at knee joint Unilateral sciatic neurectomy	30 h–42 d	189
Rat (male)	200 g	Series of three experiments to determine whether immobilization acts directly on bone by altering load or systemically; tibial nerve transection to immobilize, demineralized bone implants placed subcutaneously	3–7 weeks	190
		Casting/ Taping		
Canine, mongrel	1–2 years	Control Immobilized with bandage for 16 weeks Immobilized for 16 weeks, then mobile for 16 weeks, then treadmill for 16 weeks	16–48 weeks	191
Rat, Sprague-Dawley (female)	9 mo, 310 g	Control at T = 0 Age-matched control One-leg immobilization, leg taped to abdomen	2–26 weeks	192
Primate (*Macaca mulatto*, male)	Juvenile	Control Immobilization in body cast	2 weeks	193
		Internal Fixation		
Canine, Labrador	10 mo, 20 kg	Control Internal immobilization: left knee, extra-articular	12 weeks	194
		Hind-Limb Suspension (HLS)		
Mouse	Adult, both sexes	—	2 weeks	195
Rat, Fisher (female)	6 mo	Control HLS	2–4 weeks	196
		Confinement		
Primate (*Macaca nemestrina*)	Adult	Control Semirecumbent	10 weeks–7 mo	197
Rat, kangaroo versus white (male and female)	Adult	Pretreatment control, kangaroo vs. white Posttreatment control, kangaroo vs. white Extreme confinement, kangaroo vs. white Confinement, kangaroo vs. white Exercised	6 weeks	198

[a] Kangaroo rat (*Dipodomys ordii*) is a bipedal rodent.

Loading Models

Skeletal-loading experiments have attempted to characterize changes in bone structure and bone metabolism during application of mechanical force. Information in this area has clinical relevance in osteoporosis research and in the prevention of bone loss that occurs with immobilization, paralysis, space flight, menopause, and extreme physical activity. Numerous animal models have been described with force applied using exercise (Table 10.5) or exogenous devices (Table 10.6).

Exercise models have attempted to reproduce human activities, including running, swimming, high-impact training such as jumping, and resistance exercise through training the animal to squat or forcing the animal to eat and drink while standing on its hind limbs. Experimental results vary, depending on animal species, age, hormone status, and exercise regimen, as reviewed in Table 10.5. Regimens are designed to be voluntary or forced, high-impact or low-impact, aerobic or resistance-type training. Exercise may occur during a single daily session or may be divided into shorter sessions throughout the day. The duration of training may be days or several weeks, and a period of increasing activity is often included to gradually teach the animal to perform the desired task. Given the variability of study designs, comparison of any two studies may be difficult. An experimental protocol with carefully planned controls and well-defined outcome measures must be clearly established.

Swimming provides forced activity with minimal impact. Buoyancy counteracts the force of gravity, and therefore muscle contraction exerts the dominant mechanical influence on bone. A swim tank should be sufficiently deep to prevent the animal from balancing on its tail. Water temperature must be carefully controlled because of potential impact on animal behavior.

Running may be voluntary or forced. Voluntary running occurs through placement of a running wheel in the cage. Voluntary running is quantified using video monitoring or a wheel from which data can be recorded. Forced running is performed with a motorized treadmill set to a particular speed (in meters per second) and incline (in degrees). Studies include a brief training period, and the speed and daily duration of exercise are gradually increased.

Jump training usually begins by placing animals in a specially designed box that delivers an electrical stimulus, forcing the animal to jump to avoid an unpleasant sensation. With time, the animal learns to jump when placed in the box. The height that the animal must jump to grab the side of the box gradually increases, allowing larger jump distances. A second type of jump training involves dropping the animal from a specified height to achieve greater impact on landing. Judex and Zernicke described a rooster model in which the animals were dropped from 50 to 60 cm with an *in vivo* strain gauge in place to quantify the mechanical environment.[66]

Resistance training requires teaching the animal to perform a task that includes the desired posture changes. A squatting-type exercise was used in studies by Westerlind et al.[67] to determine the effect of resistance training on tibial cortical and cancellous bone. Animals were conditioned to press a high lever on one side of the cage and a lower lever on the opposite side of the cage. This squatting exercise was then performed, with the animal wearing a weight vest to increase resistance. Notomi and colleagues[68] modified climbing exercises initially developed to study muscle.[69,70] In this model, rats must climb a mesh tower to obtain food and water, making this a voluntary-resistance exercise model.

Bipedal stance leads to a shift in weight distribution and increased loading of the hind limbs in quadripedal animals. A raised-cage model was used in studies by Yao et al.[71] and Chen et al.[72] to evaluate the effect of bipedal stance on bone structure. The raised cage includes placement of the food supply at a specified height to force the animal to feed while standing on its hind limbs. Food must be within reach of the animal, or else weight loss begins to occur.

A number of devices that apply a controlled load to bone have been developed (Table 10.6). Noninvasive loading techniques include the rat tibia model described by C.H. Turner and colleagues.[73] The loading device applies four-point bending to the tibia in a medial-lateral direction, causing compression on the lateral surface and tension on the anteromedial surface. This model

Table 10.5   Exercise Studies

Animal	Age	Groups	Exercise Regimen	Ref.
Swimming				
Rat, Sprague-Dawley (female)	12–24 mo	OVX + normal cage activity or swim	Swim 60 min/d, 5 d/week; 12-week study	199
Rat, Wistar-Kyoto (WKY), stroke-prone hypertensive (SHRSP)	7 wks	Sedentary control WKY Sedentary control SHRSP Swim-trained SHRSP	Swim 60 min/d, 5 d/week; 12-week study	200
Rat, Sabra (female)	5 or 12 wks	Control or swim ± weight	Swim 1 h/d, 5 d/week; 12- to 20-week study	201, 202
Running — Forced				
Mouse, DDY strain (female)	7 wks	Sham and OVX ± genistein ± exercise	Treadmill: 12 m/min, 30 min/d, 7 d/week (10° slope); 4-week study	203
Rat, Sprague-Dawley (female)	4 wks	8 or 12 weeks of exercise 8 or 12 weeks as sedentary control	Treadmill: 24 m/min, 60 min/d, 5 d/week; 8- and 12-week studies	204
Rat, Sprague-Dawley (female)	4 wks	Same as above + 8 weeks of exercise, then 4 weeks sedentary	Treadmill: 24 m/min, 60 min/d; 5 d/week (5° slope); 8- to 12-week study	205
Rat, Wistar (female)	5 mo	1. Exercise 30 min/d 2. Exercise ± 50 g of weight	Treadmill: 20 m/min (duration based on group); 5 d/week; 17-week study	206
Rat, Wistar (female)	3 mo	Similar to previous, run 15 min/d + 40 g of weight	Treadmill: 16.6 m/min, 15 min/d; 5 d/week (5° slope); 6-week study	207
Rat, Wistar (female)	15 wks	Sham and OVX mice ± etidronate ± exercise	Treadmill: 30 m/min, 60 min/d; 5 d/week; 10-week study	208
Rat, Wistar (female)	15 wks, 252 g	Sham and OVX, ± Ca-supplemented diet, ± exercise	Treadmill: 1080 m/d at 8 /min; 15 min exercise, 30-min rest; 5 d/week; 12-week study	209
Rat, Wistar diabetic (female)	13 wks	Running + unilateral sciatic neurectomy	Treadmill: 60 m/min, 60 min/d; 5 d/week; 8-week study	210
Rooster	9 wks	Normal activity High-speed running	Treadmill: 1.84 m/sec, 5 min, three times per day; 6 d/week; 8-week study	211
Running — Voluntary				
Rat, virgin F344 (female)	14 mo	Baseline control Solvent vehicle Growth hormone Voluntary exercise Growth hormone + exercise Food restricted	18-week study Running wheel: 35-cm diameter attached to plastic cage, running activity noninvasively monitored 24 h/d, silent magnetic counter attached to wheel	212
Rat, F344 (female)	13 mo	Similar study to previous (same research group)		213
Jump Training				
Rooster, White Leghorn	12 wks	Normal activity or jump	Jumps: 200 drop-jumps per d (2.5 min/d); 5 d/week (dropped from 50–60 cm); 3-week study	214
Rat, F344 (female)	4 wks	Control, and 5, 10, 20, 40, 100 jumps per day	Jumps: 5 d/week (height gradually increased to 40 cm); 8-week study *Trained to jump using board box with electric stimulus	215

(continued)

Table 10.5 (continued) Exercise Studies

Animal	Age	Groups	Exercise Regimen	Ref.
		Resistance Training		
Rat, Sprague-Dawley (male)	10 wks	Control, sedentary, and resistance groups evaluated at 4 weeks and 8 weeks	Water placed at top of mesh tower; tower gradually raised from 20 cm to 200 cm; rat voluntarily climbed tower to reach water; 4-week study	68
Rat, Sprague-Dawley (female)	21 d; 28 wks	Control Young/exercise + tail weight Mature/exercise + tail weight	Custom-designed racks, 41 cm high with vertical rungs 1.46 cm or 0.9 cm apart, platform at top, animals trained to climb, 3x/week; 10-week study	216
		Bipedal Stance		
Rat, Sprague-Dawley (male)	6 mo	Sham and OVX ± raised cage	Raised cage: food gradually raised to 35.5 cm, bipedal stance necessary for feeding in RC group; 12-week study	71
Rat, Sprague-Dawley (female)	6 mo	Sham and OVX ± raised cage ± estrogen	Similar to previous; 4–8 week study	217
		Sudden Impact Loading		
Rat, Sprague-Dawley (male)	13 wks	Sedentary control Low-intensity exercise control Low intensity exercise + sudden impact load	Exercise: walking mill at 10 cm/sec, 20 min/d; 5 d/week (50 impacts per session, gradually increased to 200 impacts; 9-week study	218

Note: OVX, ovariectomy.

Table 10.6   Loading Devices

Animal	Structure Loaded	Invasive/Noninvasive	Technique	Ref.
Mouse	Tibia	Noninvasive	Cantilever bending	75
Pig	Radius	Invasive	Ulnar osteotomy	81
Rat	Tail vertebra	Percutaneous pin	Vertebral compression	76, 77
Rat, sheep	Whole body	Noninvasive	Vibration	80
Rat	Tibia	Noninvasive	Four-point bending	73
Rooster	Ulna	Invasive	Axial loading	78
Sheep	Radius	Invasive	Removal of ulna	82
Turkey	Ulna	Invasive	Axial loading	79, 219

applies relatively small loads (<40 N) to achieve desired strains (1000–3000 microstrain), and its padded design minimizes any damage to soft tissues. Criticism of the tibial-loading model included the potential effect of direct pressure on the periosteum as a stimulus for bone formation. To establish a model of *in vivo* loading without periosteal pressure, Torrance et al.[74] developed a device for axial loading of the rat ulna. The loading device consists of two padded brass cups that hold the olecranon proximally and the flexed carpus distally, avoiding periosteal pressure in the bone areas of interest. Gross and colleagues[75] have recently developed a method of noninvasive loading of the mouse tibia. A loading device applies cantilever-like bending by fixing the proximal tibia and applying loads to the distal tibia just proximal to the ankle. Bending occurs with the medial surface in compression and the lateral surface in tension. A murine-loading device is particularly valuable given its potential use with GEM. These bending models are primarily used to evaluate the effect of load on cortical bone dynamics.

Chambers et al.[76] and Chow et al.[77] have developed a more invasive rat vertebral-loading model. Stainless steel pins are percutaneously inserted in the seventh and ninth tail vertebrae. The pins are attached to an external loading device that applies dynamic compression to the eighth vertebra. The eighth vertebra is not surgically altered, and therefore the effects of mechanical loading can be evaluated. This compression model is different from the previously mentioned bending models. The vertebral body has a greater amount of trabecular bone, and the load is received at the epiphysis rather than middiaphysis. It can be used to evaluate the effects of load on trabecular bone remodeling.

An ulnar axial-loading model has been used in studies involving the rooster[78] and the turkey.[79] The procedures require parallel transverse submetaphyseal osteotomies. Ends of the bone shaft are covered with stainless steel caps and pierced with parallel stainless steel pins. The pins are held with an external fixator that is removed during the loading procedure. This avian model results in a functionally isolated, externally loadable ulna preparation. The advantage of an avian model is the potential for haversian remodeling. Relative to developing haversian remodeling systems in mammals, these avian models are less expensive, and there are reduced animal welfare issues.

Whole-body vibration has been described for both small and large animals using an oscillating plate or other device that generates low-magnitude, high-frequency mechanical stimuli.[80] Although further study is required, this involuntary, minimal-impact stimulus has possible clinical application in the prevention and treatment of human osteoporosis in those who are unable to exercise.

Quantitative studies of functional adaptation of bone have sought to demonstrate the relationship between increases in compressive strain and bone formation. Classic experiments in this area were performed by Goodship and colleagues in 1979[81] and by Lanyon and colleagues in 1982.[82] Experimental design included removal of the sheep ulna, followed by a period of excess loading of the radius. New bone formation in the radius was then characterized and quantified.

The isolated effect of growth factors and mechanical loading on bone formation can be studied using *in vivo* bone chamber models.[83–85] A hydraulic-loading design was used in studies by Moalli et al.,[86] with the bone chamber placed in the proximal tibial metaphysis of adult male canines. After 8 weeks of infiltration, the loading mechanism was activated to apply a controlled compressive load to woven trabecular bone. Advantages of bone chamber models include potential for repeated harvesting of bone infiltrating the chamber, ability to mechanically isolate the bone while growth occurs in an *in vivo* system, ability to deliver growth factors to a targeted location, and survival of the animals at the end of the experiment.

Models of Fracture Healing

Bone fractures are a common cause of pain and disability. In general, bone has a high regenerative capacity. Although bone regeneration mimics healing of other tissues, the process is more complex. Depending on the degree of stability, a fracture site contains many different tissue types (cartilage, old bone, new bone, fibrous marrow, blood vessels, hematopoiesis, inflammatory cells). The biological processes governing this complex reparative program are poorly understood, and fracture nonunion is relatively common.

The study of fracture healing requires animal models in which fractures can be reliably reproduced from animal to animal, both within a study and from study to study. In an attempt to meet this need, numerous animal models using both open- and closed-fracture techniques have evolved (Table 10.7). Open-fracture models generally include a surgical incision and sharp osteotomy or fracture under direct visualization. An osteotomy can be performed in almost any bone in any animal species. Closed-fracture models involve targeted injury to the bone, usually a long bone, using external force. Advantages of open techniques include more exact placement of the fracture site, nearly identical fractures in all experimental animals, controlled effects on adjacent structures, and the opportunity for open operative reduction and fixation. Disadvantages of open-fracture models include disruption of the hematoma, increased infection risk, and dissection of soft tissues

Table 10.7   Closed-Fracture Models

Animal	Bone	Fracture Technique	Fixation	Ref.
Mouse	Tibia	Guillotine	Intramedullary wire	94
Rat	Tibia	Manual	None	88, 220
Rat	Femur	Three-point bending	None	89
Rat	Femur	Pneumatically driven guillotine	Intramedullary wire	90
Rat	Tibia	Guillotine	Intramedullary wire	91
Rat	Femur, tibia	Weight-driven guillotine	Intramedullary wire	92, 93

surrounding the fracture site. For models in which a sharp osteotomy is created, the smooth bone ends do not interdigitate like most physiologic fractures and therefore may affect bony healing. Thermal damage from surgical power tools may also confound experimental results. With closed-fracture techniques, advantages include lower infection risk, a simpler procedure, and no need for surgical dissection or disruption of the fracture hematoma. Disadvantages of closed-fracture models include a less uniform fracture pattern, damage or crush injury to adjacent skin and soft tissues, need for stabilization, and need for additional surgical access for operative intervention.

Selection of the appropriate fracture model is based on experimental objectives and experimental design. For studies in which hardware is to be used for fixation or tested for potential human use, larger animals with bone structure similar to that of humans must be considered. Cortical thickness and structure of the marrow cavity vary across species, making screws, plates, and intramedullary nailing impossible in some small animal models. The dog is a popular animal model for the study of fracture fixation techniques. The tubular structure and cortical thickness of long bones in rabbit and cat models have also led to their use in studies involving hardware placement. Rats are used in numerous studies involving intramedullary fixation with thin steel wires; however, rigid fixation is difficult and the bones are too small for use with plates and screws, but an external fixator can be used instead. Other animal models that have been described include chicken, pigeon, sheep, goat, horse, pig, and non-human primates (for review, see Nunamaker, 1998[87]). Because of cost, animal size, housing requirements, and animal cooperation, these animal models are impractical and rarely used.

If the main objective is a histological or molecular study of fracture healing under experimental conditions, a large-animal model is usually not necessary. Use of small animals or rodents will allow an increase in sample size, reduce costs, and enable molecular and genetic analysis, given the availability of antibodies and genetic information for the rat and mouse. For studies of haversian remodeling in fracture healing, the dog, cat, rabbit, and avian models are more appropriate.

Several investigators have used closed-fracture models, with the simplest and most reproducible techniques used for the majority of studies (Table 10.7). Fracture production can occur through manual pressure,[88] three-point bending,[89] or use of guillotine-like devices. Manual techniques do not produce a uniform fracture location or pattern and as a result are infrequently used. Three-point bending devices generally do not apply a standard force and result in variable crush injury and a less reproducible fracture pattern than guillotine techniques. In recent years, the majority of closed-fracture models have used a guillotine. In 1970, Jackson and colleagues[90] described a pneumatically driven guillotine used to fracture the rat femur after intramedullary wiring. The wire bridges the fracture defect and provides intramedullary fixation to minimize displacement and angulation. In a similar investigation, Greiff[91] demonstrated a reproducible guillotine fracture of the rat tibia after intramedullary wiring. Bonnarens and Einhorn[92] described a method of closed rat femur fracture using a weight-driven guillotine ramming system. An intramedullary Kirchner wire was placed percutaneously before fracture. This technique was modified in 1994 by An and colleagues[93] to include the rat tibia instead of the femur. The subcutaneous location of the tibia with minimal overlying soft tissue allowed easier placement in the fracture device and creation of a nondisplaced transverse midshaft tibia fracture. Closed-fracture models in the mouse provide a smaller amount of fracture tissue but have the advantage of application using transgenic mouse strains. Hiltunen

Table 10.8   Distraction Osteogenesis

Animal	Age Indicator	Structure	Regimen	Ref.
Canine, mongrel	5 mo	Mandible	10-d latency; 1 mm/d, 20 d	221
Goat, Spanish-cross (M)	Immature, 9–10 mo	Tibia	5 d latency; automatic distracter; 0.75 mm/d total, divided over 1 to 720 times	222
Mouse, MF1 (M)	Adult, 30–40 g	Tibia	7-d latency; 0.25 mm, twice per day, for 10 d	96
Rat, Sprague-Dawley (M)	400- to 500-g breeder	Femur	3-d latency, 0.5 mm/d, 4 d; weight bearing alters the expression of collagen types I and II, BMP2/4, and osteocalcin	223
Rat, Sprague-Dawley (M)	1 yr; 500 g	Femur (bilateral)	6-d latency; 0.5 mm/d, 12 d OR 1.5 mm/d, 4 d — 6 mm total	224
Rat, Sprague-Dawley	4–24 mo, 350–700 g	Tibia	1-d latency; 0.2 mm, twice per day, for 14 or 20 d; 5.6- or 8-mm gap	225
Rat, Sprague-Dawley	Adult, 350–400 g	Mandible	Variable latency, rate, rhythm; 5-mm total distance	226
Sheep, Wethers	Growing	Mandible	Variable latency; 0.5 mm, twice per day, 20 d	227

and colleagues[94] described a mouse model of intramedullary wiring and guillotine fracture of the tibia. This model has been used with alpha-1 integrin knockout mice to demonstrate that alpha-1 integrins are required for progenitor cell proliferation after fracture.[95]

Distraction Osteogenesis

Since its initial description by Ilizarov, distraction osteogenesis (DO) has become an important research topic. Clinically, DO is used for bone lengthening and for closure of segmental bony defects. Animal models include studies in dogs, sheep, goats, rats, and mice (Table 10.8). DO has been applied to long bones as well as bones of the craniofacial skeleton in humans and animals. Although hardware placement is more challenging in mouse models, Isefuku and colleagues[96] described a murine model of DO using a ring fixator and tibial osteotomy. This unique model of DO will provide valuable information when applied to GEM models.

Special Considerations

Losses and gains of bone mass, as well as healing responses, can be visualized in whole bone, either *ex vivo* or *in vivo*, using a variety of nondestructive methods.[97,98] Radiography and microradiography permit the two-dimensional visualization of the skeleton using relatively inexpensive, easy-to-operate equipment. Dual-energy x-ray absorptiometry (DEXA) is used to determine quantitative changes in bone density in two dimensions. DEXA differs from traditional radiographs in that bone is differentiated from soft tissue based on the x-ray penetration from two different radiation sources, a high-energy and a low-energy source. In this manner, an image is generated that excludes soft tissue, and the content of bone in two dimensions is analyzed digitally. Computerized tomography (CT) is arguably the most sensitive method to evaluate alterations in bone geometry and loss and gains. Specifically, microcomputerized tomography (microCT) can be used at less than 10-μm resolution to digitally reconstruct a scanned bone in three dimensions. Unfortunately, because of the extremely high radiation dose, high-resolution CT can only be used *ex vivo*. As well, high-resolution micro-CT devices are extremely expensive and require extensive training to operate. A lower resolution CT instrument referred to as *peripheral quantitative CT* (pQCT) can be used at ~100-μm resolution to examine longitudinal changes in bone geometry. In addition to DEXA, pQCT is used in humans for the evaluation of osteoporosis. The choice of imaging modality is dependent on the size of the animal and the time course, as well as the desired resolution. The two methods most commonly used for quantitative assessment are DEXA and micro-CT. If an investigator is primarily interested in changes in bone density over time, without examining changes in geometry, then DEXA is probably appropriate. However, if an investigator is most interested in single-time-point, high-resolution comparisons, then micro-CT is the instrument of choice.

Determining changes in bone structure, geometry, and density is not sufficient to understand the *in vivo* function of the bone. In most cases, a study of geometry should be accompanied by a determination of mechanical function. Bone can be loaded under compression, tension, or torsion.[99,100] Each loading regimen can be used to generate a stress–strain curve that provides different characteristics about the mechanical function of bone.

Two additional techniques that provide dynamic data include histomorphometry of undecalcified bone and serum- and urine-based assays for systemic factors. Both of these assay types provide a greater degree of detail concerning cellular functionality than do the static measurements previously discussed. Dynamic histomorphometry is the gold standard for evaluating bone formation and was developed in the 1960s.[101] Serum- and urine-based bioassays can be used to demonstrate both bone resorption and formation (bone turnover) over a time course; however, these assays generally lack a high degree of sensitivity.[102] In general, these assays are based on the liberation of specific collagen degradation products, or OCL enzymes (i.e., TRAP), to measure bone resorption; or on collagen fragments that are generated during collagen maturation (amino propeptide) or osteocalcin, which are measured to determine bone formation.

CARTILAGE

Overview

There are three types of cartilage — hyaline, fibrous, and elastic. Herein, we focus on abnormalities associated with hyaline cartilage because of its importance in the development of bone and in the function of joints. Hyaline cartilage is morphologically amorphous, relatively acellular, and contains abundant extracellular matrix that is composed of type II, rather than type I, collagen, as well as secondary collagens such as IX, X, and XI. Cartilage also contains a large amount of negatively charged polysulfated glycosaminoglycans. The most prevalent polysulfated glycosaminoglycan is aggrecan. The matrix of cartilage entombs cartilage cells, termed *chondrocytes*. Relative to bone, cartilage is avascular and typically nonmineralized. These two distinctions are essential to fully appreciate cartilage biology, pathology, healing, and repair.

Hyaline cartilage is found at two primary sites: articular surfaces and sites of endochondral ossification. On the joint surface, cartilage absorbs and distributes load to prevent damage to bone and provides a gliding surface for joint motion. Endochondral ossification is the process by which bone is formed from a cartilage precursor. Condensations of cartilage undergo mineralization and then vascular invasion leading to bone formation. Growth plates represent a specialized type of endochondral ossification responsible for longitudinal bone growth.

Endochondral Ossification Defects

The generation of bone occurs via two distinct processes. Intramembranous bone growth — which encompasses neoplastic, trabecular remodeling, craniofacial development, and diaphyseal growth — is not be considered in this section. Rather, endochondral ossification, a process using a cartilaginous anlage to direct growth, is the subject of this discussion.

A tight interrelationship of genes and the microenvironment governs the development of long bones.[4,5] The shaping of the bony precursors during skeletal patterning occurs in undifferentiated mesenchyme. Gene expression results in intracellular signals that induce site-dependent liberation of morphogens, such as BMP. These extracellular mediators are distributed in a gradient that directs target cells in a concentration-dependent manner.[103,104] During embryonic development, cellular condensations transdifferentiate into cartilage segment and branch into rudimentary limbs. After the development of cartilage in limb rudiments, the cartilage anlage undergoes vascular invasion. Blood vessel ingrowth initiates bone formation by providing ingress for OBs, which develop from MSC. The process by which the cartilage skeleton develops into bone is not completely understood; however, the process requires two essential OB transcription factors, cbfa1 and osterix, for the induction of OB development and activity.[105]

Growth plates are formed at the metaphyseal regions of the developing long bone and act as sites of longitudinal bone growth. Growth plates are highly structured cartilage condensations. At least four morphologic zones are recognized in the growth plate: (1) resting (progenitor cells), (2) proliferative, (3) hypertrophic, and (4) mineralized. Vessels invade calcified cartilage to initiate bone formation in a process similar to that observed in embryonic endochondral bone formation.

Endochondral ossification is a complex developmental process that requires the coordination of chondrocyte proliferation and hypertrophy, vascular ingrowth, chondroclastic activity, and OB development. Defects in endochondral ossification are common and represent a spectrum of human disorders referred to as osteochondrodysplasias (OC).[106] These conditions are manifested by abnormal modeling of the cartilage anlage, resulting in abnormally shaped bones and shortened limb length and generally lead to dwarfism and craniofacial malformation. OC may develop because of errors in cell-to-cell or hormonal signaling, embryonic organization, gene expression, cellular replication, or ECM structure. Through detailed molecular and genetic analysis of human OC, a number of themes have been revealed regarding the genetics of abnormal skeletal development: (1) conditions are often autosomal dominant; (2) when the conditions are associated with haploinsufficiency, there are graded phenotypic alterations; (3) the principal abnormality is the appearance of an abnormal protein or the absence of a necessary protein in the cellular milieu; and (4) the quality of ECM molecules can be affected by various defects in posttranslational maturation.[103,107,108] The vast majority of identified OC have generalized defects in either chondrocyte differentiation and proliferation or in the matrix produced by the cells. It should be emphasized that growth and development of the cartilaginous skeleton is not only affected by the intricate interplay of morphogens and the ECM but also by mechanical stresses; thus, mechanical strain on the cartilage can result in significant disruption of molecular signaling.[109]

Animal models are important tools in the evolution of our understanding of the specific alterations that initiate aberrant skeletal development. There are a number of acquired OC mutations observed in animals such as the dog, pig, rat, and chicken (Table 10.9). As well, numerous GEM and spontaneous mutant mice have been identified that have OC defects. Mouse models of OC are highlighted in a number of reviews.[54,106,110,111] A number of these models, many of which mimic human disease, are highlighted in Table 10.9. In at least one case, "knock-in" mice have been generated that have a targeted mutation that recapitulates a mutation found in the human disease achondrodysplasia (FGFR3-targeted mutations).[112] Other models have used a transgenic approach to overexpress a gene that may code for a protein that acts in a dominant-negative manner (collagen X mutants).[113] Finally, a number of GEM models with targeted disruptions reveal the absolute requirement of a given gene for endochondral bone formation. In fact, a number of the null models show haploinsufficiency (Sox9).[114] Caveats to the use of GEM models for studying OC include the fact that these models often show reduced life span and that potential functional overlap of genes may lead to erroneous conclusions. In addition to genetic models of OC, defects in endochondral ossification have been induced using various methods, including trauma, retinoid administration, and radiation exposure (Table 10.10).

Table 10.9   Representative Chondrodysplasias

Animal, Model Type	Model (Gene Mutation)	Modeled Human Condition	Pathology Description	Ref.
Canine, spontaneous	Canine: miniature poodles (autosomal recessive)	Pseudoachondroplastic dysplasia	Lamellar inclusions of rough endoplasmic reticulum in physeal chondrocytes; metaphyseal flaring; decreased longitudinal growth of long bones	228
Chick, spontaneous	nanomelia (absent aggrecan)	Chondrodystrophy	Cleft palate; shortened limbs/tail/snout; die at birth; NL type II collagen levels	229
Murine, spontaneous	cmd/cmd (autosomal recessive; absent aggrecan)	Chondrodystrophy	Cleft palate; shortened limbs/tail/snout; die at birth	230
Murine, spontaneous	ocd/ocd (autosomal recessive)	Osteochondral dysplasia	Short domed head; decreased trunk length; shortened bones; decreased GAG content	231
Murine, targeted disruption	(Link protein-null)	Unknown	Die at birth; delayed bone formation; short limbs; craniofacial abnormality; small epiphyses; flared metaphyses of long bones	232
Murine, targeted disruption	(Perlecan-null)	Similar to thanatophoric dysplasia	Die at birth; micromelia; bowed long bones; severely disorganized physes; decreased chondrocyte proliferation; decreased collagen fibers and GAGs	233, 234
Murine, targeted disruption	(MMP9-null)	Chondrodysplasia	Decreased invasion of growth plate by vasculature, compensates by maturity	235
Murine, targeted disruption	(PTHrP-null)	Blomstrand chondrodysplasia	Decreased chondrocyte proliferation; increased differentiation; die at midgestation	236
Murine, targeted disruption	(PTHrP/PTH receptor-null)	Unknown	Early death; accelerated differentiation; increased cortical bone; decreased trabecular bone; defective mineralization	237
Murine, targeted disruption	sox9 ± on CD-1 (autosomal dominant)	Campomelic dysplasia	Die at birth; decreased col2a1; increased hypertrophic zone; premature mineralization; skeletal hypoplasia; bowing/angulation of limbs	114
Murine, targeted disruption	Atf-2 ± (autosomal dominant)	Hypochondroplasia	Short limbs and spine — more severe in proximal segments; clustered chondrocytes in physes; decreased vascularity of physes	238
Murine, targeted disruption	Collagen II null (Col2a1)	Achondrogenesis type II	Dwarfism; shortened long bones; misshapen axial skeleton; soft bones; disorganized hyaline cartilage and physes	239
Murine, targeted disruption	Type X collagen	Schmid metaphyseal chondrodysplasia	Coxa vara; reduced resting zone thickness; ECM abnormalities in growth plate	240

(continued)

Table 10.9 (continued)   Representative Chondrodysplasias

Animal, Model Type	Model (Gene Mutation)	Modeled Human Condition	Pathology Description	Ref.
Murine, targeted mutation	(Constitutively active FGFR3; missense mutations at K644)	Achondroplasia or thanatophoric dysplasia	Decreased long bone growth; overgrowth of cartilage in nasal septum, ribs, and trachea; bowed long bones; decreased maturation and ossification of physes	112
Murine, transgenic	HKrk-H223R (autosomal dominant; PPR constitutively active)	Jansen-type metaphyseal chondrodysplasia	Decreased differentiation of chondrocytes; delayed vascular invasion	241, 242
Murine, transgenic	(GDF5 driven from Col II and Col IX promoters)	Hunter-Thompson	Shortened limbs; joint malformations; chondrodysplasia; expanded physes; increased hypertrophic zone; decreased proliferative zone	243
Murine, transgenic	FVB/NCr (increased IFN gamma)	Osteochondral dysplasia	Short, wide deformed long bones; thickened physes; irregular metaphyseal borders; spontaneous fractures; degeneration of articular cartilage	244
Murine, transgenic	(Collagen X dominant interference)	Schmid metaphyseal chondrodysplasia	Dwarfism; compression of hypertrophic zone of chondrocytes	110, 113
Porcine, spontaneous	(Type X collagen deficiency; missense mutation)	Schmid metaphyseal chondrodysplasia	Dwarfism; metaphyseal chondrodysplasia of long bones	245
Rat, spontaneous	ocd/ocd (autosomal recessive)	Osteochondral dysplasia	Short domed head; decreased trunk length; shortened bones; decreased GAG content	246

Table 10.10   Induced Osteochondrodysplasias

Model Type	Model	Modeled Human Condition	Pathology Description	Ref.
Chicken	Chick: radiation exposure	Associated morbidities of radiation therapy	Increased intracellular calcium of chondrocytes; increased apoptosis; increased caspase-3	247
Guinea pig	Retinoid agonist via osmotic pump or intraperitoneal injection for 10–14 d	Side effect of retinoid therapy	Dose-dependent stunting; loss of basophilic staining of ECM; OCL invasion into physes	248
Murine	Mechanical/surgical: insult to proximal tibial metaphysis	Physeal trauma	Ossified bridge	249
Ovine	Surgical grafting of transphyseal bony tether	Physeal trauma	Premature ossification	250
Rat	Mechanical/surgical: transection of foveal artery	Perthe's disease	Necrotic bone with resorption; neovascularization and fibrogenesis of epiphysis; flattened femoral head; osseous bridging of physis	251

Note: ECM, extracellular matrix; OCL, osteoclast.

Arthritis

Articular cartilage lacks the highly ordered structure of growth plate cartilage, but specific zones that show differing chondrocyte morphology and matrix-staining characteristics have been identified. Chondrocytes are isolated in the matrix in aggregates referred to as chondrons. Like growth plate cartilage, specific patterns of gene expression and proteoglycan synthesis are observed in articular cartilage dependent on the morphologic zone. For instance, a protein referred to as *superficial zone protein* is produced by superficial zone chondrocytes. The importance of the various morphologic zones of articular cartilage in function and disease is virtually unknown, relative to the more well-defined roles in growth plate cartilage. The purpose of articular cartilage is to absorb and dissipate load and to provide a gliding surface for joint motion.

Arthritis is a generalized term used to refer to inflammation of a synovial joint. Although tissues other than cartilage are affected in arthritis, such as joint capsule and ligaments, the end result of chronic arthritis is cartilage damage. In arthritis, the quantity of proteoglycan and cartilage ECM decreases, leading to a loss of cartilage function. Because of the avascular nature of cartilage and the paucity of chondrocytes, damaged cartilage is unable to mount an effective healing response. Thus, early damage inevitably progresses to severe, chronic damage; loss of function; and chronic pain. There are a number of different classifications for arthritis, and models for these conditions are presented.

Osteoarthritis

Osteoarthritis (OA) is the most common arthritic condition and the second-most common cause of disability in the United States. The occurrence of OA increases exponentially with advancing age. OA occurs secondary to incidental macrotrauma, repetitive microtrauma, underlying systemic conditions, and joint deformity. In many cases, a causative factor in OA cannot be discerned; thus, the development of OA is affected by genetic factors working in concert with environmental effects. The process is thought to be modulated by autocrine and paracrine cytokines (TNF-alpha, IL-1), which induce a cascade of events leading to decreased synthesis of ECM constituents, chondrocyte apoptosis, and matrix degradation by metalloproteinases.[115] Gross examination of the articular surface reveals superficial-to-deep fibrillation. These morphologic irregularities occur coincident with a loss of glycosaminoglycans (GAGs). The articular surface ulcerates, leading to eburnation and crepitus. Radiographic hallmarks of OA include cysts, bony sclerosis of the subchondral plate, osteophyte growth, and a narrowing of the joint space.

A number of animal models have been developed to investigate the pathogenesis of OA (Table 10.11; reviewed by Schwartz[116] and van den Berg et al.[117]) Historically, rabbits, guinea pigs, and dogs have been the animals of choice, although rodents and birds have been used as well. Methods of induction include direct surgical damage, biomechanical alterations, and chemical exposure of the articular cartilage. A number of GEM models develop spontaneous OA. For instance, collagen IX knockout mice, mice lacking a single collagen II allele, and MMP13-overexpressing mice all develop degenerative arthritis with increased age. As well, certain inbred strains of mice are more prone to develop chronic OA.

A number of the models presented use direct cartilage injury to induce OA (Table 10.11). Although the pathogenesis of OA development secondary to injury is different from the primary (idiopathic) human OA, which is a generalized defect and not a focal injury, the reproducibility, predictability, and similarity of outcomes support the use of these models. Variations in cartilage permeability and Poisson's ratio can drastically affect the mechanical behavior of cartilage. As well, alterations in the subchondral bone can impact the response of cartilage to direct trauma.[118] Because these three parameters differ among species, they must be considered when using an injury model to study OA.

Table 10.11   Osteoarthritis Models

Animal, Model Type	Model Description	Time Course	Pathology Description	Ref.
Canine (beagle), induced	Knee, direct injury; condylar cartilage grooves	10 wks	Increased MMP; mild osteophytes; loss of matrix proteoglycan; increased denatured collagen	252
Canine, induced	Knee, ACL transection	10 wks	Increased collagenolysis	253
Canine, induced	Knee, transarticular load	6 mo	Initially an osteochondral fracture; progression to decreased collagen thickness; fibrillation of articular cartilage	53
Guinea pig, induced	MCL/ACL-deficient knee	16–18 wks	Decreased cartilage PG; osteophytes; decreased link protein	254
Guinea pig, induced	Knee, altered biomechanics by unilateral resection of gluteal muscle, or transection of infrapatellar ligament	10–24 wks	Increased cartilage water content; narrow joint space; sclerosis of subchondral bone; osteophytes; loss of chondrocytes and matrix	255
Guinea pig, spontaneous	Knee arthritis	12–30 mo	Predilection for medial compartment of tibio-femoral joint; cartilage fibrillation	256
Murine (B6C3F1), spontaneous	Ankle arthritis	Not available	Loss of articular cartilage; erosions; osteophytes; eventual ankylosis	257
Murine (STR/ORT), spontaneous	Medial compartment secondary to medial patellar displacement	15 mo	Erosion; osteophytes; subchondral bony sclerosis; loss of proteoglycan; affects 100%	258
Murine, targeted disruption	Absent type IX collagen; Col9alpha3-null; spontaneous knee arthritis	At least 4 mo	After 4 mo, develops severe noninflammatory arthritis	259
Murine, transgenic	Overexpression of truncated Col9alpha1 chain from collagen II promoter; spontaneous knee arthritis	6 wks	Opaque corneas; early OA changes; mild proportionate dwarfism	260
Murine, targeted disruption	Collagen II-null Col2alpha1 hetero- and homozygous null mice ± voluntary running	15 mo	Inactivation of a single allele results in softer collagen with greater OA changes; exercise improves OA	261
Murine, transgenic	MMP13 driven from a tetracycline-controlled collagen II promoter	5 mo	MMP13 induced after doxycycline removal; loss of cartilage; focal erosions	262
Rabbit, induced	Knee; chemical exposure - intra-articular estradiol injection	9–12 wks	Erosion; cysts; thinning and fibrillation of cartilage	263
Rabbit, induced	Knee; lateral meniscus and LCL deficient	12 wks	Fibrillation; ulceration; erosion of cartilage; osteophytes; chondrocyte loss	264
Rabbit, induced	Knee; ACL, PCL, MCL, flexor digitorum longus, and meniscus deficient	6 mo	Decreased chondrocyte number; decreased proteoglycan; fibrillation of cartilage; increased degradative enzymes	265
Rabbit, induced	Knee, repetitive impulse loads	Not available	Subchondral bone sclerosis before cartilage changes	138
Rabbit, induced	Knee; chemical exposure — intra-articular collagenase injection	Not available	Degenerative cartilage; transient degeneration of synovium	266
Rat, induced	Knee, partial meniscectomy with high-impact loading	60 d	Increased MMP-3; apoptosis of chondrocytes	267
Rat (Wistar), induced	Knee; injury from continual strenuous running	6 wks	Dose-dependent effect of running on OA development; increased MMP-3;	268
Sheep, Induced	Knee; meniscus deficient; post-operative loading or unloading	16 wks	Effusions, synovial hyperplasia, erosion and fibrillation of medial compartment in active animals	269
Sheep, induced	Hip; denuded articular cartilage ± subchondral bone penetration	12 wks	Acute onset of destructive disease subchondral fracture; osteophytes; cysts; erosions	270

Rheumatoid Arthritis

Rheumatoid arthritis (RA) affects 1% of the world's population, with women having a three- to fivefold greater risk. RA is an immune-mediated symmetric polyarthritis. The disease is chronic and progressively destructive. Bony erosions, periarticular osteopenia, inflammation, and ultimately, joint disintegration are characteristic. Most RA patients have autoimmunity to type II collagen as well as polyclonal anti-Fc IgG. Early in the disease, a dense perivascular (CD4+ T-cell population) infiltrate develops as the synovium thickens and neovascularizes. The hyperproliferative synovial lining, or pannus, begins to creep over the articular surface. Nodular aggregates of polyclonal T cells direct the inflammatory process, liberating inflammatory mediators. These molecules, IL-1, TNF-alpha, and TGF-beta, elicit collagen and proteoglycan degradation, activate OCL-directed resorption of bone, and stimulate fibrogenesis.

The study of RA has progressed significantly since the inception of collagen-sensitization techniques in mice, rats, and primates. These models have been used extensively to investigate the pathogenesis of RA (Table 10.12). In the collagen-sensitization model, heterologous type II collagen is injected, and the development of autoimmunity drives the arthritic process.[119] Collagen-induced arthritis (CIA), although differing slightly from RA, supports the biological plausibility that an autoimmune reaction to a cartilage component (specifically, type II collagen) leads to chronic, destructive polyarthritis.[120] Similar to the case with RA, synovitis and erosions are the hallmarks of CIA.[121] CIA can be induced across species with similar result; affected animals exhibit a chronic autoimmunity to collagen, exemplified by changes in major histocompatibility complex (MHC) and the induction of rheumatoid factor titers (anti-Fc IgG).[122] Generally, rats are more susceptible than mice to CIA.[123] Use of these models has been extensively reviewed; and although we have provided a few examples in Table 10.12, the reader is referred to the aforementioned articles for more detail.[119,120,122–127]

Another model of RA is adjuvant-induced arthritis (AIA; Table 10.12). Animals injected with adjuvant display a classic T-cell-dependent arthritis. The AIA reaction, at a histological level, is equivalent to CIA.[128] This reactivity often proceeds to involve an inflammatory response within various joints.

Transgenic models are particularly useful in the study of RA because of the known link between disease and class II MHC haplotypes. The HLA-DR (HLA = human leukocyte antigen) association has led to the development of mice that express human MHC. These mice have been used to determine the association between suspect alleles and RA development (Table 10.12). By studying these models, the association between genetic determinants of immunity and the appearance of disease is now well understood. In addition, these models have been useful for testing various RA treatment modalities. Current research is focused on elucidating the inciting events in RA.

Reactive Arthritis

Reactive arthritis occurs secondary to a predisposing infection — typically a gastrointestinal or genitourinary (GI or GU) bacterial infection. The arthritic event is sterile, and there is no evidence of residual infectious agent. However, polymorphonuclear leukocytes and macrophages with intracellular inclusions can be found within the synovial fluid.[129] Reactive arthritis often develops 2 to 4 weeks after the original infection. The presentation is asymmetrical and oligoarticular, most commonly affecting the joints of the lower extremity and lumbar spine. The joint disease is usually self-limiting (3 to 12 months), but 15% of cases possess chronic or destructive features, and another 10 to 15% are relapsing.[129] There does appear to be an immunologic link to MHC class I allele human leukocyte antigen (HLA) B27, but its significance is not fully understood.[130]

When evaluating potential models for reactive arthritis, several factors must be considered. Not only is the pathogenesis important, but the temporal course of disease should be similar to the human clinical disease.[131] The anatomical sites that are frequently affected should correspond across

Table 10.12   Rheumatoid Arthritis Models

Animal, Model Type	Immunizing Agent	Disease Parameters	Pathology Description	Ref.
Canine (Shetland sheep dog), spontaneous	NA	Chronic; progressive; symmetric polyarthritis	Pannus; synovial proliferation; lymphocyte infiltrate	271
Mouse (many strains)	FCA injection into footpad	Chronic; progressive	RF not increased; synovial thickening and villus; formation with erosions	272
Mouse (many strains), CIA	Native CII	Chronic; progressive; variable joints affected	Consult seminal reference	273
Mouse (NZB/KN), spontaneous	NA	2-month onset; chronic; progressive; fore/hindpaws affected	AutoAb deposits on collagen fibers; high titers of anti-CII and RF	274
Mouse (MRL/Mp-lpr/lpr), spontaneous	NA	5- to 6-months onset; chronic; progressive; symmetric polyarthritis	Decreased life span due to systemic immune disease (lupus-like syndrome); destructive arthritis; 75% mice affected	275
Mouse (HLA-DQ8± H-2Ab0), transgenic, CIA sensitive	Bovine CII with booster 28 d later	25- to 40-d onset; chronic; progressive; fore/hindpaws affected	Strong Ab response to murine CII; symmetric polyarthritis; mononuclear infiltrate; pannus; cartilage erosions	276, 277
Mouse (HLA-DQ8+/ DR4/Ab0), transgenic, CIA sensitive	Porcine CII with booster	Chronic; progressive; fore/hindpaws affected	Strong Ab response to murine CII; symmetric polyarthritis; mononuclear infiltrate; pannus; cartilage erosions.	127
Mouse (DBA1/TCR-beta Tg), transgenic, CIA sensitive	Bovine CII	19-d onset; chronic, relapsing; progressive; fore/hindpaws affected	Extensive pannus; PMN and lymphocytic infiltrate; periarticular erosions, necrotic chondrocytes	278
Mouse (KRN X NOD), transgenic cross of NOD and T-cell receptor, spontaneous	NA	25- to 35-d onset; chronic; progressive; symmetric polyarthritis: knee, ankle, fore/hindpaws, not in hip	Hyperplastic synovitis; mostly macrophage with some T-cell infiltrate; pannus and fibrosis; cartilage erosions; IgG deposits	279
Murine (DBA/1), transgenic, spontaneous	NA	TNF-alpha transgene constitutively expressed; knee, spontaneous OA	Severe erosive arthritis; hyperplastic synovium; few viable chondrocytes; lethal at 9–10 weeks	280
Primate, CIA	CII in Freund's complete adjuvant (FCA)	3–6 weeks onset; acute; transient; phalangeal joints affected	Spontaneous remission with minor deformities; high anti-C2 titer; high death rate	281
Sheep, CIA	Native bovine CII, subcutaneous injection with FCA, booster after 14 d	21-d onset; hock joint affected	anti-CII Ab; synovial T-cells; macrophage and CD4+ T-cells infiltrate; thickened synovium	282
Rat (many strains), AIA	Pristane, single intradermal injection	2- to 3-week onset; chronic; progressive; severity varies with haplotype; ankles and paws are the affected joints	Joint inflammation; pannus; T-cell infiltrate; joint erosions; relapsing; gradual deformation	283
Rat (Wistar), AIA	FCA footpad injection	9- to 10-d onset; chronic; progressive	RF absent, macrophage and PMN infiltrate, synovial hyperplasia, cartilage and bone destruction	284

(continued)

Table 10.12 (continued)   Rheumatoid Arthritis Models

Animal, Model Type	Immunizing Agent	Disease Parameters	Pathology Description	Ref.
Rat (Sprague-Dawley, Wistar), CIA	Native chicken CII from xiphoid, intradermal injection; booster after 21d.	20-d onset; chronic; progressive; bilateral ankle, tarsus, paws affected	40% develop inflammatory polyarthritis; severe, complete destruction of joint with eventual ankylosis; 20% relapsing or transient variety	122
Rat (env-pX on LTR promoter), transgenic spontaneous	NA	5-week onset; chronic; progressive; fore/ hindpaws affected	Bilateral ankle inflammation; synovial hyperplasia; pannus; erosion of cartilage; bone destruction	285

Note: CIA, collagen-induced arthritis; AIA, adjuvant-induced arthritis; CII, collagen type II; NOD, Non-obese diabetic; RF, rheumatoid factor; NA, not applicable.

species, and the nature of inflammation at the discrete locations should be similar. As well, because the time frame for development of the reactive arthritis is important, a 2- to 4-week gap between primary infection with the GI/GU bacteria and the development of arthritis should be present. In recognition of the association between HLA-B27 and reactive arthritis, a number of studies have used HLA-B27 transgenic mice to study disease pathogenesis.[132] Several different examples of reactive arthritis models are provided in Table 10.13.

Septic Arthritis

Septic arthritis is caused by the entry of an infectious agent into the normal sterile environment of a diarthroidal joint space. It causes significant morbidity in both pediatric and joint-replacement populations. In pediatric patients, premature degenerative-joint disease results from a rapid consumption of articular cartilage. Once bacteria gain entry into the joint, they form microabscesses, alter chondrocyte metabolism, and generate an autoimmune response by the antigenic conversion of native articular cartilage.[133]

Appropriate animal models of septic arthritis should recapitulate the natural pathogenesis of the human disease. A wide variety of models have been used, and they involve either the injection of an infectious agent into the joint or the systemic administration of an agent to evaluate hematogenous spread. Several examples are highlighted in Table 10.13. These highlighted studies and others have been useful in identifying bacterial virulence factors as well as host-associated risk factors. Specifically, the use of hematogenously disseminated *Staphylococcus aureus* (LS-1) in rodents has increased our knowledge of septic arthritis secondary to staphylococcal infection. Rats, hamsters, and non-human primates have been used to study the development of arthritis secondary to *Borellia burgdorferi* infection (Lyme disease), as listed in Table 10.13.

Hemorrhagic Arthritis

Although high-energy trauma, osteochondral fractures, and even anterior cruciate ligament (ACL) tears provide dramatic examples of hemarthroses, hemophilia is the leading cause in humans. Eighty percent of bleeding events in hemophiliacs occur in the joints, usually the knee, ankle, and elbow.[134] High intra-articular pressure results in a decreased range of motion and pain. Although the pain typically resolves with clotting factor replacement, the stiffness remains as a function of the turgid joint capsule.[135] These symptoms often lead to ligamentous laxity and muscle weakness, predisposing the joint to further damage.[135] Repeated or prolonged exposure to blood products leads to iron-laden macrophages and synoviocytes. Inflammation is stimulated and the synovium becomes

Table 10.13   Miscellaneous Arthritis

Animal, Model Type	Model Description[a]	Disease Parameters	Pathology Description	Ref.
		Reactive		
Hamster	*E. coli* lipopolysaccharide; subcutaneous injection for 5 to 21 d	3-d onset; acute transient course; 3-week persistence; recovery 1 week after stopping injections	Symmetric polyarthritis symptoms; ankle joint most prominent; exudative synovitis; juxta-articular periostitis	286
Mouse (DBA/2 and BDF1)	*Y. enterocolitica* intravenously; injection of 10^8 organisms	3-d onset, peaks at 7 d, resolved 21 d; acute; transient course	Hindpaws more severely affected than forepaws; mononuclear infiltrate	287
Mouse (HLA-B27), transgenic	Requires exposure to pathogenic organisms and environmental antigens	Acute	Spontaneous tarsal ankylosis; enthesitis	132, 288, 289
Rat (LEW)	Intravenous injection of *Y. enterocolitica*	1- to 2-week onset; acute, relapsing	Sterile arthritis in 70%	290
Rat (several lines on LEW and F344)	Spontaneous occurrence; HLA-B27 with hB_2m	6- to 10-week onset; acute; progressive	50% affected; systemic inflammatory disorder; destructive synovitis; peri-articular osteogenesis; enthesitis at vertebral endplate	291, 292
		Infectious		
Hamster (LSH/SsLak)	Hindpaw injection of 10^6 *B. burgdorferi*; some hamsters preirradiated with doses of 100–700 rads	5- to 11-d onset, shorter time with higher radiation dose; transient infection, but can persist up to 50 d with higher doses of radiation	Acute transient synovitis; diffuse PMN infiltrate in synovium; effusion; symptoms increase with pre-irradiation	293
Mouse (Swiss and Balb/C)	Intravenous administration of 10^7 *S. aureus* cells (LS-1); isolated from spontaneous arthritis in NZB/W	3-d onset; acute; progressive	80–90% affected; early PMN infiltrate followed by monocytic infiltrate; increased interleukin-6 and tumor necrosis factor-alpha, severe peri-articular bone erosions	131
Mouse (C3H/He)	Inoculated with skin biopsy from infected human	Chronic	Severe inflammation of ankle joint; widespread spirochete dissemination	294
Primate (rhesus monkey)	*B. burgdorferi* inoculation via tick vector	6 months	Necrosis of articular cartilage; knee and elbow most consistently affected; synovial hyperplasia; mononuclear/lymphocyte infiltrate	295
Rabbit (NZW)	Intra-articular injection of *S. aureus*	3-week onset; acute arthritis	50% loss GAG and 33% loss collagen, persists for 7 weeks	296
Rat (LEW/N)	Intraperitoneal injection of *B. burgdorferi*	Onset 14 d; chronic	Arthritis associated with presence of spirochetes; polyarthritis	297
		Hemarthrosis		
Canine (beagle)	Intra-articular injection of autologous blood into the knee	16-d follow-up; acute arthritis	Decreased proteoglycan synthesis and content by 4 d (more severe in young); at 16 d PG synthesis has partially recovered (better recovery in older cartilage)	117
Canine (immature mongrel)	Popliteal artery anastamosis with knee joint	1–8 d; acute; progressive arthritis	Total destruction of articular cartilage and subchondral bone; transient arthritis in 6%	298

(continued)

Table 10.13 (continued)   Miscellaneous Arthritis

Animal and Model Type	Model Description	Disease Parameters	Pathology Description	Ref.
		Hemarthrosis		
Rabbit (NZW)	Autologous blood injected intra-articularly in knee	1–10 d	Decreased PG content; thickened synovium; hemosiderin-laden macrophages; mild surface fibrillation	300
Rabbit (NZW)	Intra-articular injection of autologous blood into the ankle	10–28 d; acute arthritis	Increased joint stiffness at 10 d; hypertrophic synovium; hemosiderin-laden macrophages; darkened articular cartilage	301

[a] *E. coli, Escherichia coli; Y. enterocolitica, Yersinia enterocolitica; B. burgdorferi, Borellia burgdorferi; S. aureus, Staphylococcus aureus.*

proliferative. Villous extension of the synovium can predispose to further injury and bleeding. Over time, the joint becomes fibrotic.

There are few reports of animal models of hemarthrosis (HA) (Table 10.13). The majority have used exogenous blood injected directly into the joint cavity. Although this does in part mimic human HA, it does not recapitulate the bleeding that occurs over time into the joint. Although there are a number of animal models that develop hemophilia, reports of hemarthrosis in those animals are lacking. Perhaps the exploitation of an animal model of hemophilia by inducing chronic bleeding into the joint would more successfully mimic human HA.

Articular Cartilage Defects

Articular cartilage has very low healing potential.[136] If repair tissue does form, it usually consists of fibrous tissue, fibrocartilage, and small amounts of low-proteoglycan-content hyaline cartilage.[137] One factor that contributes to the lack of regeneration is the avascularity of articular cartilage. When a defect is made that extends into the subchondral bone, there is a greater healing response, although the repair tissue remains abnormal. This second finding suggests that there may be an inherent defect in the ability of chondrocytes to repair. Skeletally immature individuals seem to have a greater capacity for regeneration of the joint surface, and adult chondrocytes, *in vivo* and *in vitro,* have a limited capacity for self-replication. Thus, an inability to generate sufficient new chondrocytes for repair may be an additional factor limiting healing. Investigators have proposed that if chondrocyte precursors could be obtained from extracartilaginous sources, then healing could be improved. The focus of current research on the healing of articular cartilage defects is validation of cells, matrices, and treatment regimens that may promote the engraftment, proliferation, and chondrogenic differentiation of exogenous precursor cells.

Although it would seem relatively simple to induce an injury in articular cartilage, the use of animal models to investigate defect healing presents a unique challenge. Species differences in the content of subchondral bone, the effect that subchondral bone has on overlying cartilage, the nature of chondral lesions, and biped vs. quadriped biomechanics are all confounding factors. Any of these considerations may adversely impact the use of a cartilage injury model.[138] As well, histo-logical, biochemical, and material properties of cartilage can vary significantly between species. Humans have thicker articular cartilage with a decreased cell density; in addition, permeability of the matrix and its Poisson's ratio are quite different from those of other frequently used animal models.[139] Even within the same species, different anatomical sites may exhibit distinct mechanical properties because variations in water content can translate into changes in hardness and perme-ability of the cartilage layer.[140] Thus, the anatomic site of investigation must be carefully considered.

Table 10.14   Articular Cartilage Defects

Animal, Model Type	Model Protocol	Time Course	Pathological Observations	Ref.
Canine (mongrel), adult, knee	4-mm diameter × 2-in femoral trochlea; 10-d postoperative immobilization	15 d	Unpredictable healing (partial at best); some hyaline cartilage; ± seams at margins; mostly fibrous ingrowth; some developed osseous injury	137
Canine, adult, knee	Used ceramic chisel; osteochondral fragments: 19 × 6.5 × 6-mm defects; replaced after hemostasis	200 d	Unstable fragments (33%) — fatty necrosis and fibrous invasion of marrow, all with fibrocartilage bridge; stable fragments (67%) — sclerosis of bony segment with no discernable interface	137
Canine, adult, knee	Chondral abrasion	6 mo	Repair cartilage with decreased PG, hydroxyproline, cellularity, types II, IX, XI collagen; increased types I and IV collagen	302
Goat, adult, knee	4 osteochondral defects per joint; no immobilization	1 yr	<50% with complete regeneration (defect filled)	303
Horse, 9-d-old foal, knee	12-mm diameter defect; femoral trochlea; subchondral infraction; limit postoperative exercise	4–8 mo	At 8 months, some bone still exposed; no synovitis; decreased synovial fluid GAGs and chondroitin	304
Mini-pig (Goettinger), adult, knee	5-mm cubic defect; femoral trochlea; partial thickness	6 wk	Sporadic patches of fibrous mesenchymal cells; no chondrogenesis	305
Rabbit (NZW), adult, knee	6-mm diameter drill, 5- to 6-mm depth into femoral trochlea; subchondral injury; immobilized 3 weeks	2–44 wk	2 weeks — fibrous/cellular clot; bony in-growth into clot; fibrocartilage at margins 6 weeks — sparse hyaline nests; progressive fibrous in-growth weeks 44 weeks — full fibrous coverage; no hyaline cartilage, subchondral sclerosis	306
Rabbit (NZW), adult, knee	3-mm diameter; full-thickness patellar "punch" defect; subchondral bone preserved; no immobilization	6 wk	No healing evident; synovitis; "cell nests" at margins of defect; about 15% healing (located at periphery); 30% osteophyte and cartilage color change	307
Rabbit (NZW), adult, knee	4-mm diameter; 8-mm depth cores into medial femoral condyle; subchondral infringement; no immobilization	12 wk	Degenerative changes: osteophytes, focal fibrillation; thin layer of soft repair tissue; partial coverage; no neocartilage; bone core necrotic	308
Rabbit (NZW), adult, knee	1-mm wide, 2-mm deep, 4- to 6-mm-long defects; custom instrumentation; femoral trochlea; partial thickness	48 wk	Sporadic patches of fibrous mesenchymal cells; no chondrogenesis	309
Sheep, knee	Denuded femoral trochlea	2 yr	Chondral erosion; early degenerative changes; profound resorption of subchondral bone plate; patchy resurfacing with loose fibrous or fibrocartilaginous tissue	310

Despite these drawbacks, animal models represent a vital tool in the development of therapeutic options for lesions of articular cartilage. A variety of animal models of chondral injury are presented in Table 10.14 (reviewed by Hunziker[141]). By and large, the most common animal model that has been used is the rabbit. Rabbits have been the traditional small-animal model of choice for research on articular defects; mice and rats have greater anatomic variation in articular cartilage and sub-chondral bone thickness (relative to humans). As well, experimental surgeries to create reliable, large-scale defects are more difficult with mice and rats because of their small size and the limited articular cartilage surface area.

FUTURE PERSPECTIVES

Over the past 10 years, significant progress has been made in understanding the development and biology of musculoskeletal tissues. Much of this has been derived from studies of GEM models. Targeted gene disruptions and transgenics have revealed key regulators in OCL development and function, and have validated the functional significance of known gene mutations in the development of osteogenesis imperfecta, osteopetrosis, osteochondrodysplasias, and rheumatoid arthritis. Despite these advances, appropriate GEM models for a number of skeletal abnormalities are either unde-veloped or incompletely characterized.

A thorough understanding of the complex interactions that occur during fracture healing has yet to be revealed by animal models; thus, reliable biologically based treatments to improve fracture healing have not been devised. As well, molecular mechanisms that enhance OB performance to restore bone mass in osteopenia are poorly described. This is partly governed by our inability to fully comprehend the complex process of OB development from osteoprogenitors. Although genetic elements that control osteoprogenitor number and differentiation have been explored, there is a paucity of information that seeks to fully describe the complex processes governing OB develop-ment and function. The molecular mechanisms that seek to explain a bone's response to loading and unloading are also not well described. It is postulated that osteocytes respond to mechanical signals, and that the signals are processed and then transferred to the osteoprogenitor, but the molecules that are involved in this process have not been revealed. One hopes that with the recent development of *in vivo* loading and fracture models in mice, as well as of GEM models of osteopenia and osteosclerosis, novel genes controlling OB biology will be elucidated.

Although GEM models have provided key insight into the process of endochondral ossification and have revealed the significant role of molecules such as FGF receptor (FGFR), vascular endo-thelial growth factor (VEGF), and matrix metalloproteinase 9 (MMP9), there is still much to be learned about the process and the role of various components. For instance, humans with a mutation in cartilage oligomeric matrix protein (COMP) have a dwarfing syndrome, pseudoachondrodyspla-sia (PSACH);[142] however, mice with the COMP gene deleted have no reported phenotype. Thus, a complete understanding of the significance of the human mutation will only be revealed by a targeted mutation in the mouse gene that mimics the known human mutation. In this way, the significance of mutations in FGFR3 in human chondrodsyplasia was revealed. Iwata et al.[112] created a targeted mutation in FGFR3 that recapitulated a single amino acid shift at position 644. In a similar manner, a murin- targeted gene mutation (*knockin*) that mimics the mutation found in COMP may reveal crucial mechanistic information concerning PSACH.

One of the biggest problems that the musculoskeletal research community faces is developing treatment options for cartilage repair, either in chronic OA or in acute injuries. Unfortunately, animal models have provided few answers. By exploiting common models of OA and cartilage injury that have been used in the rat, rabbit, and dog for use in GEM models, novel genes (or novel gene functions) that govern cartilage healing will likely be revealed.

Although GEM models are powerful tools when used to explore gene function and disease mechanism, in many cases mice may not be the best model for many human skeletal disease conditions because of physiological differences in cartilage and bone when comparing mice and humans. In that respect, studies with larger mammals are still quite useful and often more appropriate. The development of transgenic technology for use in larger animal species will likely be beneficial for future skeletal studies. As well, traditional knockouts and constitutively overexpressing mice ignore the importance of temporal and spatial relationships in gene function. Ablating a locus early may have a dominant effect, suppressing an important gene function that is not necessary until a later time point. However, this caveat can be addressed using transgenes that are inducible or expressed in a tissue-specific manner. As well, using Cre/*LoxP* technology, targeted mice can be generated with a mutation (deletion, nucleotide shift, etc.) that occurs in a tissue- and temporal-specific manner.

REFERENCES

1. World Health Organization, The Bone and Joint Decade, consensus document, 1998.
2. An, Y.H. and Friedman, R.J., *Animal Models in Orthopaedic Research,* 1st ed., CRC Press, Boca Raton, FL, 1998.
3. Laberge, M. and Powers, D.L., Scientific basis for bilateral animal models in orthopaedics, *J. Invest. Surg.,* 4(2), 109, 1991.
4. Olsen, B.R. et al., Bone development, *Annu. Rev. Cell Dev. Biol.,* 16, 191, 2000.
5. Cancedda, R. et al., Developmental control of chondrogenesis and osteogenesis, *Int. J. Dev. Biol.,* 44(6 Spec. No.), 707, 2000.
6. Manolagas, S.C., Birth and death of bone cells: basic regulatory mechanisms and implications for the pathogenesis and treatment of osteoporosis, *Endocr. Rev.,* 21(2), 115, 2000.
7. Raisz, L.G., Physiology and pathophysiology of bone remodeling, *Clin. Chem.,* 45(8 Pt. 2), 1353, 1999.
8. Parfitt, A.M. et al., Relationship between surface, volume, and thickness of iliac trabecular bone in aging and in osteoporosis: implications for the microanatomic and cellular mechanism of bone loss, *J. Clin. Invest.,* 72, 1396, 1998.
9. Erben, R.G., Trabecular and endocortical bone surfaces in the rat: modeling or remodeling?, *Anat. Rec.,* 246(1), 39, 1996.
10. Frost, H.M., Bone "mass" and the "mechanostat": a proposal, *Anat. Rec.,* 219(1), 1, 1987.
11. McCarthy, T.L. et al., Links among growth factors, hormones, and nuclear factors with essential roles in bone formation, *Crit. Rev. Oral Biol. Med.,* 11(4), 409, 2000.
12. Canalis, E. et al., Skeletal growth factors, *Crit. Rev. Eukaryot. Gene Expr.,* 3(3), 155, 1993.
13. Owen, M. and Friedenstein, A.J., Stromal stem cells: marrow-derived osteogenic precursors, *Ciba Found. Symp.,* 136, 42, 1988.
14. Bianco, P. and Gehron Robey, P., Marrow stromal stem cells, *J. Clin. Invest.,* 105(12), 1663, 2000.
15. Hock, J.M. et al., Osteoblast apoptosis and bone turnover, *J. Bone Miner. Res.,* 16(6), 975, 2001.
16. Horowitz, M.C. et al., Control of osteoclastogenesis and bone resorption by members of the TNF family of receptors and ligands, *Cytokine Growth Factor Rev.,* 12(1), 9, 2001.
17. Balemans, W. et al., Localization of the gene for sclerosteosis to the van Buchem Disease-gene region on chromosome 17q12-q21, *Am. J. Hum. Genet.,* 64(6), 1661, 1999.
18. Little, R.D. et al., A mutation in the LDL receptor-related protein 5 gene results in the autosomal dominant high-bone-mass trait, *Am. J. Hum. Genet.,* 70(1), 11, 2002.
19. Kato, M. et al., Cbfa1-independent decrease in osteoblast proliferation, osteopenia, and persistent embryonic eye vascularization in mice deficient in Lrp5, a Wnt coreceptor, *J. Cell Biol.,* 157(2), 303, 2002.
20. Boyce, B.F. et al., Recent advances in bone biology provide insight into the pathogenesis of bone diseases, *Lab. Invest.,* 79(2), 83, 1999.
21. McCauley, L.K., Transgenic mouse models of metabolic bone disease, *Curr. Opin. Rheumatol.,* 13(4), 316, 2001.
22. Ducy, P. et al., Increased bone formation in osteocalcin-deficient mice, *Nature,* 382, 448, 1996.

23. Hankenson, K.D. et al., Increased marrow-derived osteoprogenitor cells and endosteal bone formation in mice lacking thrombospondin 2, *J. Bone Miner. Res.,* 15(5), 851, 2000.

24. Ducy, P. et al., Leptin inhibits bone formation through a hypothalamic relay: a central control of bone mass, *Cell,* 100(2), 197, 2000.

25. de Vernejoul, M.C. and Benichou, O., Human osteopetrosis and other sclerosing disorders: recent genetic developments, *Calcif. Tissue Int.,* 69(1), 1, 2001.

26. Wiktor-Jedrzejczak, W. et al., Total absence of colony-stimulating factor 1 in the macrophage-deficient osteopetrotic (op/op) mouse, *Proc. Natl. Acad. Sci. U.S.A.,* 87(12), 4828, 1990.

27. Simonet, W.S. et al., Osteoprotegerin: a novel secreted protein involved in the regulation of bone density, *Cell,* 89(2), 309, 1997.

28. Brady, K.P. et al., A novel putative transporter maps to the osteosclerosis (oc) mutation and is not expressed in the oc mutant mouse, *Genomics,* 56(3), 254, 1999.

29. Hodgkinson, C.A.F. et al., Mutations at the mouse microphthalmia locus are associated with defects in a gene encoding a novel basic-helix-loop-helix-zipper protein, *Cell,* 74(2), 395, 1993.

30. Marks, S.C., Jr et al., The osteopetrotic rabbit: general and skeletal features of a new outbred stock, *Bone,* 7(5), 359, 1986.

31. Reddy, S.V. et al., Cell biology of Paget's disease, *J. Bone Miner. Res.,* 14(Suppl. 2), 3, 1999.

32. Reddy, S.V. et al., Osteoclasts formed by measles virus-infected osteoclast precursors from hCD46 transgenic mice express characteristics of Pagetic osteoclasts, *Endocrinology,* 142(7), 2898, 2001.

33. Peacock, M. et al., Genetics of osteoporosis, *Endocr. Rev.,* 23(3), 303, 2002.

34. Ralston, S.H., Genetic control of susceptibility to osteoporosis, *J. Clin. Endocrinol. Metab.,* 87(6), 2460, 2002.

35. Turner, R.T.F. et al., Animal models for osteoporosis, *Rev. Endocr. Metab. Disord.,* 2(1), 117, 2001.

36. Jerome, C.P.F. and Peterson, P.E., Nonhuman primate models in skeletal research, *Bone,* 29(1), 1, 2001.

37. Miller, S.C. et al., Available animal models of osteopenia — small and large, *Bone,* 17 (4 Suppl.), 117S, 1995.

38. Thompson, D.D. et al., FDA guidelines and animal models for osteoporosis, *Bone,* 17 (4 Suppl.), 125S, 1995.

39. Mosekilde, L., Assessing bone quality — animal models in preclinical osteoporosis research, *Bone,* 17 (4 Suppl.), 343S, 1995.

40. Bain, S.D. et al., High-dose estrogen inhibits bone resorption and stimulates bone formation in the ovariectomized mouse, *J. Bone Miner. Res.,* 8(4), 435, 1993.

41. Wronski, T.J. et al., Skeletal alterations in ovariectomized rats, *Calcif. Tissue Int.,* 37(3), 324, 1985.

42. Kalu, D.N., Evaluation of the pathogenesis of skeletal changes in ovariectomized rats, *Endocrinology,* 115(2), 507, 1984.

43. Faugere, M.C. et al., Bone changes occurring early after cessation of ovarian function in beagle dogs: a histomorphometric study employing sequential biopsies, *J. Bone Miner. Res.,* 5(3), 263, 1990.

44. Newman, E. et al., The potential of sheep for the study of osteopenia: current status and comparison with other animal models, *Bone,* 16 (4 Suppl.), 277S, 1995.

45. Yoshitake, H. et al., Osteopontin-deficient mice are resistant to ovariectomy-induced bone resorption, *Proc. Natl. Acad. Sci. U.S.A.,* 96(14), 8156, 1999.

46. Stroup, G.B. et al., Changes in bone turnover following gonadotropin-releasing hormone (GnRH) agonist administration and estrogen treatment in cynomolgus monkeys: a short-term model for evaluation of antiresorptive therapy, *Bone,* 28(5), 532, 2001.

47. Hock, J.M. and Gera, I., Effects of continuous and intermittent administration and inhibition of resorption on the anabolic response of bone to parathyroid hormone, *J. Bone Miner. Res.,* 7(1), 65, 1992.

48. Hirano, T. et al., Anabolic effects of human biosynthetic parathyroid hormone fragment (1-34), LY333334, on remodeling and mechanical properties of cortical bone in rabbits, *J. Bone Miner. Res.,* 14(4), 536, 1999.

49. Xu, J. et al., Cloning, sequencing, and functional characterization of the rat homologue of receptor activator of NF-kappaB ligand, *J. Bone Miner. Res.,* 15(11), 2178, 2000.

50. Li, M. et al., Skeletal response to corticosteroid deficiency and excess in growing male rats, *Bone,* 19(2), 81, 1996.

51. Movsowitz, C. et al., Cyclosporin-A *in vivo* produces severe osteopenia in the rat: effect of dose and duration of administration, *Endocrinology,* 123(5), 2571, 1988.

52. Jiang, Y. et al., Long-term changes in bone mineral and biomechanical properties of vertebrae and femur in aging, dietary calcium restricted, and/or estrogen-deprived/-replaced rats, *J. Bone Miner. Res.,* 12(5), 820, 1997.

53. Weinreb, M. et al., Immobilization-related bone loss in the rat is increased by calcium deficiency, *Calcif. Tissue Int.,* 48(2), 93, 1991.

54. McLean, W. and Olsen, B.R., Mouse models of abnormal skeletal development and homeostasis, *Trends Genet.,* 17(10), S38, 2001.

55. Jilka, R.L. et al., Linkage of decreased bone mass with impaired osteoblastogenesis in a murine model of accelerated senescence, *J. Clin. Invest.,* 97(7), 1732, 1996.

56. Beamer, W.G. et al., Genetic variability in adult bone density among inbred strains of mice, *Bone,* 18(5), 397, 1996.

57. Rosen, C.J. et al., Circulating and skeletal insulin-like growth factor-I (IGF-I) concentrations in two inbred strains of mice with different bone mineral densities, *Bone,* 21(3), 217, 1997.

58. Kuivaniemi, H. et al., Mutations in fibrillar collagens (types I, II, III, and XI), fibril-associated collagen (type IX), and network-forming collagen (type X) cause a spectrum of diseases of bone, cartilage, and blood vessels, *Hum. Mutat.,* 9(4), 300, 1997.

59. Forlino, A. et al., Use of the Cre/*lox* recombination system to develop a non-lethal knock-in murine model for osteogenesis imperfecta with an alpha1(I) G349C substitution. Variability in phenotype in BrtlIV mice, *J. Biol. Chem.,* 274(53), 37923, 1999.

60. Pereira, R.F. et al., Marrow stromal cells as a source of progenitor cells for nonhematopoietic tissues in transgenic mice with a phenotype of osteogenesis imperfecta, *Proc. Natl. Acad. Sci. U.S.A.,* 95(3), 1142, 1998.

61. Niyibizi, C. et al., Transfer of proalpha2(I) cDNA into cells of a murine model of human osteogenesis imperfecta restores synthesis of type I collagen comprised of alpha1(I) and alpha2(I) heterotrimers *in vitro* and *in vivo,* *J. Cell Biochem.,* 83(1), 84, 2001.

62. Morey, E.R., Spaceflight and bone turnover: correlation with a new rat model of weightlessness, *Biol. Sci.,* 29, 168, 1979.

63. Wronski, T.J. and Morey, E.R., Skeletal abnormalities in rats induced by simulated weightlessness, *Metab. Bone Dis. Relat. Res.,* 4, 69, 1982.

64. Wronski, T.J. and Morey-Holton, E.R., Skeletal response to simulated weightlessness: a comparison of suspension techniques, *Aviation Space Environ. Med.,* 58, 63, 1987.

65. Morey-Holton, E. and Wronski, T.J., Animal models for simulating weightlessness, *Physiologist,* 24 (6 Suppl.), S45, 1981.

66. Judex, S. and Zernicke, R.F., High-impact exercise and growing bone: relation between high strain rates and enhanced bone formation, *J. Appl. Physiol.,* 88, 2183, 2000.

67. Westerlind, K.C. et al., Effect of resistance exercise training on cortical and cancellous bone in mature male rats, *J. Appl. Physiol.,* 84(2), 459, 1998.

68. Notomi, T. et al., Effects of tower climbing exercise on bone mass, strength, and turnover in growing rats, *J. Bone Miner. Res.,* 16(1), 166, 2001.

69. Yarasheski, K.E., Effect of heavy-resistance exercise training on muscle fiber composition in young rats, *J. Appl. Physiol.,* 69, 434, 1990.

70. Duncan, N.D. et al., Adaptation in rat skeletal muscle following long-term resistance exercise training, *Eur. J. App. Physiol.,* 77, 372, 1998.

71. Yao, W. et al., Erect bipedal stance exercise partially prevents orchidectomy-induced bone loss in the lumbar vertebrae of rats, *Bone,* 27(5), 667, 2000.

72. Chen, J.L. et al., Bipedal stance exercise enhances antiresorption effects of estrogen and counteracts its inhibitory effect on bone formation in sham and ovariectomized rats, *Bone,* 29(2), 126, 2001.

73. Turner, C.H. et al., A noninvasive, *in vivo* model for studying strain adaptive bone modeling, *Bone,* 12, 73, 1991.

74. Torrance, A.G. et al., Noninvasive loading of the rat ulna *in vivo* induces a strain-related modeling response uncomplicated by trauma or periosteal pressure, *Calcif. Tissue Int.,* 54, 241, 1994.

75. Gross, T.S. et al., Noninvasive loading of the murine tibia: an *in vivo* model for the study of mechanotransduction, *J. Bone Miner. Res.,* 17(3), 493, 2002.

76. Chambers, T.J. et al., Induction of bone formation in rat tail vertebrae by mechanical loading, *Bone Miner.,* 20, 167, 1993.

77. Chow, J.W. et al., Characterization of osteogenic response to mechanical stimulation in cancellous bone of rat caudal vertebrae, *Am. J. Physiol.,* 265, E340, 1993.

78. Rubin, C.T. and Lanyon, L.E., Regulation of bone formation by applied dynamic loads, *J. Bone Joint Surg.,* 66A, 397, 1984.

79. Lanyon, L.E. and Rubin, C.T., Static vs. dynamic loads as an influence on bone remodelling, *J. Biomechanics,* 17(12), 897, 1984.

80. Rubin, C.T. et al., Inhibition of osteopenia by low magnitude, high-frequency mechanical stimuli, *Drug Discuss. Today,* 6(16), 848, 2001.

81. Goodship, A.E. et al., Functional adaptation of bone to increased stress, *J. Bone Joint Surg.,* 61A, 539, 1979.

82. Lanyon, L.E. et al., Mechanically adaptive bone remodelling, *J. Biomechanics,* 15(3), 141, 1982.

83. Winet, H. and Albrektsson, T., Wound healing in the bone chamber. 1. Neoosteogenesis during transition fron the repair to the regenerative phase in the rabbit tibial cortex, *J. Orthoped. Res.,* 6, 531, 1988.

84. Guldberg, R.E. et al., Mechanical stimulation of tissue repair in the hydraulic bone chamber, *J. Bone Miner. Res.,* 12, 1295, 1997.

85. Aspenberg, P. et al., Local application of growth-factor IGF-1 to healing bone, *Acta Orthoped. Scand.,* 60, 607, 1989.

86. Moalli, M.R. et al., An *in vivo* model for investigations of mechanical signal transduction in trabecular bone, *J. Bone Miner. Res.,* 15(7), 1346, 2000.

87. Nunamaker, D.M., Experimental models of fracture repair, *Clin. Orthoped.,* 355S, S56, 1998.

88. Urist, M.R. and McLean, F.C., Calcification and ossification. I. Calcification in the callus in healing fractures in normal rats, *J. Bone Joint Surg.,* 23, 1, 1941.

89. Ekeland, A. et al., Mechanical properties of fractured and intact rat femora evaluated by bending, torsional and tensile tests, *Acta Orthoped. Scand.,* 52, 605, 1981.

90. Jackson, R.W. et al., Production of a standard experimental fracture, *Can. J. Surg.,* 13, 415, 1970.

91. Greiff, J., A method for the production of an undisplaced reproducible tibial fracture in the rat, *Injury,* 9, 278, 1978.

92. Bonnarens, F. and Einhorn, A., Production of a standard closed fracture in laboratory animal bone, *J. Orthoped. Res.,* 2, 97, 1984.

93. An, Y. et al., Production of a standard closed fracture in the rat tibia, *J. Orthoped. Trauma,* 8(2), 111, 1994.

94. Hiltunen, A. et al., A standardized experimental fracture in the mouse tibia, *J. Orthoped. Res.,* 11, 305, 1993.

95. Ekholm, E. et al., Diminished callus size and cartilage synthesis in alpha1beta1 integrin-deficient mice during bone fracture healing, *Am. J. Pathol.,* 160(5), 1779, 2002.

96. Isefuku, S. et al., A murine model of distraction osteogenesis, *Bone,* 27(5), 661, 2000.

97. Barou, O. et al., High-resolution three-dimensional micro-computed tomography detects bone loss and changes in trabecular architecture early: comparison with DEXA and bone histomorphometry in a rat model of disuse osteoporosis, *Invest. Radiol.,* 37(1), 40, 2002.

98. Paulus, M.J. et al., A review of high-resolution x-ray computed tomography and other imaging modalities for small animal research, *Lab. Anim.,* 30(3), 36, 2001.

99. Turner, C.H. and Burr, D.B., Basic biomechanical measurements of bone: a tutorial, *Bone,* 14(4), 595, 1993.

100. Athanasiou, K.A. et al., Fundamentals of biomechanics in tissue engineering of bone, *Tissue Eng.,* 6(4), 361, 2000.

101. Villanueva, A.R. et al., Bone and cell dynamics in the osteoporoses: a review of measurements by tetracycline bone labeling, *Clin. Orthoped.,* 49, 135, 1966.

102. Calvo, M.S. et al., Molecular basis and clinical application of biological markers of bone turnover, *Endocr. Rev.,* 17(4), 333, 1996.

103. Mundlos, S. and Olsen, B.R., Heritable diseases of the skeleton. Part I. Molecular insights into skeletal development-transcription factors and signaling pathways, *FASEB J.,* 11(2), 125, 1997.

104. Erlebacher, A. et al., Toward a molecular understanding of skeletal development, *Cell,* 80(3), 371, 1995.

105. Nakashima, K. et al., The novel zinc finger-containing transcription factor osterix is required for osteoblast differentiation and bone formation, *Cell,* 108(1), 17, 2002.

106. Jacenko, O. et al., Of mice and men: heritable skeletal disorders, *Am. J. Hum. Genet.,* 54(2), 163, 1994.

107. Mundlos, S. and Olsen, B.R., Heritable diseases of the skeleton. Part II. Molecular insights into skeletal development-matrix components and their homeostasis, *FASEB J.,* 11(4), 227, 1997.

108. Cohn, D.H., Defects in extracellular matrix structural proteins in the osteochondrodysplasias, *Novartis Found. Symp.,* 232, 195, 2001.

109. Rauch, F. and Schoenau, E., The developing bone: slave or master of its cells and molecules?, *Pediatr. Res.,* 50(3), 309, 2001.

110. Chan, D. and Jacenko, O., Phenotypic and biochemical consequences of collagen X mutations in mice and humans, *Matrix Biol.,* 17(3), 169, 1998.

111. Olsen, B.R., Mutations in collagen genes resulting in metaphyseal and epiphyseal dysplasias, *Bone,* 17(2 Suppl.), 45S, 1995.

112. Iwata, T. et al., Highly activated Fgfr3 with the K644M mutation causes prolonged survival in severe dwarf mice, *Hum. Mol. Genet.,* 10(12), 1255, 2001.

113. Jacenko, O. et al., Spondylometaphyseal dysplasia in mice carrying a dominant negative mutation in a matrix protein specific for cartilage-to-bone transition, *Nature,* 365(6441), 56, 1993.

114. Bi, W. et al., Haploinsufficiency of Sox9 results in defective cartilage primordia and premature skeletal mineralization, *Proc. Natl. Acad. Sci. U.S.A.,* 703(12), 6698, 2001

115. Fukui, N. et al., Cell biology of osteoarthritis: the chondrocyte's response to injury, *Curr. Rheumatol. Rep.,* 3(6), 496, 2001.

116. Schwartz, E.R., Animal models: a means to study the pathogenesis of osteoarthritis, *J. Rheumatol.,* 14, 101, 1987.

117. van den Berg, W.B., Lessons from animal models of osteoarthritis, *Curr. Opin. Rheumatol.,* 13(5), 452, 2001.

118. Athanasiou, K.A. et al., Interspecies comparisons of *in situ* intrinsic mechanical properties of distal femoral cartilage, *J. Orthoped. Res.,* 9(3), 330, 1991.

119. Cremer, M.A. et al., The cartilage collagens: a review of their structure, organization, and role in the pathogenesis of experimental arthritis in animals and in human rheumatic disease, *J. Mol. Med.,* 76(3-4), 275, 1998.

120. Myers, L.K. et al., Collagen-induced arthritis, an animal model of autoimmunity, *Life Sci.,* 61(19), 1861, 1997.

121. Stuart, J.M. et al., Nature and specificity of the immune response to collagen in type II collagen-induced arthritis in mice, *J. Clin. Invest.,* 69(3), 673, 1982.

122. Trentham, D.E. et al., Autoimmunity to type II collagen: an experimental model of arthritis, *J. Exp. Med.,* 146(3), 857, 1977.

123. Wilder, R.L., Hormones and autoimmunity: animal models of arthritis, *Baillieres Clin. Rheumatol.,* 10(2), 259, 1996.

124. Anthony, D.D. and Haqqi, T.M., Collagen-induced arthritis in mice: an animal model to study the pathogenesis of rheumatoid arthritis, *Clin. Exp. Rheumatol.,* 17(2), 240, 1999.

125. Bendele, A. et al., Animal models of arthritis: relevance to human disease, *Toxicol. Pathol.,* 27(1), 134, 1999.

126. Joe, B. et al., Animal models of rheumatoid arthritis and related inflammation, *Curr. Rheumatol. Rep.,* 1(2), 139, 1999.

127. Taneja, V. and David, C.S., HLA transgenic mice as humanized mouse models of disease and immunity., *J. Clin. Invest.,* 101(5), 921, 1998.

128. Caulfield, J.P. et al., Morphologic demonstration of two stages in the development of type II collagen-induced arthritis, *Lab. Invest.,* 46(3), 321, 1982.

129. Arnett, F.C. and Chakraborty, R., Ankylosing spondylitis: the dissection of a complex genetic disease, *Arthritis Rheum.,* 40(10), 1746, 1997.

130. Khare, S.D. et al., HLA-B27 and other predisposing factors in spondyloarthropathies, *Curr. Opin. Rheumatol.,* 10(4), 282, 1998.

131. Bremell, T. et al., Experimental *Staphylococcus aureus* arthritis in mice, *Infect. Immunol.*, 59(8), 2615, 1991.

132. Khare, S.D. et al., Animal models of human leukocyte antigen B27-linked arthritides HLA-B27 and other predisposing factors in spondyloarthropathies, *Rheum. Dis. Clin. North Am.*, 24(4), 883, 1998.

133. Patti, J.M. et al., The *Staphylococcus aureus* collagen adhesin is a virulence determinant in experimental septic arthritis, *Infect. Immunol.*, 62(1), 152, 1994.

134. Avina-Zubieta, J.A. et al., Rheumatic manifestations of hematologic disorders, *Curr. Opin. Rheumatol.*, 10(1), 86, 1998.

135. Jean-Baptiste, G. and De Ceulaer, K., Osteoarticular disorders of haematological origin, *Baillieres Best Pract. Res. Clin. Rheumatol.*, 14(2), 307, 2000.

136. O'Driscoll, S.W., The healing and regeneration of articular cartilage, *J. Bone Joint Surg. Am.*, 80(12), 1795, 1998.

137. Breinan, H.A. et al., Effect of cultured autologous chondrocytes on repair of chondral defects in a canine model, *J. Bone Joint Surg.*, 79(10), 1439, 1997.

138. Radin, E.L. et al., Effects of mechanical loading on the tissues of the rabbit knee, *J. Orthoped. Res.*, 2(3), 221, 1984.

139. Buckwalter, J.A., Evaluating methods of restoring cartilaginous articular surfaces, *Clin. Orthoped.*, (367 Suppl.), S224, 1999.

140. Akizuki, S. et al., Tensile properties of human knee joint cartilage. II. Correlations between weight bearing and tissue pathology and the kinetics of swelling, *J. Orthoped. Res.*, 5(2), 173, 1987.

141. Hunziker, E.B., Biologic repair of articular cartilage. Defect models in experimental animals and matrix requirements, *Clin. Orthoped.*, (367 Suppl.), S135, 1999.

142. Hecht, J.T. et al., Mutations in exon 17B of cartilage oligomeric matrix protein (COMP) cause pseudoachondroplasia, *Nat. Genet.*, 10(3), 325, 1995.

143. Yoshitake, H. et al., Osteopontin-deficient mice are resistant to ovariectomy-induced bone loss, *Proc. Natl. Acad. Sci. U.S.A.*, 96(14), 8156, 1999.

144. Ishijima, M. et al., Enhancement of osteoclastic bone resorption and suppression of osteoblastic bone formation in response to reduced mechanical stress do not occur in the absence of osteopontin, *J. Exp. Med.*, 193(3), 399, 2001.

145. Spurney, R.F. et al., Anabolic effects of a G protein-coupled receptor kinase inhibitor expressed in osteoblasts, *J. Clin. Invest.*, 109(10), 1361, 2002.

146. Sabatakos, G. et al., Overexpression of DeltaFosB transcription factor(s) increases bone formation and inhibits adipogenesis, *Nat. Med.*, 6(9), 985, 2000.

147. Jochum, W. et al., Increased bone formation and osteosclerosis in mice overexpressing the transcription factor Fra-1, *Nat. Med.*, 6(9), 980, 2000.

148. Zhao, G. et al., Targeted overexpression of insulin-like growth factor I to osteoblasts of transgenic mice: increased trabecular bone volume without increased osteoblast proliferation, *Endocrinology*, 141(7), 2674, 2000.

149. Gardiner, E.M. et al., Increased formation and decreased resorption of bone in mice with elevated vitamin D receptor in mature cells of the osteoblastic lineage, *FASEB J.*, 14(13), 1908, 2000.

150. Rajapurohitam, V. et al., The mouse osteopetrotic grey-lethal mutation induces a defect in osteoclast maturation/function, *Bone*, 28(5), 513, 2001.

151. Soriano, P. et al., Targeted disruption of the c-src proto-oncogene leads to osteopetrosis in mice, *Cell*, 64(4), 693, 1991.

152. Wang, Z.Q. et al., Bone and haematopoietic defects in mice lacking c-fos, *Nature*, 360(6406), 741, 1992.

153. Gowen, M. et al., Cathepsin K knockout mice develop osteopetrosis due to a deficit in matrix degradation but not demineralization, *J. Bone Miner. Res.*, 14(10), 1654, 1999.

154. Kong, Y.Y. et al., OPGL is a key regulator of osteoclastogenesis, lymphocyte development and lymph-node organogenesis, *Nature*, 397(6717), 315, 1999.

155. Dougall, W.C. et al., RANK is essential for osteoclast and lymph node development, *Genes Dev.*, 13(18), 2412, 1999.

156. Hayman, A.R. et al., Mice lacking tartrate-resistant acid phosphatase (Acp 5) have disrupted endochondral ossification and mild osteopetrosis, *Development*, 122(10), 3151, 1996.

157. Lomaga, M.A. et al., TRAF6 deficiency results in osteopetrosis and defective interleukin-1, CD40, and LPS signaling, *Genes Dev.,* 13(8), 1015, 1999.

158. McHugh, K.P. et al., Mice lacking beta3 integrins are osteosclerotic because of dysfunctional osteo-clasts, *J. Clin. Invest.,* 105(4), 433, 2000.

159. Dai, X.-M. et al., Targeted disruption of the mouse colony-stimulating factor 1 receptor gene results in osteopetrosis, mononuclear phagocyte deficiency, increased primitive progenitor cell frequencies, and reproductive defects, *Blood,* 99(1), 111, 2002.

160. Hsu, H.L. et al., Tumor necrosis factor receptor family member RANK mediates osteoclast differen-tiation and activation induced by osteoprotegerin ligand, *Proc. Natl. Acad. Sci. U.S.A.,* (7), 3540, 1999.

161. Dobbins, D.E. et al., Mutation of macrophage colony stimulating factor (Csf1) causes osteopetrosis in the tl rat, *Biochem. Biophys. Res. Commun.,* 294(5), 1114, 2002.

162. Marks, S.C., Jr., Osteopetrosis in the IA rat cured by spleen cells from a normal littermate, *Am. J. Anat.,* 146(3), 331, 1976.

163. Marks, S.C., Jr. and Popoff, S.N., Osteoclast biology in the osteopetrotic (op) rat, *Am. J. Anat.,* 186(4), 325, 1989.

164. Cielinski, M.J. and Marks, S.C., Jr., Neonatal reductions in osteoclast number and function account for the transient nature of osteopetrosis in the rat mutation microphthalmia blanc (mib), *Bone,* 15(6), 707, 1994.

165. Oz, O.K. et al., Bone has a sexually dimorphic response to aromatase deficiency, *J. Bone Miner. Res.,* 15(3), 507, 2000.

166. Sims, N.A. et al., Deletion of estrogen receptors reveals a regulatory role for estrogen receptors-[beta] in bone remodeling in females but not in males, *Bone,* 30(1), 18, 2002.

167. Mizuno, A. et al., Severe osteoporosis in mice lacking osteoclastogenesis inhibitory factor/osteopro-tegerin, *Biochem. Biophys. Res. Commun.,* 247(3), 610, 1998.

168. Li, B. et al., Mice deficient in Abl are osteoporotic and have defects in osteoblast maturation, *Nat. Genet.,* 24(3), 304, 2000.

169. Ogata, N. et al., Insulin receptor substrate-1 in osteoblast is indispensable for maintaining bone turnover, *J. Clin. Invest.,* 105(7), 935, 2000.

170. Xu, T. et al., Targeted disruption of the biglycan gene leads to an osteoporosis-like phenotype in mice, *Nat. Genet.,* 20(1), 78, 1998.

171. Delany, A.M. et al., Osteopenia and decreased bone formation in osteonectin-deficient mice, *J. Clin. Invest.,* 105(7), 915, 2000.

172. Kawaguchi, H. et al., Independent impairment of osteoblast and osteoclast differentiation in klotho mouse exhibiting low-turnover osteopenia, *J. Clin. Invest.,* 104(3), 229, 1999.

173. Holmbeck, K. et al., MT1-MMP-deficient mice develop dwarfism, osteopenia, arthritis, and connective tissue disease due to inadequate collagen turnover, *Cell,* 99(1), 81, 1999.

174. Armour, K.E. et al., Defective bone formation and anabolic response to exogenous estrogen in mice with targeted disruption of endothelial nitric oxide synthase, *Endocrinology,* 142(2), 760, 2001.

175. Montero, A. et al., Disruption of the fibroblast growth factor-2 gene results in decreased bone mass and bone formation, *J. Clin. Invest.,* 105(8), 1085, 2000.

176. Bikle, D. et al., The skeletal structure of insulin-like growth factor I-deficient mice, *J. Bone Miner. Res.,* 16(12), 2320, 2001.

177. Zimmerman, D. et al., Impaired bone formation in transgenic mice resulting from altered integrin function in osteoblasts, *Dev. Biol.,* 220(1), 2, 2000.

178. Liu, W. et al., Overexpression of Cbfa1 in osteoblasts inhibits osteoblast maturation and causes osteopenia with multiple fractures, *J. Cell Biol.,* 155(1), 157, 2001.

179. Corral, D.A. et al., Dissociation between bone resorption and bone formation in osteopenic transgenic mice, *Proc. Natl. Acad. Sci. U.S.A.,* 95(23), 13835, 1998.

180. Angel, N.Z. et al., Transgenic mice overexpressing tartrate-resistant acid phosphatase exhibit an increased rate of bone turnover, *J. Bone Miner. Res.,* 15(1), 103, 2000.

181. Erlebacher, A. and Derynck, R., Increased expression of TGF-beta 2 in osteoblasts results in an osteoporosis-like phenotype, *J. Cell Biol.,* 132 (1–2), 195, 1996.

182. Bonadio, J. et al., Transgenic mouse model of the mild dominant form of osteogenesis imperfecta, *Proc. Natl. Acad. Sci. U.S.A.,* 87(18), 7145, 1990.

183. Chipman, S.D. et al., Defective pro alpha 2(I) collagen synthesis in a recessive mutation in mice: a model of human osteogenesis imperfecta, *Proc. Natl. Acad. Sci. U.S.A.,* 90(5), 1701, 1993.

184. Sillence, D.O. et al., Fragilitas ossium (fro/fro) in the mouse: a model for a recessively inherited type of osteogenesis imperfecta, *Am. J. Med. Genet.,* 45(2), 276, 1993.

185. Stacey, A. et al., Perinatal lethal osteogenesis imperfecta in transgenic mice bearing an engineered mutant pro-alpha 1(I) collagen gene, *Nature,* 332(6160), 131, 1988.

186. Khillan, J.S.F. et al., Transgenic mice that express a mini-gene version of the human gene for type I procollagen (COL1A1) develop a phenotype resembling a lethal form of osteogenesis imperfecta, *J. Biol. Chem.,* 266(34), 23373, 1991.

187. Zerath, E. et al., Spaceflight inhibits bone formation independent of corticosteroid status in growing rats, *J. Bone Miner. Res.,*15(7), 1310, 2000.

188. Turner, R.T. et al., Evidence for arrested bone formation during spaceflight, *Physiologist,* 24 (6 Suppl.), S97, 1981.

189. Weinreb, M. et al., Osteopenia in the immobilized rat hind limb is associated with increased bone resorption and decreased bone formation, *Bone,* 10(3), 187, 1989.

190. Turner, R.T. and Bell, N.H., The effects of immobilization on bone histomorphometry in rats, *J. Bone Miner. Res.,* 1(5), 399, 1986.

191. Kaneps, A.J. et al., Changes in canine cortical and cancellous bone mechanical properties following immobilization and remobilization with exercise, *Bone,* 21(5), 419, 1997.

192. Li, X.J. et al., Adaptation of cancellous bone to aging and immobilization in the rat: a single photon absorptiometry and histomorphometry study, *Anat. Rec.,* 227, 12, 1990.

193. Wronski, T.J. and Morey, E.R., Inhibition of cortical and trabecular bone-formation in the long bones of immobilized monkeys, *Clin. Orthoped.,* (181), 269, 1983.

194. Klein, L. et al., Isotopic evidence for resorption of soft tissues and bone in immobilized dogs, *J. Bone Joint Surg.,* 64A(2), 225, 1982.

195. Simske, S.J. et al., Age dependent development of osteopenia in the long bones of tail-suspended mice, *Biomed. Sci. Instrum.,* 26, 87, 1990.

196. Garber, M.A. et al., Bone loss during simulated weightlessness: a biomechanical and mineralization study in the rat model, *Aviation Space Environ. Med.,* 71(6), 586, 2000.

197. Young, D.R. et al., Immobilization-associated osteoporosis in primates, *Bone,* 7(2), 109, 1986.

198. Muths, E. and Reichman, O.J., Kangaroo rat bone compared to white rat bone after short-term disuse and exercise, *Comp. Biochem. Physiol.,* 114A, 355, 1996.

199. Hart, K.J. et al., Swim-trained rats have greater bone mass, density, strength, and dynamics, *J. Appl. Physiol.,* 91, 1663, 2001.

200. Kim, C. et al., Prolonged swimming exercise training induce hypophosphatemic osteopenia in stroke-prone spontaneously hypertensive rats (SHRSP), *J. Physiol. Anthropol. App. Hum. Sci.,*19(6), 271, 2000.

201. Swissa-Sivan, A. et al., Effect of swimming on bone growth and development in young rats, *Bone Miner.,* 7, 91, 1989.

202. Swissa-Sivan, A. et al., The effect of swimming on bone modeling and composition in young adult rats, *Calcif. Tissue Int.,* 47, 173, 1990.

203. Wu, J. et al., Cooperative effects of exercise training and genistein administration on bone mass in ovariectomized mice, *J. Bone Miner. Res.,* 16(10), 1829, 2001.

204. Iwamoto, J. et al., Differential effect of treadmill exercise on three cancellous bone sites in the young growing rat, *Bone,* 24(3), 163, 1999.

205. Iwamoto, J. et al., Effect of deconditioning on cortical and cancellous bone growth in the exercise trained young rats, *J. Bone Miner. Res.,* 15(9), 1842, 2001.

206. Van Der Wiel, H.E. et al., Additional weight-bearing during exercise is more important than duration of exercise for anabolic stimulus of bone: a study of runnung exercise in female rats, *Bone,* 16(1), 73, 1995.

207. Bravenboer, N. et al., The effect of exercise on systemic and bone concentrations of growth factors in rats, *J. Orthoped. Res.,* 19, 945, 2001.

208. Tamaki, H. et al., Effects of exercise training and etidronate treatment on bone mineral density and trabecular bone in ovariectomized rats, *Bone,* 23(2), 147, 1998.

209. Gala, J. et al., Short- and long-term effects of calcium and exercise on bone mineral density in ovariectomized rats, *Br. J. Nutr.,* 86, 521, 2001.

210. Verhaeghe, J. et al., Effects of exercise and disuse on bone remodeling, bone mass, and biomechanical competence in spontaneously diabetic female rats, *Bone,* 27(2), 249, 2000.

211. Judex, S. and Zernicke, R.F., Does the mechanical milieu associated with high-speed running lead to adaptive changes in diaphyseal growing bone?, *Bone,* 26(2), 153, 2000.

212. Mosekilde, L.I. et al., Additive effect of voluntary exercise and growth hormone treatment on bone strength assessed at four different skeletal sites in an aged rat model, *Bone,* 24(2), 71, 1999.

213. Banu, J. et al., Analysis of the effects of growth hormone, exercise, and food restriction on cancellous bone in different bone sites in middle-aged female rats, *Mech. Ageing Dev.,* 122, 849, 2001.

214. Judex, S. and Zernicke, R.F., High-impact exercise and growning bone: relation between high strain rates and enhanced bone formation, *J. Appl. Physiol.,* 88, 2183, 2000.

215. Umemura, Y. et al., Five jumps per day increase bone mass and breaking force in rats, *J. Bone Miner. Res.,* 12(9), 1480, 1997.

216. Bennell, K. et al., Effects of resistance training on bone paramaters in young and mature rats, *Clin. Exp. Pharmacol. Physiol.,* 27, 88, 2000.

217. Chen, J.L. et al., Bipedal stance exercise enhances antiresorption effects of estrogen and counteracts its inhibitory effect on bone formation in sham and ovariectomized rats, *Bone,* 29(2), 126, 2001.

218. Jarvinen, T.L. et al., Randomized controlled study of effects of sudden impact loading on rat femur, *J. Bone Miner. Res.,* 13(9), 1475, 1998.

219. Rubin, C.T. and Lanyon, L.E., Regulation of bone mass by mechanical strain magnitude, *Calcif. Tissue Int.,* 37, 411, 1985.

220. Slatis, P. and Rokkanen, P., The normal repair of experimental fractures, *Acta Orthoped. Scand.,* 36, 221, 1965.

221. Karp, N.S. et al., Membranous bone lengthening: a serial histologic study, *Ann. Plast. Surg.,* 29(1), 2, 1992.

222. Welch, R.D. et al., Histomorphometry of distraction osteogenesis in a caprine tibial lengthening model, *J. Bone Miner. Res.,* 13(1), 1, 1998.

223. Radomisli, T.E. et al., Weight-bearing alters the expression of collagen types I and II, BMP 2/4 and osteocalcin in the early stages of distraction osteogenesis, *J. Orthoped. Res.,* 19(6), 1049, 2001.

224. Richards, M. et al., Increased distraction rates influence precursor tissue composition without affecting bone regeneration, *J. Bone Miner. Res.,* 15(5), 982, 2000.

225. Aronson, J. et al., The effect of aging on distraction osteogenesis in the rat, *J. Orthoped. Res.,* 19(3), 421, 2001.

226. Paccione, M.F. et al., Rat mandibular distraction osteogenesis: latency, rate, and rhythm determine the adaptive response, *J. Craniofac. Surg.,* 12(2), 175, 2001.

227. Tavakoli, K. et al., Expression of growth factors in the mandibular distraction zone: a sheep study, *Br. J. Plast. Surg.,* 52, 434, 1999.

228. Riser, W.H. et al., Pseudoachondroplastic dysplasia in miniature poodles: clinical, radiologic, and pathologic features, *J. Am Vet. Med. Assoc.,* 176(4), 335, 1980.

229. Vertel, B.M. et al., The chondrodystrophy, nanomelia: biosynthesis and processing of the defective aggrecan precursor, *Biochem. J.,* 301(Pt. 1), 211, 1994.

230. Watanabe, H. et al., Mouse cartilage matrix deficiency (cmd) caused by a 7 bp deletion in the aggrecan gene, *Nat. Genet.,* 7(2), 154, 1994.

231. Sweet, H.O. and Bronson, R.T., Osteochondrodystrophy (ocd): a new autosomal recessive mutation in the mouse, *J. Hered.,* 82(2), 140, 1991.

232. Watanabe, H. and Yamada, Y., Mice lacking link protein develop dwarfism and craniofacial abnormalities, *Nat. Genet.,* 21(2), 225, 1999.

233. Arikawa-Hirasawa, E. et al., Perlecan is essential for cartilage and cephalic development, *Nat. Genet.,* 23(3), 354, 1999.

234. Costell, M. et al., Perlecan maintains the integrity of cartilage and some basement membranes, *J. Cell Biol.,* 147(5), 1109, 1999.

235. Vu, T.H. et al., MMP-9/gelatinase B is a key regulator of growth plate angiogenesis and apoptosis of hypertrophic chondrocytes, *Cell,* 93(3), 411, 1998.

236. Karaplis, A.C. et al., Lethal skeletal dysplasia from targeted disruption of the parathyroid hormone-related peptide gene, *Genes Dev.*, 8(3), 277, 1994.

237. Lanske, B. et al., PTH/PTHrP receptor in early development and Indian hedgehog-regulated bone growth, *Science*, 273(5275), 663, 1996.

238. Reimold, A.M. et al., Chondrodysplasia and neurological abnormalities in ATF-2-deficient mice, *Nature,* 379(6562), 262, 1996.

239. Li, S.W. et al., Transgenic mice with targeted inactivation of the Col2 alpha 1 gene for collagen II develop a skeleton with membranous and periosteal bone but no endochondral bone, *Genes Dev.,* 9(22), 2821, 1995.

240. Kwan, K.M. et al., Abnormal compartmentalization of cartilage matrix components in mice lacking collagen X: implications for function, *J. Cell Biol.,* 136(2), 459, 1997.

241. Schipani, E. et al., Targeted expression of constitutively active receptors for parathyroid hormone and parathyroid hormone-related peptide delays endochondral bone formation and rescues mice that lack parathyroid hormone-related peptide, *Proc. Natl. Acad. Sci. U.S.A.,* 94(25), 13689, 1997.

242. Calvi, L.M. and Schipani, E., The PTH/PTHrP receptor in Jansen's metaphyseal chondrodysplasia, *J. Endocrinol. Invest.,* 23(8), 545, 2000.

243. Tsumaki, N. et al., Role of CDMP-1 in skeletal morphogenesis: promotion of mesenchymal cell recruitment and chondrocyte differentiation, *J. Cell Biol.,* 144(1), 161, 1999.

244. Nii, A. et al., Osteochondrodysplasia occurring in transgenic mice expressing interferon-gamma, *Vet. Pathol.,* 34(5), 431, 1997.

245. Nielsen, V.H. et al., Abnormal growth plate function in pigs carrying a dominant mutation in type X collagen, *Mamm. Genome*, 11(12), 1087, 2000.

246. Kikukawa, K. et al., Electron microscopic observations and electrophoresis of the glycosaminoglycans in the epiphyseal cartilage of the congenital osteochondrodysplasia rat (ocd/ocd), *Matrix,* 10(6), 378, 1990.

247. Pateder, D.B. et al., The role of autocrine growth factors in radiation damage to the epiphyseal growth plate, *Radiat. Res.,* 155(6), 847, 2001.

248. Standeven, A.M. et al., Retinoid-induced epiphyseal plate closure in guinea pigs, *Fundam. Appl. Toxicol.,* 34(1), 91, 1996.

249. Lee, M.A. et al., Utilization of a murine model to investigate the molecular process of transphyseal bone formation, *J. Pediatr. Orthoped.,* 20(6), 802, 2000.

250. Johnstone, E.W. et al., The effect of osteogenic protein-1 in an *in vivo* physeal injury model, *Clin. Orthoped.,* 395, 234, 2002.

251. Peskin, B. et al., Transphyseal osseous bridges in experimental osteonecrosis of the femoral head of the rat. Histologic study of the bony bridges connecting the epiphyseal with the metaphyseal bony trabeculae through gaps in the physeal cartilage, *J. Pediatr. Orthoped.,* 10(3), 214, 2001.

252. Marijnissen, A.C. et al., The canine "groove" model, compared with the ACLT model of osteoarthritis, *Osteoarthritis Cartilage,* 10(2), 145, 2002.

253. Pond, M.J. and Nuki, G., Experimentally-induced osteoarthritis in the dog, *Ann. Rheum. Dis.,* 32(4), 387, 1973

254. Schwartz, E.R. et al., Experimentally induced osteoarthritis in guinea pigs: metabolic responses in articular cartilage to developing pathology, *Arthritis Rheum.,* 24(11), 1345, 1981.

255. Arsever, C.L. and Bole, G.G., Experimental osteoarthritis induced by selective myectomy and tendotomy, *Arthritis Rheum.,* 29(2), 251, 1986.

256. de Bri, E. et al., Primary osteoarthrosis in guinea pigs: a stereological study, *J. Orthoped. Res.,* 13(5), 769, 1995.

257. Yamamoto, H. and Iwase, N., Spontaneous osteoarthritic lesions in a new mutant strain of the mouse, *Exp. Anim.,* 47(2), 131, 1998.

258. Mason, R.M. et al., The STR/ort mouse and its use as a model of osteoarthritis, *Osteoarthritis Cartilage,* 9(2), 85, 2001.

259. Fassler, R. et al., Mice lacking alpha 1 (IX) collagen develop noninflammatory degenerative joint disease, *Proc. Natl. Acad. Sci. U.S.A.,* 91(11), 5070, 1994.

260. Nakata, K. et al., Osteoarthritis associated with mild chondrodysplasia in transgenic mice expressing alpha 1(IX) collagen chains with a central deletion, *Proc. Natl. Acad. Sci. U.S.A.,* 90(7), 2870, 1993.

261. Lapvetelainen, T. et al., More knee joint osteoarthritis (OA) in mice after inactivation of one allele of type II procollagen gene but less OA after lifelong voluntary wheel running exercise, *Osteoarthritis Cartilage,* 9(2), 152, 2001.

262. Neuhold, L.A. et al., Postnatal expression in hyaline cartilage of constitutively active human colla-genase-3 (MMP-13) induces osteoarthritis in mice, *J. Clin. Invest.,* 107(1), 35, 2001.

263. Tsai, C.L. and Liu, T.K., Estradiol-induced knee osteoarthrosis in ovariectomized rabbits, *Clin. Orthoped.,* 291, 295, 1993.

264. Colombo, C. et al., A new model of osteoarthritis in rabbits. I. Development of knee joint pathology following lateral meniscectomy and section of the fibular collateral and sesamoid ligaments, *Arthritis Rheum.,* 26(7), 875, 1993.

265. Ehrlich, M.G. et al., Biochemical confirmation of an experimental osteoarthritis model, *J. Bone Joint Surg.,* 57(3), 392, 1975.

266. Kikuchi, T. et al., Intra-articular injection of collagenase induces experimental osteoarthritis in mature rabbits, *Osteoarthritis Cartilage,* 6(3), 177, 1998.

267. Lozoya, K.A. and Flores, J.B., A novel rat osteoarthrosis model to assess apoptosis and matrix degradation, *Pathol. Res. Pract.,* 196(11), 729, 2000.

268. Pap, G. et al., Development of osteoarthritis in the knee joints of Wistar rats after strenuous running exercise in a running wheel by intracranial self-stimulation, *Pathol. Res. Pract.,* 194(1), 41, 1998.

269. Ghosh, P. et al., The influence of weight-bearing exercise on articular cartilage of meniscectomized joints. An experimental study in sheep, *Clin. Orthoped.,* 252, 101, 1990.

270. Phillips, T.W. and Gurr, K., A preconditioned arthritic hip model, *J. Arthrop.,* 4(3), 193, 1989.

271. Allen, H.L. and Newton, C.D., Animal model of human disease. Juvenile rheumatoid arthritis. Animal model: rheumatoid arthritis in the dog, *Am. J. Pathol.,* 81(3), 699, 1975.

272. Knight, B. et al., Induction of adjuvant arthritis in mice, *Clin. Exp. Immunol.,* 90(3), 459, 1992.

273. Courtenay, J.S. et al., Immunisation against heterologous type II collagen induces arthritis in mice, *Nature,* 283(5748), 666, 1980.

274. Nakamura, K. et al., Spontaneous degenerative polyarthritis in male New Zealand black/KN mice, *Arthritis Rheum.,* 34(2), 171, 1991.

275. Hang, L. et al., A spontaneous rheumatoid arthritis-like disease in MRL/l mice, *J. Exp. Med.,* 155(6), 1690, 1982.

276. Cosgrove, D. et al., Mice lacking MHC class II molecules, *Cell,* 66(5), 1051, 1991.

277. Nabozny, G.H. et al., HLA-DQ8 transgenic mice are highly susceptible to collagen-induced arthritis: a novel model for human polyarthritis, *J. Exp. Med.,* 183(1), 27, 1996.

278. Mauri, C. et al., Treatment of a newly established transgenic model of chronic arthritis with nonde-pleting anti-CD4 monoclonal antibody, *J. Immunol.,* 159(10), 5032, 1997.

279. Kouskoff, V. et al., Organ-specific disease provoked by systemic autoimmunity, *Cell,* 87(5), 811, 1996.

280. Butler, D.M. et al., DBA/1 mice expressing the human TNF-alpha transgene develop a severe, erosive arthritis: characterization of the cytokine cascade and cellular composition, *J. Immunol.,* 159(6), 2867, 1997.

281. Cathcart, E.S. et al., Experimental arthritis in a nonhuman primate. I. Induction by bovine type II collagen, *Lab. Invest.,* 54(1), 26, 1986.

282. Thorp, B.H. et al., Type II collagen-immune complex arthritis in sheep: collagen antibodies in serum, synovial fluid and afferent lymph, *Clin. Exp. Rheumatol.,* 10(2), 143, 1982.

283. Vingsbo, C. et al., Pristane-induced arthritis in rats: a new model for rheumatoid arthritis with a chronic disease course influenced by both major histocompatibility complex and non-major histocom-patibility complex genes, *Am. J. Pathol.,* 149(5), 1675, 1996.

284. Geiler, V.G. et al., Comparative histology of adjuvant arthritis in rats, mice and hamsters. *Allerg. Immunol.,* 20-21(2), 251, 1974.

285. Yamazaki, H. et al., HTLV-I env-pX transgenic rats: prototype animal model for collagen vascular diseases, *Leukemia,* 11 (Suppl 3), 258, 1997.

286. Gruys, E. et al., Polyarthritis and periostitis induced by *Escherichia coli.* Lipopolysaccharide injection in young male hamsters, *J. Rheum.,* 25(4), 748, 1998.

287. Yong, Z. et al., An experimental mouse model of Yersinia-induced reactive arthritis, *Microb. Pathol.,* 4(4), 305, 1988.

288. Taurog, J.D. et al., HLA-B27 in inbred and non-inbred transgenic mice. Cell surface expression and recognition as an alloantigen in the absence of human beta 2-microglobulin, *J. Immunol.*, 141(11), 4020, 1988.

289. Khare, S.D. et al., Spontaneous inflammatory arthritis in HLA-B27 transgenic mice lacking beta 2-microglobulin: a model of human spondyloarthropathies, *J. Exp. Med.*, 182(4), 1153, 1995.

290. Zhang, Y. et al., Antibiotic prophylaxis and treatment of reactive arthritis. Lessons from an animal model, *Arthritis Rheum.*, 39(7), 1238, 1996.

291. Hammer, R.E. et al., Spontaneous inflammatory disease in transgenic rats expressing HLA-B27 and human beta 2m: an animal model of HLA-B27-associated human disorders, 63(5), 1099, 1990.

292. Taurog, J.D. et al., Susceptibility to inflammatory disease in HLA-B27 transgenic rat lines correlates with the level of B27 expression, *J. Immunol.*, 150(9), 4168, 1993.

293. Schmitz, J.L. et al., Induction of lyme arthritis in LSH hamsters, *Infect. Immunol.*, 56(9), 2336, 1998.

294. Oteo, J.A. et al., Use of the C3H/He Lyme disease mouse model for the recovery of a Spanish isolate of *Borrelia garinii* from erythema migrans lesions, *Res. Microb.*, 149(1), 39, 1998.

295. Roberts, E.D. et al., Chronic Lyme disease in the rhesus monkey, *Lab. Invest.*, 72(2), 146, 1995.

296. Smith, R.L. and Schurman, D.J., Comparison of cartilage destruction between infectious and adjuvant arthritis, *J. Orthoped. Res.*, 1(2), 136, 1983.

297. Barthold, S.W. et al., An animal model for Lyme arthritis, *Ann. N.Y. Acad. Sci.*, 539, 264, 1988.

298. Roosendaal, G. et al., Blood-induced joint damage: a canine in vivo study, *Arthritis Rheum.*, 42(5), 1033, 1999.

299. Sancho, F.G., Experimental model of haemophilic arthropathy with high pressure haemarthrosis, *Int. Orthoped.*, 4(1), 57 1980.

300. Parsons, J.R. et al., Mechanical and histological studies of acute joint hemorrhage, *Orthopedics*, 10(7), 1019, 1987.

301. Safran, M.R. et al., The effect of experimental hemarthrosis on joint stiffness and synovial histology in a rabbit model, 303, 280, 1984.

302. Altman, R.D. et al., Preliminary observations of chondral abrasion in a canine model, *Ann. Rheum. Dis.*, 51(9), 1056, 1992.

303. Shahgaldi, B.F. et al., Repair of cartilage lesions using biological implants. A comparative histological and biomechanical study in goats, *J. Bone Joint Surg.*, 73B(1), 57, 1991.

304. Hendrickson, D.A. et al., Chondrocyte-fibrin matrix transplants for resurfacing extensive articular cartilage defects, *J. Orthoped. Res.*, 12(4), 485, 1994.

305. Hunziker, E.B. et al., Chondrogenesis in cartilage repair is induced by members of the transforming growth factor-beta superfamily, *Clin. Orthoped.*, (391 Suppl.), S171, 2001.

306. Speer, D.P. et al., Enhancement of healing in osteochondral defects by collagen sponge implants, *Clin. Orthoped.*, 144, 326, 1979.

307. Grande, D.A. et al., The repair of experimentally produced defects in rabbit articular cartilage by autologous chondrocyte transplantation, *J. Orthoped. Res.*, 7(2), 208, 1989.

308. Amiel, D. et al., Rib perichondrial grafts for the repair of full-thickness articular-cartilage defects. A morphological and biochemical study in rabbits, *J. Bone Joint Surg.*, 67(6), 911, 1985.

309. Hunziker, E.B. and Rosenberg, L.C., Repair of partial-thickness defects in articular cartilage: cell recruitment from the synovial membrane, *J. Bone Joint Surg.*, 78(5), 721, 1996.

310. Rothwell, A.G., Synovium transplantation onto the cartilage denuded patellar groove of the sheep knee joint, *Orthopedics*, 13(4), 433, 1990.

CHAPTER **11**

Animal Models in Cancer Research

Jørgen Rygaard

CONTENTS

INTRODUCTION

Cancer is a common term for all malignant tumors. Cancers can be divided into main groups, depending on their origin. Tumors originating from the mesenchyme are called sarcomas. They comprise malignancies arising from connective tissue, muscle, endothelial and related tissues, and blood. Carcinomas are derived from epithelial cells. They contribute the main part of malignancies in humans, such as tumors of the skin, breast, lungs, and the gastrointestinal and urinary tracts. Also, malignant melanomas are usually included in this group, which poses the most serious problems in the clinic and therefore is given special emphasis in the experimental laboratory.

Basic characteristics of cancers in humans and in other vertebrates are the same. They show autonomous growth, disregarding the social order of the multicellular organism from which they arise. They invade locally, destroying neighbor cells and tissues; and most seriously, they can spread in the organism and form metastases. If left untreated, cancers will almost inevitably lead to the death of the individual that they form part of. Humans and animals alike fall victim to this. Therefore, animal models of cancer can be considered relevant tools in biomedical research. They can help us understand what causes cancers, how cancers develop, and, one hopes, how they can be treated. It should be stressed that much of our present-day knowledge has been achieved in the test tube or tissue culture flask, thanks to the fact that cell lines can be propagated in such circumstances and will respond to cancer-provoking stimuli, carcinogens, and therapeutic agents in much the same way as they do in the intact organism. One important aspect is lost, however, namely the interaction between the tumor and the host organism. This can be remedied by working with transplantable animal tumors in animals. But still, laboratory animals *are* animals and extrapolations have to be made from the animal model to the human situation.

This dilemma can be solved midway by using human tumor material heterotransplanted into and maintained in animals with spontaneous or induced immunodeficiencies, primarily the athymic nude mouse and rat and the severely combined immunodeficiency (SCID) mouse.

After giving a brief outline of the roots of experimental cancer research, this presentation focuses on the laboratory mouse, thereby omitting some animal models such as rat, hamster, rabbit, and dog often used in long-term carcinogenesis studies because these applications may be of more interest in toxicology.

As pointed out by Sivak,[1] "the single most cogent reason for the use of mice is the availability of a wide variety of inbred strains of markedly different properties. The use of these inbred strains, with their wide range of properties relevant to the induction of cancer, and the ability to obtain genetically known hybrid strains of mice to examine the hereditary basis for these properties, make available a unique animal resource among the small rodents that are used in carcinogenesis research." The same arguments can be expressed in relation to tumor biology studies and experimental cancer therapy. Since the statement was made, the mouse-based models have been supplemented with transgenic mice, some of which are of major interest in cancer research.

Also, successful research is strongly dependent on ready access to relevant chemicals, which today mean well-defined monoclonal antibodies and reagents to demonstrate mediators such as cytokines, probes for *in situ* hybridization, etc. The range of such reagents directed against mouse cells and molecules by far outdoes what is available against the cells and molecules of other animal species, which is another pragmatic argument for focusing on the mouse in cancer research.

ORIGIN OF EXPERIMENTAL CANCER RESEARCH

Chemical Carcinogenesis

Experimental cancer research using laboratory animal models started in 1914 with the observation by Yamagiwa and Ichakawa[2] that repeated painting of rabbits' ears with tar would lead to the formation of carcinomas of the skin, similar to squamous cell carcinomas in humans. Those investigators may have gotten their inspiration from the finding by Pott[3] 140 years earlier that former chimney-sweeper boys who had been exposed to tar and soot during infancy would in many cases develop cancers of the scrotum, again squamous cell carcinomas. The knowledge of chemical carcinogens increased over the next few years, leading to the identification of various carcinogens, such as the polycyclic hydrocarbon compound DMBA (7,12-diimethylbenz(a)anthracene), which is still one of the most used chemical carcinogens, and showing that mice also would develop skin tumors after exposure to tar products.[4] This initiated the leading role of the laboratory mouse in cancer research. Further experiments demonstrated that the efficiency of chemical carcinogens could be increased if the exposed skin was pretreated with a substance that could induce hyperplasia but that was not necessarily carcinogenic itself.[5] One such promoter that is still widely used is croton oil, which contains 12-o-tetradecanoylphorbol-13-acetate (TPA). This finding led to the establishment of the so-called two-stage or initiation–promotion model.[6]

Viral and Other Carcinogens

Today we know a range of viruses that can cause cancer in vitro and in vivo.[1,7] They comprise both DNA and RNA viruses in many species, ranging from frog to chicken, mouse, rabbit, dog, cow, and man. Although the evidence for viral carcinogenesis in man is weak, Burkitt's lymphoma is associated with the presence of Epstein-Barr virus, and some types of human papilloma virus are suspected of causing cancer of the uterine cervix.

Other well-known techniques for inducing cancers in laboratory animals include irradiation and hormone treatment.

Spontaneous Tumors

A wide range of spontaneous tumors are known to arise in laboratory animals, with the highest frequency in some inbred strains of mice,[8] but also in the laboratory rat, again showing some strain difference.[9] Spontaneous animal tumors metastasize with a species- and strain-dependent frequency that is generally lower than that of tumors in man. A large number of well-defined cultured cell lines has been established from spontaneous animal tumors and forms an important tool in experimental cancer research. The scope of this chapter does not allow detailed information on spontaneous and induced tumors in mouse and rat; that must be sought elsewhere.[8,9]

The latest addition to the field of cancer research is the demonstration of oncogenes and techniques for producing transgenic animal models with defined genetic changes that may enhance or inhibit the development of cancer. This, combined with the recently acquired knowledge of the human genome and the mouse genome, will offer research opportunities limited only by human imagination.

Readers who are particularly interested in these aspects will find ample general information in textbooks on pathology and cancer as well as on the Internet; see recommendations at the end of this chapter.

Oncogenes

In the late 1970s, a prominent group of cancer-related genes, the proto-oncogenes, was discovered; and during the next decades, several members of this group were identified. Today, more than 100 such proto-oncogenes have been described. Most oncogenes were discovered in one of the following two ways: they were the transforming genes of certain viruses able to cause cancer in laboratory animal models[10,11] or they were genes identified in DNA extracts from cancer cells that could be shown to transform mouse fibroblasts in vitro into cells with certain malignant characteristics.[12,13] The oncogenes were later shown to have a normal counterpart, called a proto-oncogene, present in all nucleated normal cells. They appear over a wide span of evolution, indicating that their functions are essential for the survival of cells.

The next step was the discovery in the early 1980s that many of the proto-oncogenes are, in fact, identical, with genes coding for growth factors, such as platelet-derived growth factor and epidermal growth factor receptor. Other proto-oncogene products have been identified as membrane-bound kinases, signal transducers, or regulators of transcription. Also, genes with a growth restriction function, which may indirectly promote growth when inactivated, have been foreseen and later described. The first member of this group, the retinoblastoma gene, *Rb,* was molecularly cloned in 1986.[14] Genes belonging to this group are also termed *anti-oncogenes* and *tumor-suppressor* genes; the latter is a somewhat misleading designation as it implies that the main role of such genes is to prevent tumors from arising. For a review, see Bishop.[15]

The genetic mutations most frequently described in human cancers occur in the p53 tumor-suppressor gene. This mutation has been constructed in transgenic mice, which have become of great importance in cancer research, as have several other transgenics.

Again, readers wanting details about these models are referred to the library services via the Internet, where one can find frequently updated lists of publications and available models.

HETEROTRANSPLANTATION MODELS

In early attempts to transplant human malignant tumors into animal hosts, the anterior eye chamber of the rabbit or the brain of heterologous species[16] and the hamster cheek pouch[17] were used for implantation. Success was reasonable as regards take, but growth time was limited, and observation of the implant was difficult. Whole-body-irradiated animals[18] or corticosteroid-treated hosts[19] rendered better possibilities for implantation in places in which the fate of the implant could be monitored, but both irradiated and hormone-treated animals were affected by the treatment, which could also influence the growth of the implants. The introduction of the athymic nude mouse in the late 1960s, of the athymic nude rat, and the SCID mouse in the early 1980s, followed by the development of the SCID-hu model, has provided important animal model possibilities for cancer research.

The following discussion describes immunomodulated and spontaneously immunodeficient models and comments on their applicability in cancer research.

Immunomodulation

Immunomodulation is an urgent issue in experimental cancer research, in part as a tool in tumor immunologic intervention but also for the establishment of heterotransplantation models.

X-Ray and Cytostatic Treatment

Agents that have a general inhibitory effect in the multicellular organism will also possess immunosuppressive characteristics. X-ray irradiation is a potent proliferation inhibitor and was — and to some extent still is — widely used as an immunosuppressant. In laboratory animal models, lethal or sublethal irradiation can be combined with transplantation of bone marrow or selected lymphocyte subpopulations. In this respect, irradiated animals are similar to animals with some congenital immunodeficiencies; see below. Side effects may occur because of irradiation of tissues or organs other than the immune system.

Drugs with a wide spectrum of action, such as cytostatic drugs and corticosteroids, will affect immune responsiveness. Their action is dose dependent within certain limits. They may however, as is the case of x-irradiation, have undesirable side effects.

Therefore, more specific approaches, depending on the part of the system that one wishes to influence, can be recommended. Such procedures will be described in relation to the cellular components of the immune system.

T-Cell Modulation

T cells are responsible for cell-mediated immune responses and are necessary to initiate B-cell responses to thymus-dependent antigens. Because T cells mature in neonatal life in the thymus (although some extrathymic development may take place), neonatal thymectomy can delete T-cell responses, as demonstrated by Miller;[20] foreign grafts are accepted; and immune responses to many antigens are poor, resulting in wasting and death at a young age. In the adult mouse (or other laboratory animal), T cells have spread to the whole organism. Adult thymectomy must therefore be combined with irradiation to remove mature T cells. Because the irradiation, as already mentioned, will damage not only T cells but other cells, including B cells, irradiation must be followed by the transfer of B-cell-containing bone marrow to establish B competence.

A more specific removal of T cells can be achieved by treatment with anti-lymphocyte serum or better, anti-thymocyte serum — polyclonal sera from rabbits or other species. Also, drug treatment can be used to abort T-cell responses. The most promising example of this category is cyclosporin A, which has a pronounced anti–T-cell activity and fewer side effects on other components of the immune system, although not totally free of side effects in other organs, such as the kidneys. The introduction of monoclonal antibodies in experimental and clinical work may offer an improved treatment. Using monoclonal antibodies, highly specific subsets of lymphocytes can be defined (the CD system) and isolated.

Because thymus is the organ responsible for T-cell maturation, thymic hormonal factors have been introduced under various names. Results from experimental and clinical investigations are discordant; and with a more detailed knowledge of the processes involved in maturation of T cells in the thymus, the research in this area has lost impetus but is still active.[21] More steady results can be obtained with lymphokines (e.g., interleukins, interferon), which can now be produced in large amounts using recombinant techniques. A wide range of interleukines has been isolated and their actions identified, providing biomedical research with unique tools for both *in vitro* and *in vivo* work.

Specific T-cell potentiation in the experimental setup can be obtained with transfer of specific T cells, educated and sorted, or selected by cloning procedures. Priming with tumor cells can be used to specifically boost T-cell responses and dendritic cell action.

B-Cell Modulation

B-cell responses in the neonatal mouse can be suppressed totally or to a wide extent by treatment with anti-μ immunoglobulin directed against heavy chains of IgM immunoglobulin. Potentiation of B cells follows the same general line as that of T cells: priming and lymphokine treatment.

Spontaneous Immunodeficiency Models

Immunodeficient laboratory animal mutants have been known for more than 30 years. Their genetically determined deficiency does not include the side effects seen in irradiated or heavily drug-treated models. They are highly susceptible to microorganisms from the environment and therefore call for optimal housing conditions. In the following, some immunodeficient mutants are described, with primary emphasis on the athymic *nude* mouse and the SCID mouse.

The Athymic (nude) Mouse

The athymic (*nude*) mouse has been used in biomedical research since 1968.[22–24] The athymic condition is due to a recessive autosomal mutation, *nude,* the symbol for which is *nu*. On the basis of the genetics of the mutation, various breeding schemes can be set up. In proper microbiological conditions, *nude* females are fertile but they have difficulty in weaning their young. *Nude* males are generally fertile, although infections in the genital tract may cause infertility.

Breeding of *nude* mice can be based on the mating of heterozygous males and females, or, preferably, on the mating of homozygous males with heterozygous-haired females, which will give a 50% *nude* offspring in contrast to heterozygous–heterozygous matings, in which only an average of 25% are athymic.

Because of its lack of T-cell responses, the *nude* mouse accepts grafts of allogeneic and xenogeneic tissue, including malignant tumors. Full immunocompetence can be established with a thymus graft, and partial immunocompetence with spleen cells or selected T-cell subpopulations.

The natural killer (NK) cell was first described in the *nude* mouse. In 1975, Kiessling et al.[25] and Herberman et al.[26] gave simultaneous descriptions of this cell type, which appears in various percentages in *nude* mice, depending on their genetic background. Much interest has focused on NK cells and their suggested anti-cancer potential. The *hypothesis of immunological surveillance*[27] predicted that thymus-dependent cell-mediated immune responses were responsible for the constant removal of malignant cells, which were postulated to be generated continuously in the organism, in mouse as well as in man. Observations in athymic *nude* mice, which do not develop malignant tumors with a higher frequency than do normal mice of the same genetic background,[28] strongly advocated against the immune surveillance hypothesis. Today, despite much conflicting experimental evidence, and although by definition not belonging to the immune system *sensu stricte,* the NK cell seems to have taken over the role of immune surveillance from the T lymphocyte.

The Athymic (nude) Rat

The athymic (*nude*) rat[29,30] has characteristics similar to those of the *nude* mouse, including the ability to host human malignant tumors. Immunocompetence can be established in part or totally with thymus grafts or selected T-cell subpopulations. See also the "Discussion and Recommendations" section near the end of this chapter.

The beige Mouse

The *beige* mouse[31] has no NK-cell activity. Double mutants of *nude* and *beige* mice can be bred, lacking both NK- and T-cell functions.

The xid Mouse

The *xid* mouse[32] has an x-linked immunodeficiency with a partly impaired B-cell function.

The SCID Mouse

The SCID mutation[33] has a *s*evere *c*ombined *i*mmuno*d*eficiency involving both T and B cells. A low percentage of SCID mice are leaky; that is, they have polyclonal B-cell activation, leading to the production of high levels of (nonsense) immunoglobulin. The SCID mouse accepts grafts of human malignant tumors and — most important — also grafts of normal human lymphoid cells so that a human immune system can be constructed in it (SCID-hu).[34] This combination of mouse and human offers highly interesting possibilities for immunomodulatory studies and not least for the study of specific cell-mediated immune responses against (even) autologous tumor tissue.

HETEROTRANSPLANTATION

Human malignant tumors transplanted into *nude* mice and later into SCID mice have been widely used in many areas of cancer research. For an early review, see Boven and Winograd[35] and consult the Internet for updates. Tumors retain their human characteristics: histological and cytological morphology, karyotype, molecular structures including oncogenes,[36] and the ability to express clonal evolution. These heterotransplantation models have found widespread application. During an 18-month period starting in January 2001, some 700 and 230 publications for transplants into *nude* and SCID mice, respectively, have been included in the PubMed database (http://www.ncib.nlm.nih.gov/PubMed), documenting the continued interest in these models despite the availability of highly specific transgenic models.

Transplantation Techniques

Since the first human malignant tumor was implanted subcutaneously in *nude* mice in 1969, the subcutaneous tissue seems to have been the most popular site for implantation,[23] as based on a survey of the literature, and this seems to hold also for the limited experience in SCID mice. Tumors can be implanted s.c. (subcutaneous) as solid blocks, as needle biopsies by use of a trochar, or as cell suspensions. In all instances, a space is easily prepared, either by surgical procedures or by the pressure of the trocar or the inoculated cell suspension. The area is richly vascularized so that blood supply and lymph drainage can be easily established. The free mobility of the skin allows expansion over the growing tumor.

Mode of Growth and Metastases

In the *nude* mouse, tumors implanted s.c. will in nearly all cases grow locally, encapsulated in a connective tissue capsule, thus mimicking the growth mode of benign tumors in humans. Only in rare instances have metastases been observed. In the SCID mouse, tumors will be locally invasive; and a few weeks after implantation, metastases can be demonstrated in the peritoneum, spleen, lymph nodes, and lungs.[37] This difference in growth pattern between the *nude* and SCID mouse is a striking feature that must be taken into consideration when choosing a heterotransplantation model. A recently identified *nude* mutant substrain on a partly BALB/cA background allows a range of human malignant tumors to metastasize with a frequency close to that of SCID mice. Early results indicate that the ability to accommodate metastases is due to a recessive gene, presently under study in our laboratory.

When looking for metastases, one must use a higly sensitive detection system because metastases in lungs or lymph nodes are usually very small. Even small metastases from tumors tagged with the lacZ gene[38–40] or with the green fluorescent protein (gfp) gene[41] are easily detected, as are lymph node micrometastases using contrast-enhanced magnetic resonance imaging.[42]

Regional Growth Differences

Tumors implanted into *nude* mice show pronounced regional growth rate differences. This fact was also noticed in murine tumors grown in their syngenic hosts by Aurbach et al.[43] There seems to be a significant predeliction for tumor growth in the anterior (occipital) region of the mouse trunk as opposed to the posterior (caudal) region. Anterior tumors may grow three to four times as rapidly as posterior tumors. Also, there is a growth difference between tumors transplanted in the dorsal and in the ventral region, with ventral tumors developing more rapidly than dorsal tumors. There are no differences between the right side and left side of the mouse trunk. The reason for the difference in growth in the various regions is not known. Obviously, immunological factors cannot account for the difference. It is important to be aware of this phenomenon, particularly when comparing tumor sizes.

Age-Dependent Differences in Tumor Take

Tumor grafts are more readily accepted in young animals than in older animals. It has been shown that cancer cell lines were accepted significantly more often in young compared with adult animals, and the maximum tumor size in young mice was found to be twice that in adult mice. In *nude* mice, lymphoid cells with T-cell markers are found with increasing frequency with age, but it is not clear whether this phenomenon accounts for the difference in take rate between young and old. The difference should be kept in mind when working with tumor transplantation in this model.

Tumorigenicity

On the basis of observations of extensive materials, it is obvious that some tumor types are extremely difficult to establish in *nude* mice and also that several factors such as background strain of the mice, age of host, site of inoculation, addition of feeder cells with the implant, etc., may influence the outcome. This is of importance because tumorigenicity in *nude* mice is used as a characteristic of tumor cell lines, for instance in the American Tissue Culture Collection Catalog and also in oncogene studies. From what has been mentioned, it becomes obvious that tumorigenicity in the unadulterated *nude* mouse is not an absolute value. A more well-defined model for tumorogenicity may be needed. The SCID mouse may actually represent a better tumorigenesis model; but at the present time, evidence is still too scarce to allow final conclusions.

Monitoring Tumor Growth

Traditionally, the size of subcutaneously implanted tumors has been described by measurement with a slide caliper in two, or in some instances, three dimensions. There can be several objections to this. The measurement in only two dimensions (length × width) does not, of course, mathematically describe the volume of the tumor but only the two measured dimensions. By using suitable formulas, the two measurements can be transformed into an approximation of tumor volume. For discussion of this, see Boven and Winograd.[35]

TRANSGENIC ANIMAL MODELS

Mutations in the p53 tumor-suppressor gene are the most frequently observed genetic lesions in human cancers. The normal physiological role of the gene seems to be in the regulation of the cell cycle. Donehower et al.[44] introduced a null mutation into the gene by homologous recombination in murine embryonic cells. Mice homozygous for the mutation appeared normal but developed a variety of neoplasms by 6 months of age. Those investigators concluded that the absence of the p53 gene predisposes to neoplastic disease and further that an oncogenic mutant form of the p53 gene is not obligatory for the genesis of many types of tumors.

Tumors have been observed already from the age of 8 weeks in these transgenic mice, and the spectrum is very wide, most tumors observed so far having been sarcomas. These mice, GenPharm® TSG-p53 transgenic mice, are commercially available and of great interest in both toxicology and cancer research. Heterozygous TSG-p53 mice are also available. They have a low spontaneous level of tumorigenesis but a shorter latency period in carcinogenesis experiments compared with nontransgenic mice. Several types of transgenic mice of interest to cancer research have appeared, supplying cancer research with more refined tools "than dreamt of in our philosophy."

DISCUSSION AND RECOMMENDATIONS

Is it reasonable in a presentation of animal models in cancer research to focus so relatively narrow-mindedly on heterotransplantation models? In the author's opinion, such models represent the closest approximation to the human situation when used with due consideration. After more than 30 years in laboratory use, they have not given definitive clues to an overall understanding of cancer or to a miracle cure — nor has any other model or test system during the same period.

Since this handbook first appeared, two major events have made research in general much easier and much more complicated: the access to an overwhelming amount of information via the Internet and the mapping of the human and the murine genomes. What can an unexperienced cancer researcher do to benefit from these opportunities? The PubMed database (http://www.ncib.nlm. nih.gov/PubMed) allows searching for several parameters at the same time, giving all available references to, for instance, *nude mouse tumor transplant metastasis*. By carefully selecting, it is possible to have an update on the area in which one is interested. When it comes to laboratory animals, the databases of the Jackson Laboratory (Bar Harbor, ME)[46] include the laboratory's own data — updated weekly — and links to other databases, also including material on rats. The Jackson Laboratory also maintain the list, "Mouse Models for Cancer Research," which by Spring 2002 included 427 different strains under headings such as "Growth Factors, Increased Tumor Incidence, Oncogenes, etc."; a special database of transgenics; and the Mouse Genome Database, which lists some 400,000 mouse DNA sequences. Various bioinformatics tools[47] are available to use these data.

The basis for experimental cancer research has never been more solid!

ACKNOWLEDGMENTS

The experimental work in our laboratory underlying this presentation was supported by the Danish Medical Research Council, the Danish Cancer Society, Ejnar Willumsens Mindelegat, Meta & Håkon Baggers Legat, and Simon Spies Fonden. My son, Kåre Rygaard, cand. med., dr. med., was a helpful sparring partner during the preparation of the manuscript.

REFERENCES

1. Sivak, A., Chemical carcinogenesis, in *The Mouse in Medical Research, Vol. 4: Experimental Biology and Oncology,* Foster, H.L., Small, J.D., and Fox, J.G., Eds., Academic Press, New York, 1982, chap. 19.
2. Yamagiwa, K. and Ichikawa, K., Über die atypische Epithelwucherung, *Gann,* 11, 1914.
3. Pott, P., Chirurgical observations relative to the cataract, the polypus of the nose, the cancer of the scrotum, the different kinds of ruptures, and mortification of the toes and feet, Hawes, Clarke and Collins, London, 1775, reprinted in *Natl. Cancer Inst. Monogr.,* 10, 7, 1963.
4. Kennaway, E.L., On the cancer-producing factor in tar, *Int. Med. J.,* 1, 564, 1924.
5. Berenblum, I., The cocarcinogenic action of croton resin, *Cancer Res.,* 1, 44, 1941.
6. Berenblum, I. and Shubik, P., A new, quantitative approach to the study of chemical carcinogenesis in mouse's skin, *Br. J. Cancer,* 1, 383, 1947.
7. zur Hausen H., Papillomaviruses and cancer: from basic studies to clinical application, *Nat. Rev. Cancer,* 2, 342, 2002 (review).

8. Murphy, E.D., Characteristic tumors, in *The Biology of the Laboratory Mouse*, Green, E.L., Ed., McGraw-Hill, New York, 1966, chap. 27.

9. Peckham, J.C., Experimental oncology, in *The Laboratory Rat, Vol. II, Research Applications*, Baker, H.J., Lindsey, J.R., and Weisbroth, S.H., Eds., Academic Press, New York, 1980, chap.6.

10. Stehelin, D., Varmus, H.E., Bishop, J.M., and Vogt, P.K., DNA related to the transforming gene(s) of avian sarcoma viruses is present in normal avian DNA, *Nature*, 260, 170, 1976.

11. Levinson, A.D., Oppermann, H., Levintow, L., Varmus, H.E., and Bishop, J.M., Evidence that the transforming gene of avian sarcoma virus encodes a protein kinase associated with phosphorylation, *Cell*, 15, 561, 1978.

12. Shih, C., Padhy, L.C., Murray, M., and Weinberg, R.A., Transforming genes of carcinomas and neuroblastomas introduced into mouse fibroblasts, *Nature*, 290, 261, 1981.

13. Blair, D.G., Cooper, C.S., Oskarsson, M.K., Eader, L.A., and Vande Woude, G.F., New method for detecting cellular transforming genes, *Science*, 218, 1122, 1982.

14. Friend, S.H., Bernards, R., Rogelj, S., Weinberg, R.A., Rapaport, J.M., Albert, D.M., and Dryja, T.P., A human DNA segment with properties of the gene that predisposes to retinoblastoma and osteosarcoma, *Nature*, 323, 643, 1986.

15. Bishop, J.M., The molecular genetics of cancer, *Science*, 235, 305, 1987.

16. Greene, H.S.N. and Lund, P.K., The heterologous transplantation of human cancers, *Cancer Res.*, 4, 24, 1944.

17. Lutz, B.R., Fulton, G.P., Patt, D.I., and Handler, A.H., The growth rate of tumor transplants in the cheek pouch of the hamster (*Mesocricetus auratus*), *Cancer Res.*, 10, 321, 1950.

18. Clemmesen, J., On transplantation of tumor cells to normal and pre-irradiated heterologous organisms, *Am. J. Cancer*, 29, 313, 1937.

19. Toolan, H.W., Growth of human tumors in cortisone-treated laboratory animals: the possibility of obtaining permanently transplantable human tumors, *Cancer Res.*, 13, 389, 1953.

20. Miller, J.F.A.P., Immunological function of the thymus, *Lancet*, 2, 748, 1961.

21. Bodey, B., Thymic hormones in cancer diagnostics and treatment, *Expert Opin. Biol. Ther.*, 1, 93, 2001 (review).

22. Pantelouris, E.M., Absence of thymus in a mouse mutant, *Nature*, 217, 370, 1968.

23. Rygaard, J. and Povlsen, C.O., Heterotransplantation of a human malignant tumour to "nude" mice, *Acta Pathol. Microbiol. Scand., Sect. A*, 77, 758, 1969.

24. Rygaard, J., Thymus and Self. Immunobiology of the Mouse Mutant *nude*, FADL, Copenhagen, 1973; John Wiley & Sons, London, 1975; Japanese ed., Tuttle-Mori, Tokyo, 1979.

25. Kiessling, R., Klein, E., and Wigzell, H., "Natural" killer cells in the mouse. I. Cytotoxic cells with specificity for mouse Moloney leukemia cells. Specificity and distribution according to genotype, *Eur. J. Immunol.*, 5, 112, 1975.

26. Herberman, R.B., Nunn, M.E., and Lavrin, D.H., Natural cytotoxic reactivity of mouse lymphoid cells against syngeneic an allogeneic tumors. Distribution of reactivity and specificity, *Int. J. Cancer*, 16, 216, 1975.

27. Burnet, F.M., *Immunological Surveillance*, Pergamon Press, Sydney, 1970.

28. Rygaard, J. and Povlsen, C.O., The nude mouse vs. the hypothesis of immunological surveillance, *Transplant. Rev.*, 28, 43, 1976.

29. Schuurman, H.-J., Rozing, J., van Loveren, H., Vaessen, L.M.B., and Kampinga, J., The athymic nude rat, in Wu, B.-Q. and Zheng, J., Eds., *Immune-Deficient Animals in Experimental Medicine*, Karger, Basel, Switzerland, 1989, p. 54.

30. Hougen, H.P., The athymic nude rat, *APMIS J.*, 99 (Suppl. 21), 1991.

31. Roder, J.C., The *beige* mutation in the mouse. I. A stem cell predetermined impairment in natural killer cell function, *J. Immunol.*, 123, 2168, 1979.

32. Amsbaugh, D.F., Hansen, C.T., Prescott, B., Stashak, P.W., Barthold, D.R., and Baker, P.J., Genetic control of the antibody response to type III pneumococcal polysaccharide in mice, *J. Exp. Med.*, 136, 931, 1972.

33. Bosma, G.C., Custer, R.P., and Bosma, M.J., A severe combined immunodeficiency mutation in the mouse, *Nature*, 301, 527, 1983.

34. Mosier, D.E., Immunodeficient mice xenografted with human lymphoid cells: new models for *in vivo* studies of human immunobiology and infectious diseases, *J. Clin. Immunol.*, 10, 185, 1990.

35. Boven, E. and Winograd, B., Eds., *The Nude Mouse in Oncology Research,* CRC Press, Boca Raton, FL, 1991.
36. Rygaard, K., Sorenson, G.D., Pettengill, O.S., Cate, C.C., and Spang-Thomsen, M., Abnormalities in structure and expression of the retinoblastoma gene in small cell lung cancer cell lines and xenografts in nude mice, *Cancer Res.,* 50, 5312, 1990.
37. Xie, X., Brünner, N., Jensen, G., Albrectsen, J., Gotthardsen, B., and Rygaard, J., Comparative studies between nude and scid mice on the growth and metastatic behavior of xenografted human tumors, *Clin. Exp. Metastasis,* 10, 201, 1992.
38. Kruger, A., Schirrmacher, V., and Khokha, R., The bacterial lacZ gene: an important tool for metastasis research and evaluation of new cancer therapies, *Cancer Metastasis Rev.,* 17, 285, 1998–1999 (review).
39. Holleran, J.L., Miller, C.J., Edgehouse, N.L., Pretlow, T.P., and Culp, L.A., Differential experimental micrometastasis to lung, liver, and bone with lacZ-tagged CWR22R prostate carcinoma cells, *Clin. Exp. Metastasis,* 19, 17, 2002.
40. Culp, L.A., Holleran, J.L., and Miller, C.J., Tracking prostate carcinoma micrometastasis to multiple organs using histochemical marker genes and novel cell systems, *Histol. Histopathol.,* 16, 945, 2001 (review).
41. Huang, M.S., Wang, T.J., Liang, C.L., Huang, H.M., Yang, I.C., Yi-Jan, H., and Hsiao, M., Establishment of fluorescent lung carcinoma metastasis model and its real-time microscopic detection in SCID mice, *Clin. Exp. Metastasis,* 19, 359, 2002.
42. Wunderbaldinger, P., Josephson, L., Bremer, C., Moore, A., and Weissleder, R., Detection of lymph node metastases by contrast-enhanced MRI in an experimental model, *Magn. Reson. Med.,* 47, 292, 2002.
43. Aurbach, R., Morrissey, L.W., and Sidky, Y.A., Regional differences in the incidence and growth of mouse tumors following intradermal or subcutaneous inoculation, *Cancer Res.,* 38, 1739, 1978.
44. Donehower, L.A., Harvey, M., Slagle, B.L., McArthur, M.J., Montgomery, C.A., Jr., Butel, J.S., and Bradley, A., Mice deficient for p53 are developmentally normal but susceptible to spontaneous tumours, *Nature,* 356, 215, 1992.
45. Available at: http://jaxmice.jax.org (look for *Mouse Models Lists, Cancer Research, and The Transgenic/Targeted Mutation Database* [TBASE: also available at http://tbase.jax.org]).
46. Edgerton, M.E., Taylor, R., Powell, J.I., Hunter, L., Simon, R., and Liu, E.T., A bioinformatics tool to select sequences for microarray studies of mouse models of oncogenesis, *Bioinformatics,* 18, 774, 2002.

CHAPTER 12

Animal Models in Oral Health Sciences

Björn Klinge and Jörgen Jönsson

CONTENTS

0-8493-1084-9/03/$0.00+$1.50

INTRODUCTION

This review describes selected animal models used in oral health sciences (OHS).

Successful research is seldom limited to an anatomical region, like the soft and hard tissues of the mouth for OHS. Relevant models are often used to answer more general biological questions. To study bone formation with application to the maxillofacial skeleton as an example, the long bones or the calvarias are often used, and not only the jawbones. Similarly, in studying inflammation of relevance for the oral cavity, often more general models are used. This of course makes the demarcation of relevant animal models for dental and other OHS somewhat artificial. Nevertheless, for this review, we have in essence limited the inclusion criteria to literature that is classified as "models, animal and dental." This is by no means a precise method. Relevant information and articles may well be excluded, but this review is not intended to represent a total vacuum-cleaning of the literature. Rather, we have aimed at selecting a representative width of models used. For specific questions, we suggest a thorough literature search in relevant databases.

Today the value as evidence for treatment often follows strict criteria. Randomization, an adequately large number of study subjects, use of tests and controls, blinding or independent researchers, adequate follow-up time, and taking confounders into account are often among the criteria to be evaluated. In this review these and additional criteria are not necessarily discussed. We have instead diverged from the principles of "evidence based" to include subjective advice from staff and scientists at recognized laboratory animal facilities. One reason for this is that the detailed background for selecting certain methods cannot often be found in the "materials and methods" section of the resulting scientific articles. This often-critical knowledge can be classified as being part of the important, so-called professional silent knowledge. We have therefore deliberately allowed ourselves to include small pieces of practical advice here and there, based on our own experience and on that of our respected colleagues.

ANIMAL MODELS IN DENTAL AND MAXILLOFACIAL RESEARCH

The use of animal models in OHS has increased significantly over the past 20 years. In 1972, around 370 articles were published according to our search criteria using the National Library of Medicine database PubMed. Using the same criteria for 2001, more than 1000 articles were found. The distribution of articles over the past 20 years is presented in Figure 12.1. Interestingly, the rat model was used in about one third of the publications at both time points, 20 years apart. The distribution of different animal species is presented in Figure 12.2.

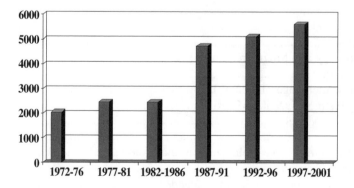

Figure 12.1   Animal models in oral health sciences: number of publications in the National Library of Medicine (1972–2001).

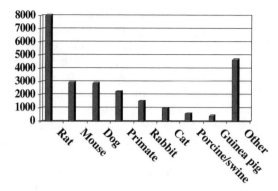

Figure 12.2   Animal species used in oral health sciences: number of publications in the National Library of Medicine (1972–2001).

ORAL HEALTH AND DISEASE TRENDS IN HUMANS

Oral health, like general health, has obviously improved in recent decades. The percentage of young children and adolescents who have never experienced dental caries in their permanent teeth continues to increase. In the age group of 18 to 34 years, these adults have less decay and fewer fillings than ever before. The percentage of people who have lost all their teeth has declined dramatically in the past 30 years. In the period 1971 to 1974, around 45% of American adults aged 65 to 74 years were edentulous. In the period 1988 to 1994, the percent edentulous was reduced to approximately 28% in this age group.[1] It is more difficult to track trends for other oral health conditions, like periodontal diseases. The majority of the adult population will have gingival inflammation of varying magnitude. About 40% of all adults above the age of 40 years will have tissue-destructive periodontal disease at single teeth. Fewer than 10% are calculated to have more generalized periodontal disease affecting most teeth and eventually leading to the loss of teeth. The genetic background of periodontal diseases has recently become more of a focus area.

Overall oral cancer rates are declining. However, certain site-specific oral cancers are on the rise. The incidence of tongue cancers among young males is climbing. The 5-year survival rate for oral cancers has remained the same for the past 25 years.

Human immunodeficiency virus–acquired immune deficiency syndrome (HIV-AIDS) and other infectious diseases having oral manifestations and other systemic diseases or conditions associated with oral pathogens are also of concern. In addition, other genetically and environmentally triggered oral diseases and disorders, such as craniofacial birth defects, are of great significance. Systemic conditions, such as diabetes, have long been known to affect oral diseases. More recently, the results from epidemiologic studies have shown an association between oral infections, especially periodontal diseases, and general health problems such as atherosclerosis, other cardiovascular diseases, stroke, chronic pulmonary disease, and additional diseases and disorders. These early findings will also require confirmation by experimental animal studies to determine whether the association between general conditions and oral diseases is actually causative in nature. In trying to understand the onset and dissemination of these diseases and in identifying and developing proper dental materials and methods to restore the damaged tissues, animal experiments are of fundamental significance.

DEVELOPING RAT TEETH

The rat incisor is the most commonly used model in the investigation of the development of dental hard tissues. This relates to its continuous growth that allows studying the whole life cycle of the ameloblasts and odontoblasts in the same tooth. In contrast to the rat incisor, the rat molar has limited growth and similar orientation of the outer prism layer to the human tooth. The molar has three major cusps, each with an enamel-free area at the tip. At day 2 of age, dentin formation has started on both the mesial and distal sides of the cusps of the first molar. After a thin layer of dentin has been deposited, the ameloblasts begin enamel deposition. Amelogenesis includes several stages of cellular activity. The secretory ameloblasts start to produce enamel matrix in the occlusal region of the cusps. The enamel matrix mineralizes to some extent immediately after deposition. In the 5- to 6-day-old rat, enamel matrix formation is almost complete at the tip of the cusps, and the ameloblasts are reduced in height. At 7 to 9 days of age, the enamel has reached its final thickness except in the cervical areas. Maturation begins at the tip of the central cusp, and a secondary stage of mineralization starts, with an increase in the mineral content of the enamel, whereas matrix production continues in the cervical part of the tooth. Between these two stages, there is a transitional stage when the ameloblasts change from tall and secretory to short and engaged in enamel maturation. This transitional zone moves from the occlusal region toward the growing end of the tooth. At 12 days of age, an increase in the mineral content is seen in the enamel of all cusps. This process proceeds cervically to involve about half of the cusp height. At this stage, the tip of the central cusp of the erupting molar reaches the overlying oral epithelium. At the age of 20 d, the enamel attains a high degree of mineralization with an even pattern. The enamel is more mineralized than the dentin along the entire height of the cusps, and the maxillary first molar is fully erupted.[2]

TOOTH ERUPTION

At 8 days of age, the first maxillary molar in the rat shows early signs of root development and begins to erupt through the alveolus. The tooth does not penetrate the submucosal and epithelial tissues until day 15. This region is therefore well suited for the study of tooth eruption and actively resorbing osteoclasts. The surrounding alveolar bone is being physiologically resorbed to accommodate the movement of the teeth throughout the alveolus.[3]

CRANIOFACIAL MALFORMATIONS

Orofacial clefting is the second-most common birth defect in humans and the most frequent of all birth defects affecting the craniofacial region. The use of animal model systems for developmental genetics has resulted in remarkable scientific advances. The evolutionary conservation of morphoregulatory pathways has revealed the homology of genes associated with human craniofacial malformations and their counterparts that regulate the morphogenesis of fruit flies.[4] Extensive research and training supported by the National Institute of Dental and Craniofacial Research (the NIDCR of the National Institutes of Health) have led to the identification and characterization of more than 100 human and animal genes and to the interrelations of the products of these genes in the signal transduction pathways that regulate the development of the form and function of the craniofacial-oral-dental complex.[5,6] Mutations in many of these genes cause characteristic defects in craniofacial development, as observed in human patients and in whole-animal assays such as transgenic mice. It deserves emphasizing that different mutations within a single gene can cause widely different clinical phenotypes. Hemifacial microsomia (HFM) is one such malformation complex with an extremely variable phenotype. The validity of the *Hfm* transgenic mouse as a model for hemifacial microsomia was presented by Cousley et al.[7] They reported observations extending the *Hfm* phenotype beyond microtia and jaw asymmetry, to include structural and positional anomalies affecting the external auditory meatus, middle ear, cranial base, maxilla, and pharyngeal structures. Temporomandibular joint development and palatal shelf fusion were also affected but in fewer cases. Human and animal studies indicate that cleft lips of multifactorial etiology may be generically susceptible because of small medial nasal prominences or other developmental alterations in medial nasal prominences, such as those found in A/J mice that make prominence contact more difficult. Another research area of immediate interest relates to cigarette smoking and developmental defects. Experimental maternal hypoxia in mice indicates that cigarette smoking may increase the incidence of cleft lip by interfering with morphogenetic movements.[8]

ORTHODONTIC TOOTH MOVEMENT

Teeth are often moved for either or both functional or aesthetic reasons. Several animal models are used to explore this research area. The dog (Beagle dog) has been suggested as a suitable experimental animal when the model should mimic tooth movement across the midpalatal suture. The dog has a straight midpalatal suture with similar appearance to that in humans.

Rodents are not suitable for studies involving anterior teeth because of their continuously erupting incisors. Cats have very small incisor teeth, making it complicated to attach the orthodontic appliance. Monkeys have an extremely winding midpalatal suture. It is noteworthy that in young dogs with open suture, the suture becomes dislocated in front of the tooth moved. This is in contrast to the case of the old dog with a closed suture, in which orthodontic tooth movement was reported to be more easily performed. However, root resorption of the teeth occurred to a greater degree in the old dog with the closed suture than in the young dog with open suture.[9]

The rabbit has been used as an experimental animal in investigating the transversal development of the dental arch and osseous remodeling at the lateral surfaces of the maxillary alveolar process and in the midpalatal suture after stretching the bucca (cheek) by use of buccal shields in the vestibulum.[10] In designing experiments involving affection of growth areas, like the sutures, it is important to be aware of the normal growth parameters. The midpalatal suture has been reported to be closed in 3-month-old rabbits. The skeletal growth in male rabbits has been reported to end at the age of 7.5 months; the variation for different strains may need validation when this parameter is of critical importance.

Tetracycline hydrochloride and Alizarine complexone, both at a dosage of 30 mg per kilogram body weight, can be used to label the mineralizing tissues. In our experience, the Alizarine seems to be quite irritating when injected i.v. in the ear veins of rabbits. It is therefore suggested that the animals are anesthetized before injection.[10] In young animals, the bone-metabolic rate may be too high for extended (over weeks) labeling intervals.

Rats and monkeys are also used for orthodontic experiments. When using rats, it should be remembered that the incisors are continuously erupting, as contrasted to the case of the molar teeth.

In monkeys, the dental anatomy, as well as chewing behavior, has been referred to as more human-like than that of other models. The relevance of these factors, all other dissimilarities unaccounted for, is open for questions.

BONE HEALING

Heat-Induced Bone Injury

Bone is a highly differentiated tissue. After injury, there is a possibility that the bone tissue will not heal as bone but as fibrous connective tissue. Undue heat injury will increase this risk for disturbed bone healing. At surgical intervention of bone, frictional energy will generate heat and thus increase the risk for fibrous bone healing. This basic knowledge is of utmost significance for all animal experiments involving bone cutting or drilling procedures.

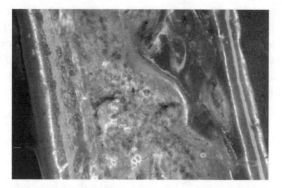

Figure 12.3   Fluorescent labeling of rabbit skull bone. The bone growth to the left appears more prominent than that to the right.

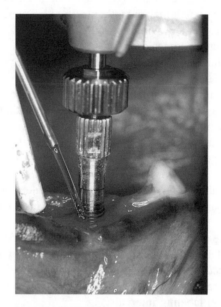

Figure 12.4   Titanium implant placed in dog jaw bone; notice cooling of the implant with profuse irrigation.

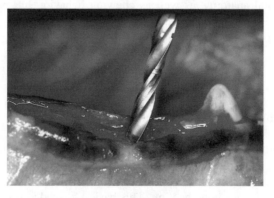

Figure 12.5   Twist drill preparation in mandibular bone for implant site.

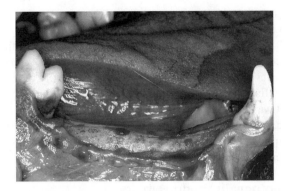

Figure 12.6   Edentulous mandible of dog.

By overheating the bone tissue, even at modest temperatures, healing may be drastically affected. This should also be taken into account when performing implant procedures. The heat sensitivity of mature bone tissue, the critical temperature for impaired bone regeneration, and temperature rise when drilling bone have all been reported.[11]

In these experiments, adult Belgian hares and New Zealand white rabbits were used. The experimental model includes the use of a bone chamber for microscopic investigation of heat-injured bone. The chamber consists of an externally threaded, hollow titanium cylinder into which two glass rods are placed and separated by a 100-μm-wide space. This space is located at the same level as a transverse canal that penetrates the chamber. This narrow passage will become invaded by bone and blood vessels after insertion of the chamber into the rabbit tibia. After incorporation in the rabbit tibia for 8 to 10 weeks, the bone, which has grown through the chamber, is subjected to thermal injury. The progression of the heat injury is observed and registered at repeated observations, from hours to several weeks, after the heat injury. This model for vital microscopic registrations may of course also be used for several other applications.

After these thorough experiments and subsequent analysis of the data, the authors[11] concluded that the blood vessels were irreversibly injured after heating to 53°C for 1 min. The morphological pattern of the vessels remained unchanged after heating to 47°C for 1 min. Bone regeneration was severely impaired after heating to 47°C, whereas a temperature of 44°C did not cause any significant adverse effect. It should thus be stressed that these findings indicate that relatively low temperatures are enough to impair bone regeneration.

Factors affecting the temperature rise in bone cutting included drill speed, drill diameter, drill geometry, drill wear, predrilling, pressure, cooling, penetration depth, blood flow, and type of bone. Drill speeds in the range of 1000 to 2000 rpm are recommended, provided that specific precautions for cooling are undertaken. Small drills give rise to lower temperatures than large drills. Twist drills are more suitable for drilling in bone than fissure burs. New or sharp drills should be used. Predrilling is an effective method for minimizing temperature flucuation. Low pressure is recommended when drilling in vital bone. Cooling the drill is important; a cooling agent (sterile saline) should be used in combination with profuse irrigation. With increased penetration depth, the effect of the cooling agent decreases, and thus more heat is generated. The blood flow will likely affect the temperature rise when drilling in living bone tissue. Cortical bone is more likely to be injured by frictional heat than cancellous bone.

Jawbone Healing in Rabbits

An experimental rabbit model for jawbone healing was developed by Lundgren.[12] Surgical defects were made in the maxillary edentulous area between the incisors and molars using 4-mm round bur under generous irrigation with saline. The defect was approximately 11 × 5 mm wide and 3 mm deep. No signs of oral infection were found for the healing period of 4 weeks. The contralateral side served as control. Radiographs and histological sections were obtained for analysis. An average loss of 17% of the total bone volume as compared to the case of the untreated control side was reported. This means that the rabbit jawbone has a considerable capacity for spontaneous healing. However, it was concluded that the surgically created defects do not show complete spontaneous healing. It was furthermore suggested that the test side could also serve as its own control because it was possible to redraw the original bone contour by interpolation between unaffected areas of bone, coronal and apical to the defect. The right and left sides of the maxilla were considered to be equivalent. This model can be used when testing different barrier materials and bone grafts and other bone substitutes.

Management of Craniotomy in Young Rabbits

In studies of cranial growth aberrations, intramembraneous bone regeneration, and bone-healing capacity, young rabbits have often been used. Young animals have an intensive craniofacial growth period. Experimental procedures, which include craniotomy, are often reported to be associated with complications. Local infections and hemorrhages after injury to the sinus system are the most often noted complications. A simple and safe procedure for craniotomy in young rabbits was reported by Alberius et al.[13]

Each mother with offspring was housed in a large plastic cage sized 1.05 × 0.55 × 0.45 m (Scanbur ApS, Denmark). Mothers with six or fewer offspring were selected. The perforated cage floor was covered with autoclaved hay bedding. The cages were thoroughly cleaned on a daily basis. Standard pelleted diet with no antibiotics added and tap water were provided *ad libitum*.

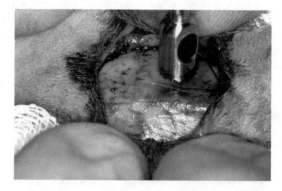

Figure 12.7   A circular drill is used to create a standardized skull bone defect.

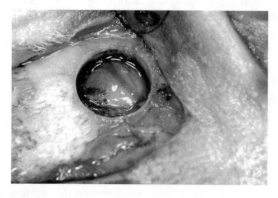

Figure 12.8   Circular skull bone defect; note vessels under the dura.

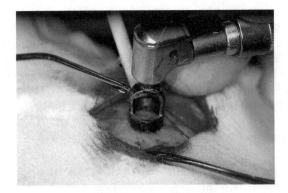

Figure 12.9   Drill preparation of skull bone defect; notice cooling and suction.

At age 7 to 8 weeks, the young rabbits were separated from their mother and placed in cages half the size of those above. One or two rabbits were housed together. The rabbits were anesthetized by i.m. neuroleptanalgesia (fluanisone, 10 mg/ml, and fentanyl, 0.2 mg/ml; 0.6 ml per kilogram body weight). No premedication was administered. After the onset of analgesia, that is, after about 10 min, the head was shaved with a high-quality electric shaver, and the surgical field was carefully cleaned with an antiseptic solution (alcoholic chlorhexidine, 5mg/ml). The animal was placed prone on a thermal blanket on the operating table. The body caudal to the occipital region was draped, allowing exposure of the craniofacial region.

Bone defects were created both in the calvarial bone plate and in the sutural areas using a diamond wheel (to produce 4×6-mm defects) or a trephine (6-mm diameter) mounted on a low-speed dental drill. To reduce thermal damage during the drilling procedure, the surgical field was continuously irrigated with cooled sterile saline. Hemostasis was secured by sterile bone wax. After suturing, the wound was finally covered with plastic spray (Nobecutan spray, Astra Meditec, Sweden). This latter procedure is essential to avoid having the mothers (or siblings) lick the wound, which is otherwise a natural behavior supposed to promote wound healing.

To compensate for dehydration, immediately after surgery, 10 ml saline was injected dorsally s.c. Antibiotic (Streptocillin vet., Novo Industry A/S, Denmark) was given i.m. in a 0.1-ml dose The antibiotic administration was continued once daily for 1 week. The animals were left to recover on a thermostatically controlled electric blanket, and a towel covered them to maintain normal body temperature.

With this procedure used for craniotomy operations on 90 young rabbits, one animal died perioperatively from hemorrhage caused by a sagittal sinus rift. The mortality and morbidity is thus extremely low.

Skull Bone Defects in Rats and Rabbits

A calvarial wound model bears many similarities to the maxillofacial region. Both calvarial and midfacial bones develop from a membrane precursor, and the calvaria and the mandible consist of two cortical tables with regions of intervening cancellous bone. It contains only modest amounts of bone marrow, which generally facilitates bone formation, although the marrow is not necessary for bone formation to occur. When the aim is to investigate the pattern of bone regeneration in growth areas, like the sutural region and the calvarial bone plate proper, young animals having an intense craniofacial growth period are preferably used.

In adult animals, the regenerative capacity of the calvarium is reduced, and therefore it constitutes a suitable site for research work on agents for enhancement of bone repair.[14]

Small defects (5-mm diameter) that would correspond to a typical operative defect between bony segments in clinical maxillofacial surgery have been produced and used in rats and rabbits.

That defect size makes spontaneous bone regeneration possible, allows evaluation of the regenerative influence stemming from the implant material and of the maturation of the newly formed bone tissue, and enables experimental testing of several implant materials in each animal.[14,15] A *critical defect size* is a defect that will not heal during the lifetime of the animal.

When using a defect large enough to preclude spontaneous healing, the osteogenic potential of an implant or graft may be considered unambiguous. The critical-size model allows assessment of whether enhancement of bony regeneration occurs.[16]

Bone Growth Chamber

At the laboratories of Experimental Biology, Department of Anatomy, University of Gothenburg, and the Institute for Applied Biotechnology, Gothenburg, several methods to study living bone tissue have been developed and evaluated. These methods can be adapted to various experiments and to different animals. The bone growth chamber (BGC) is a dividable titanium implant that is inserted in the proximal tibial metaphysis of the rabbit using a very gentle surgical technique.[17] Blood vessels and bone tissue will grow through two implant pores. After various healing periods, the implant is removed and taken apart. The tissue that has invaded the pores can be collected and analyzed.

Bone Harvest Chamber

The bone harvest chamber (BHC) builds on principles similar to the BGC. The important difference is that the animals need not be killed for the collection of the bone samples. This allows for repeated tissue harvests from the same animal at different time intervals.[18]

The Vital Microscopic Chamber, BGC, and BHC were used to study bone behavior after irradiation using rabbits as experimental animals.[17] It was concluded that mature bone and vessels are relatively resistant to irradiation trauma up to 40 Gy, whereas the bone-healing response is severely disturbed after similar doses. Irradiation of 15 Gy caused a significant early depression of the osteogenesis with a clear tendency to recovery after 1 year. The minimal irradiation dose that caused a temporary depression in bone healing was 5 Gy.

GINGIVITIS AND PERIODONTITIS

Gingivitis (gingival inflammation) and periodontitis (destructive inflammation of the supporting tissues of the teeth) are diseases initiated by bacterial infection. The mouth provides an optimal environment for bacterial growth, which is why bacteria are seen in great numbers in the saliva, mucosa, and tooth surfaces. When bacteria along the tooth surfaces grow to large numbers, they form an adhesive plaque around the edge of the gingival (the gingival margin). These bacteria release toxins that irritate and injure the gingiva and result in inflammation of the gingival tissues (gingivitis). If this bacterial plaque is left undisturbed, it can spread down into and infect the gingival pocket. The host responds with an inflammatory reaction to the infectious challenge. The tooth-supporting tissues, gingival connective tissue, and bone are destroyed as a result of the inflammatory process, and the tooth will eventually become loose and may be lost. Periodontal diseases, including gingivitis and periodontitis, are naturally of frequent occurrence in humans and animal species.[19] Unlike many other diseases with infectious background, periodontitis is widespread both in humans and in the animal kingdom. To study the etiopathology of periodontal diseases and to assess various treatment modalities, a multitude of animal models have been developed, including mouse, rat, hamster, ferret, cat, dog, and various non-human primates, among others.

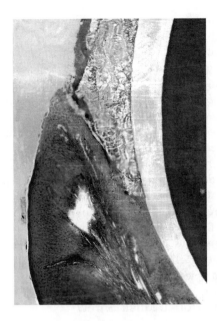

Figure 12.10   Histological section (undecalcified ground section) of gingiva with dental plaque and calculus in gingival pocket next to enamel; dentin appears darker.

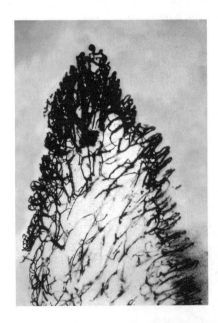

Figure 12.11   Gingiva perfused with ink after induction of gingival inflammation.

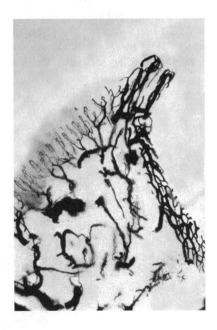

Figure 12.12   Corresponding healthy gingiva; notice difference in presence of blood vessels.

Periodontal Disease in Rats

The rat bears much resemblance to the human with respect to periodontal anatomy, development and composition of dental plaque, histopathology of periodontal lesions, and basic immunology.[20] Experimental studies in germ-free rats have confirmed the pathogenicity of several suspected periodontal pathogens *(Actinobacillus actinomycetemcomitans, Porphyromonas gingivalis, Capno-cytophaga sputigena, Eikenella corrodens,* and *Fusobacterium nucleatum).*

The incisors of rats are rootless and continuously growing teeth; therefore, they are unsuitable as model organs for human periodontal disease. The molar teeth are similar in humans and rats in relation to the structure and organization of the periodontal tissues (i.e., oral sulcular epithelium, junctional epitehelium, periodontal collagen fibers, cementum, and alveolar bone). One major difference is that the gingival sulcular epithelium of the rat is keratinized, in contrast to the corresponding human structure. The clinical and histological findings in experimental periodontal disease in rats are similar to findings in humans. Clinically, gingival bleeding on gentle probing can be observed in rats a few days after the introduction of periodontal microbial pathogens. Histologically, the junctional epithelium gradually undergoes pathologic changes, including rete peg formation, ulceration, and apical migration of epithelium.

Periodontal Disease in the House Musk Shrew

Rodents such as mice, rats, and hamsters have been widely used for periodontal research. However, the differences in anatomical structures (keratinized oral sulcular epithelium in rodents) and some histopathological features of periodontal disease in rodents are different from those of humans. Neutrophils appear to be the only infiltrating cells in periodontal lesions of rodents. This is in contrast to periodontally involved human tissues showing a more complex infiltrate of inflammatory cells like lymphocytes, plasma cells, macrophages, and neutrophils.

In the house musk shrew *(Suncus murinus),* a large number of polymorphonuclear leukocytes have been observed in areas in which bacterial plaque have accumulated. Neutrophils have been observed in the pocket epithelium and in the connective tissue. Dense infiltration of plasma cells and lymphocytes are contained in deeper connective tissue layers. Chronic periodontal lesions, similar to those in humans, have thus been demonstrated, suggesting the utility of *Suncus murinus* as a novel, interesting model for human periodontal diseases.[21]

Gingivitis and Periodontitis in the Dog

The anatomy of the free-gingival and the supracrestal portion of the periodontium of the permanent dentition in the human and the mandibular premolar region of the dog have many features in common. In both species, dental plaque accumulation results in inflammatory reactions that are

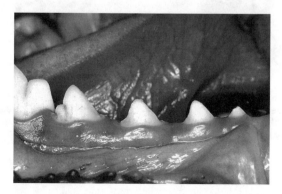

Figure 12.13   Right mandibular premolar area of a beagle dog.

initially confined to the gingiva but subsequently may develop to include all components of the periodontium proper. The location and composition of the subgingival plaque and the associated inflammatory lesions differ in some aspects between the human and the dog; but despite this, the dog (especially the Beagle) has been frequently used as a model in the study of fundamental aspects of the development, treatment and prevention of periodontal disease.[22–29] One reason for selecting larger animals like the dog is the physical dimensions of the tissues, which resemble those of human tissues, and the possibility of using all the special dental instruments that have been developed for use in humans.

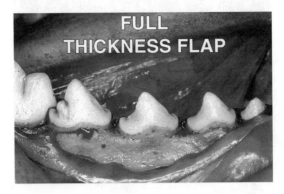

Figure 12.14   A full-thickness flap has been lifted.

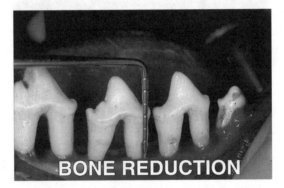

Figure 12.15   Alveolar bone has been surgically removed.

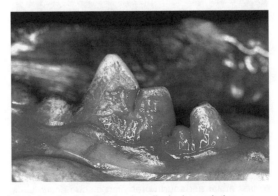

Figure 12.16   The bacterial plaque is visualized using disclosing solution.

The most commonly used method for studying gingival tissue reaction to dental plaque formation is the model originally described by Löe et al.[30] In those investigators' experiment, it was demonstrated that undisturbed plaque formation resulted in clinically detectable gingivitis within a period of 3 weeks. Gingivitis was established sooner in some individuals than in others. The onset of the gingival inflammation was related to the rate of plaque formation and to the establishment of a complex microbiota. The human model has thus been transferred to experimental animal studies. The local effect of the diet on plaque formation and development of gingivitis has been

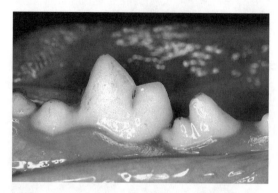

Figure 12.17   Right mandible first molar and fourth premolar; plaque accumulation after 4 weeks of soft diet without tooth cleaning.

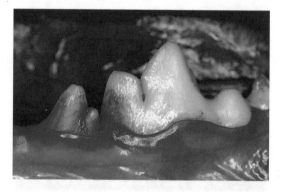

Figure 12.18   The bacterial plaque is visualized using disclosing solution.

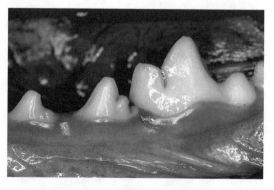

Figure 12.19   Left mandible first molar and fourth premolar; plaque accumulation after 4 weeks of hard diet without tooth cleaning.

found to be of great significance in experimental studies. A soft diet is more consistent with plaque accumulation and subsequent inflammatory reaction, as contrasted to the more healthy gingival conditions resulting from the use of a hard diet.[31] To establish more pronounced periodontal tissue destruction, a ligature of silk or cotton can be attached around the neck of the experimental tooth.[32] In studies designed to evaluate periodontal tissue regeneration, the experimental model includes surgically removing the tooth-supporting structures, including the periodontal ligament and the alveolar bone.[33] The chronic background to the destructive periodontal disease is of course lost in these more acute models. However, with the apparent variation in the defect baseline of naturally occurring periodontal disease, it is suggested that natural disease defects have limited potential in discerning treatment effects after periodontal reconstructive therapy.[34]

Periodontal Research in the Ferret

The first reports of the use of the ferret as an experimental animal in periodontal research were those made by King.[35] More recently, gingival hyperplasia has also been studied in ferrets. Periodontal disease in ferrets was found to be similar to that in humans. The lesions appear first around the carnassial teeth, normally related to the presence of calculus deposits. It may be of significance that the salivary glands of the ferret, as in the dog and cat, open into the carnassial regions of the upper jaw. Clinically, the first sign of periodontal disease is redness of the gum margin. Hyperemia, hemorrhage, hypertrophy, ulceration, involvement of the alveolar bone, and loosening of the teeth may follow. Silk ligatures have been used to promote tissue destruction. The ligature-induced periodontal breakdown has been shown to be similar in ferrets and dogs. In studying the role of pharmaceuticals on the development of periodontal lesions, the ferret may be used, being a smaller animal that requires more limited doses of the drugs than does the dog.[36]

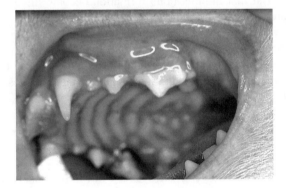

Figure 12.20 Upper left maxillary quadrant of the ferret.

GUIDED TISSUE REGENERATION

The histological healing outcome after periodontal surgery has been suggested to depend on the kinds of cells that repopulate the detached root surface during healing.

The tissues that repopulate the instrumented root surface may be epithelium, gingival connective tissue, bone, and periodontal ligament cells. It was suggested that the result of healing would predictably be new periodontal ligament attachment to the root surface, provided that the cells derived from the periodontal ligament were allowed to repopulate the root surface in an undisturbed fashion. The ingrowth of epithelium and gingival connective tissue onto the root surface was precluded during healing by means of a cell-occlusive membrane acting as a mechanical barrier.

This surgical technique is termed *guided tissue regeneration* (GTR).[37] Models to study the effect of GTR have been developed in dogs, monkeys, rats, and rabbits.

Guided bone regeneration (GBR) is a refinement of the originally developed GTR technique in situations in which, selectively, only bone healing should be promoted.[38]

The Capsule Model

The capsule model is based on the principles of GTR and allows for the evaluation of various grafting materials on bone formation. A rigid hemispherical capsule made of polytetrafluoroethylene is placed on the lateral surface of the mandibular ramus in rats. The open part of the capsule is facing the bone surface. A peripheral collar allows for a close adaptation of the device onto the bone surface. By this procedure, a secluded space is created adjacent to an essentially uninjured bone surface. At the same time, the surrounding soft connective tissue and muscles are excluded from participating in the healing process.

The capsule may be grafted (filled) with various graft materials or bioactive substances. Subsequently, the amount of bone formation is compared with that in empty control capsules placed on the contralateral side of the jaw in the same animal. It has been shown that such empty capsules will eventually be filled with newly formed bone after a period of 6 to 12 months. When choosing a shorter observation period, the bioactivity of a material regarding the formation of bone tissue can be readily discriminated. The amount of bone formed in the empty capsules during a given observation period reflects the intrinsic bone-forming potential of the model for this specific time period and may in this way serve as comparison for the evaluation of the results. Capsules with material that favors bone regeneration become filled earlier or present larger amounts of newly formed bone tissue at a given time point than do the originally empty control capsules. Conversely, capsules filled with material that inhibits bone formation become filled later or with less newly formed bone, as compared with the empty control capsules.[39,40]

Other investigators who have studied the formation of intramembraneous skull bone have used a titanium dome. Experimental studies using rats and rabbits have shown the augmentation of intramembraneous bone beyond the skeletal envelope using an occlusive titanium barrier.[12]

Wound stability seems to be critical to all tissue regeneration procedures.[41,42] When using various flap procedures, membranes, capsules, or domes, the stability of the device will most likely determine the outcome of the healing process. Micromovements of the devices have been suggested to jeopardize the regenerative event. Thus, control of the factors possibly affecting the movement of the devices is critical and will involve the creative imagination of all parties involved in these experiments, not the least of which are the animal technicians. Just lifting the animal in an inappropriate way may create unintentional movement of the tissues and related devices. As always, it is important to inform and involve all engaged staff. Do not forget to inform stand-ins or substitute staff.

Dental Implants

On the basis of animal research, dental implants for human clinical use have been developed. This is a significant contribution to restoring the human body and improving health and the quality of life. The original contributions by the Swedish scientist Brånemark are of unparalleled importance in this context.

During the 1950s, Brånemark was engaged in searching for ways to better carry out his own studies on blood microcirculation in rabbit bone and marrow. This work involved vital microscopy. Brånemark[42] developed and refined techniques of looking into living bone tissue and of studying the mechanisms by which bone repairs after damage. Chambers carrying optical equipment were inserted into the tibia of rabbits. Because of difficulties in obtaining tantalum, which was the original material for tissue chambers, an alternative design was made of titanium.[43,44] The chambers eventually became so strongly rooted in living bone that the bone would break before the titanium device could be removed.

New sets of experiments were then carried out to study the hypothesis that titanium could be successfully used over a long period of time in living bone, something that had never before been achieved. Work on inserting titanium components in living bone and other tissues has revolutionized the treatment of a wide range of dental and other medical problems, ranging from replacing lost teeth to providing high-quality facial prostheses for cancer patients, improved replacement joints for arthritis patients, and a totally new approach to attaching artificial limbs and hearing aids.

Vital Microscopy and Microcirculation

The initial concept of osseo-integration stemmed from vital microscopic studies of the bone marrow of rabbit fibula. The bone marrow and the microcirculation were uncovered for visual inspection by carefully grinding down the covering bone to a thickness of only 10 to 20 μm. Using direct microscopy of the illuminated tissue with the aid of a intravital microscope, the marrow and microcirculation could thus be studied *in vivo*. Brånemark[45] found that the blood circulation was maintained in this thin layer of bone. Very few signs of microvascular damage were recorded after the surgical procedures; such damage is an early and sensitive indication of tissue injury.[45] This atraumatic technique of dealing with bone, marrow, and circulating blood has since proven to be critical for the achievement of osseo-integration.

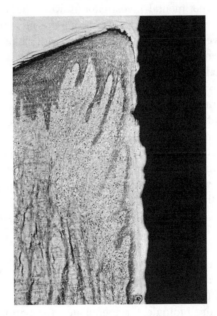

Figure 12.21   Histological section (cutting and grinding technique) of titanium implant (black) penetrating gingival soft tissue.

Tissue Integration

The vital microscopy technique was further improved when a titanium chamber of screw-shaped design was used. Long-term *in vivo* microscopic studies of bone and marrow were performed. Brånemark discovered that the optical titanium chambers could not be removed from the adjacent bone once they had healed in. It was found that the titanium chambers were inseparably incorporated within the bone tissue. The appliances were inserted by specially devised microsurgical methods involving a minimum of trauma to the tissues. The findings were considered to justify experimental investigation of the possibility of using titanium appliances for bridging experimental long-bone defects and to stabilize defective jawbones in dogs. A series of experiments were carried out with resection of mandible and tibia of the dog, followed by reconstruction with transplants of trabecular bone and marrow reinforced with titanium framework.[46,47] The results showed new formation of bone without any demonstrable undesired tissue reaction to the implanted titanium metal.

Intra-osseous Anchorage of Dental Prostheses

There have been several attempts to devise a method for permanently anchoring artificial teeth. A number of models and methods have been tried without achieving permanent retention of the attached dental appliances.[48] Two main groups of implants have been tried: subperiostal and intra-osseous. The subperiostal type is made of a meshed framework. The implant is inserted between the jawbone and the periosteum. From this framework, abutments project into the oral cavity, where they serve as anchors for the artificial appliance.

In the intra-osseous group, various types of screws, posts, or pins are anchored in the bone and project through the mucoperiosteum to the appliance. Implants used until 1969 consisted mainly of stainless steel, chromium-cobalt-molybdenum alloys, tantalum, or titanium.

Objections were raised against the investigations performed until that time. Many scientists criticized the use of animal models. The major critique was related to the fact that basically all implants had been unloaded and that the observation period was too short. Most methods used in evaluation of the results of experimental investigations were the same as those used in clinical studies, such as radiography, examination of gingival conditions, mobility testing, and histology. At the time, most studies showed that the tissues in contact with the metal implant showed histologic changes resembling those seen in common chronic unspecific inflammation, including gingivitis and chronic osteitis. The metal was rarely seen in direct contact with the bone but was separated from the bone by a connective tissue capsule. Mack[49] interpreted the tissue phenomenon after insertion of implants as indicating a moderate inflammatory reaction of the tissues when the implants are inserted. This is followed by the formation of fibrous tissue around the metal framework and by epithelial downgrowth that at the time was considered part of the healing process. The epithelial reaction will eventually enclose the entire framework in a bed of epithelium surrounded by fibrous tissue, so that the metal, in effect, is external to the body. Cherchève[50] claimed that every break of the continuity of the epithelium is against nature's law. Consequently, there would be no success in trying to achieve implants that penetrate skin or mucosa.

It is in this context that the discovery of osseo-integration and subsequent critical research by Brånemark and co-workers[43–47] should be interpreted. The older implant technologies often left a person with worse dental problems than before. It was this serious shortcoming of existing implant technologies that led to the majority of the dental profession regarding all implant techniques with scorn and that explains why any new technology relating to implants was treated with similar contempt and disbelief. Until the studies by Brånemark et al. in 1969, no objective experimental analysis had been made on the biological prerequisites for permanent anchorage of a dental prosthesis in the jawbone. Brånemark stated that "if implantation is to be applied clinically, the method should first be studied experimentally on animals and not, as now appears to be the rule, by trial and error *in homo*."[46]

In their remarkable study, the purpose of the experimental investigation was to find the factors liable to influence the stability of anchorage of an implant. Thereby, the possibility of successful clinical use of a prostheses anchored in skeletal tissue could be determined. The investigation was designed to evaluate early and late reactions to the surgical insertion of an appliance, the tissue reaction to the implant, the effect of loading, and oral hygiene measurements.[46]

Special implants of titanium were designed; these types of implants were, at the time, called *fixtures*. This nomenclature has since been used in the context of Brånemark-designed screw-shaped implants. The results from this study for the first time showed excellent stability of the anchorage

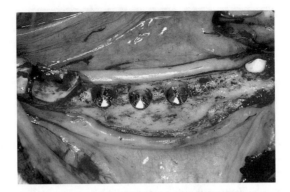

Figure 12.22   Human-size titanium implants in mandible of dog.

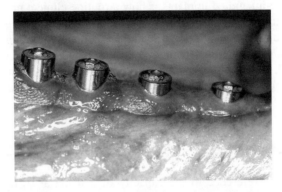

Figure 12.23   Titanium implants placed in the dog mandible; the implants are kept clean by daily toothbrushing.

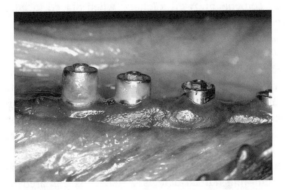

Figure 12.24   The same implants after 6 weeks of discontinued oral hygiene; dental plaque and calculus are seen on the implants.

of implants. It was concluded that atraumatic preparation of the bed for the implant was critical, as were inert, mechanically, and chemically clean titanium implants. Primary closure of the implant site from the oral cavity until the barrier functions of the tissue had recovered after the operation also seems critical, and loading of the implant by prostheses results in the remodeling of the jawbone.

On the basis of these findings, a series of clinical investigations was performed by Brånemark et al.[51] and other international research teams,[52,53] and the successful data from animal experiments were confirmed.

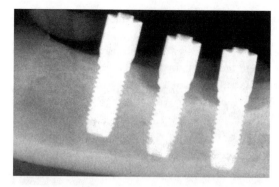

Figure 12.25   Radiograph of implants in the dog mandible. A silk ligature has been in place around the two implants to the right for 6 weeks, and a typical bone destruction can be observed.

Treatment with tissue-integrated implants is now a routine clinical procedure used globally. In current research on dental implants, the following animal models are most frequently used: rat tibiae, rabbit tibiae, and dog mandibular jaw. Rat and rabbit models are used to study tissue reactions to specially designed miniature implants, whereas the dog mandible can be used for the evaluation of standard-size clinical implants. Animal models are, however, less than ideal for measurements of clinical function and for evaluating the effects of various forces on tissue reactions to the loaded implant.

BIOCOMPATIBILITY TESTING OF DENTAL MATERIALS

Biocompatibility bears reference to the capacity of a material to respond in a biologically appropriate way in a specific application. It is clear that many materials react differently in different test sites in the body. Dental restoration materials provide a good example of this site specificity. Zinc oxide eugenol-based cements are well tolerated when placed in intracoronal cavities but are irritants if implanted directly into connective tissue.[54] It is therefore important that any test designed to assess the biocompatibility of a dental material must reproduce as closely as possible the conditions of its planned clinical use.

The tests for the biocompatibility of dental materials are often referred to as usage tests, dependent on the similarity to routine clinical procedures. In the international standard (ISO DIS 7405, "Preclinical Evaluation of Biocompatibility Medical Devices Used in Dentistry," 1994), three usage tests are recommended: the pulp and dentine usage test, the pulpotomy test, and the endodontic usage test. These tests are designed to mimic the clinical usage of current materials as liners and fillers, pulp capping, and root canal filling materials.

Often, the teeth of ferrets, dogs, or monkeys are used for these studies to allow for the physical dimension of cavities resembling human defects. A cavity is prepared in the crown of the tooth using traditional cavity preparation techniques. The test material is inserted into the experimental sites and left for intervals of time, often 3 to 6 months. Thereafter, the tooth is removed and the specimens are examined histologically. The occurrence of reactions in the pulpodentinal tissues is evaluated. A great deal of attention has been paid to the limitations to this testing method. In preparing the cavity, a so-called smear layer is formed. This layer consists of hard and soft tissue remnants and proteins and is often contaminated by saliva. The outcome of the test may vary significantly, depending on whether this smear layer is present, or partly or fully removed. There is no clinical method to detect the presence or absence of this layer. Furthermore, the pulpal reaction may be evoked by overheating the dental hard tissues in the drilling procedure. Microleakage of microbiota at the material–cavity interface is another concern. The details of the test methodologies are not always standardized between different testing centers; thus, it is difficult to compare the outcome of tests between different laboratories.

Despite the controversies in the design and interpretation of the biocompatibility testing of dental materials, animal usage tests remain the only generally recommended way of testing. In addition, human adverse reactions to dental materials are a matter of increasing concern. It is therefore essential that independent laboratories are encouraged and supported to further develop and refine adequate animal models.

DENTAL CARIES ANIMAL MODELS

Dental caries remain a major global public health problem. Despite the decline in the prevalence of coronal caries in certain age groups in most Western countries, the risk of developing caries is greatly enhanced because life expectancy is increasing and teeth are being retained longer.

In a classical study, Keyes[55] reported on the distribution of carious lesions in the molar teeth of several hundred rats maintained on various high-carbohydrate, low-fat diets. Keyes found that almost all strains of rats develop active caries on occlusal and circumferential surfaces of the molar teeth when fed the special diet. The incidence of caries lesions and the pattern of the lesions varied for each type of rat and diet used. An accurate appraisal of the caries pattern required grinding or sectioning of the teeth so that sulcal and proximal caries lesions could be diagnosed, as well as lesions on the buccal and lingual surfaces.[55]

Caries development in rats of different ages was studied.[56] The molar dentition of the rats was shown to become less susceptible to the carious process with increasing age.

A test of an animal caries model in the hands of different investigators was performed, and the results were compared. Several factors that contributed to the similarity of the results were reported. These factors included the same source of animals, same diet and drinking water, as well as the same procedures for feeding, watering, and infecting the animals. Only one investigator performed scoring of the carious lesions. This was reported to be critical in that the application of scoring criteria may vary widely among investigators. The highest number of carious lesions was always found in the sulci, and the lowest on the buccal–lingual surfaces. The animals infected with *Streptococcus mutans* showed increased lesions, largely on the proximal surfaces. Caries levels in rats seem to be influenced more by differences in bacterial challenge than by genetic differences.

Results from several studies using various rat strains as the experimental model have shown that removal of salivary glands results in more enhanced susceptibility to coronal dental caries.[57]

The influence of removal of salivary glands on coronal caries and root surface caries in rats was determined.[58] Susceptibility to coronal caries has been shown to decrease in older animals; therefore, rats aged 36 d at the start of the experiment were used. The submandibular and sublingual salivary glands were removed. The animals were fed a diet including 28% sucrose and 28% glucose, and the drinking water was sweetened with 10% sucrose. The rats were infected on two successive days with a culture of *Actinomyces viscosus* OMZ105E and *Streptococcus mutans (sobrinus)* 6715-17 (Bratthall serotype *d/g*). In addition, 0.2 ml culture was added to the drinking water for 2 d. The experiment included observations at 0, 1, 2, 3, 4, 5, and 6 weeks after exposure to the caries-promoting diet.

Smooth-surface caries developed rapidly; lesions were observed within days of the experiment. It was concluded that continuation of the investigation beyond 2 to 3 weeks in desalivated animals is undesirable because of excessive lesion development if the focus of interest is on smooth-surface caries only. Early root-surface caries lesions were also detected within days of commencing the experiment. It appears that sufficient root-surface caries lesions develop in 4 to 5 weeks. The results demonstrated the critical importance of saliva in maintaining the integrity of the oral cavity; susceptibility to caries was greatly enhanced after removal of salivary glands.

In vivo immunotherapy has recently been used as a new tool for the treatment of experimental caries in rats. Lactobacilli were used for delivery of vaccine components for active immunization *in vivo*.[59] A marked reduction both in the number of *S. mutans* bacteria and caries scores was reported after administration of scFv-expressing bacteria.

SALIVARY GLANDS

The major salivary glands consist of the paired parotid, submandibular, and sublingual glands, which together produce 95% of all saliva. The parotid glands primarily contain serous cells, whereas the submandibular gland contains a mix of serous and mucinous cells and the sublingual gland is predominantly mucinous.

The fundamentals of salivary gland physiology are largely based on experiments in dogs and cats. Today, the rat is a common laboratory animal for studies on salivary glands.

The importance of nerves in the regulation of salivary secretion was first demonstrated by Ludwig in 1850. He stimulated the chordalingual nerve and found that it caused a copious flow of saliva from the submandibular gland of the dog. A few years later, in 1858, Bernard, using the same preparation, found the blood flow through the gland to increase markedly in response to stimulation of the nerve. In 1878, Heidenhain made the observation that the flow of saliva from the mandibular gland in the dog occurring on chorda stimulation was abolished by atropine, whereas the vascular response was not. The observation in dogs by Heidenhain was confirmed in cats by Langley in 1878 (for review, see Månsson[60]).

A nonadrenergic, noncholinergic secretion of saliva in response to stimulation of the parasympathetic nerve was shown to occur in all three of the major salivary glands of the rat. The rat is not the only species showing a nonadrenergic, noncholinergic secretion of saliva in response to parasympathetic nerve stimulation. It has also been demonstrated in ferrets and sheep. The method for dissection and stimulation of autonomic parotid and submandibular gland nerves in ferrets, cats, dogs, and rats is described in detail.[61]

Experimental Autoimmune Sialadenitis in the Mouse

Experimental autoimmune sialadenitis (EAS), an animal model for Sjögren's syndrome (SS) in humans, develops spontaneously in certain mouse strains.[62] A major feature of EAS and SS is infiltration of exocrine glands by mononuclear cells and functional impairment of predominantly salivary and lachrymal glands leading to mouth and eye dryness.

One of the several murine models available for the study of systemic autoimmune diseases is that of MRL/*lpr* mice (lpr = lymphoproliferation). These mice were the first example of a single gene-accelerating locus, converting the relatively mild SLE-like syndrome of the congenic partner MRL/+ mice to a rapid-onset autoimmune syndrome associated with lymphoid hyperplasia, high accumulation of double-negative T cells, and high titers of autoantibodies specific for a variety of nuclear and surface antigens. The *lpr* mutation results in an altered Fas protein and defective lymphocyte apoptosis, and appears to cause defective clonal deletion of autoreactive T cells after response to antigen. MRL/*lpr* mice spontaneously develop inflammatory lesions of salivary and lacrimal glands.

In situ hyridization with synthetic radiolabeled oligonucleotide probes was used to examine expression of mRNA encoding pro- and anti-inflammatory cytokines in submandibular glands of 2-, 3-, 4-, and 5-month-old MRL/*lpr* mice. A major role of the proinflammatory cytokines in initiation and perpetuation of autoimmune sialoadenitis in MRL/*lpr* was suggested.[63]

Salivary Gland Transplantation in Rats

Radiation tends to result in rapid and permanent destruction of serous salivary cells more than of mucinous cells. The effects of xerostomia (dry mouth) are devastating. In addition to dry mouth, the patients experience severe difficulty with speech and swallowing and often report a burning sensation in the oral cavity. Animal models have been developed to assess the possibility of transplantation of the salivary glands.

A technique for microvascular transplantation of the rat mandibular gland has been reported.[64] The microvascular techniques were shown to be applicable to the transplantation of submandibular gland salivary tissue.

Rat Model Gene Transfer to Salivary Glands

Transferring foreign genes to different tissues *in vivo* has met with evident progress; salivary gland gene transfer has been used for the repair of hypofunctional glands and for the production of secretory transgene products. In addition, it has been suggested that salivary glands could also secrete proteins in an endocrine manner into the bloodstream. An excellent review on, above all, the rat model gene transfer to salivary glands was recently published by the Gene Therapy and Therapeutics Branch, NIDCR of the U.S. National Institutes of Health.[65] Access to the major salivary glands is relatively easy. The ductal orifices of the glands open into the mouth and can be cannulated. Intraductal retrogade infusion or direct intracapsular injection are methods used for the transfer of the vector-encoding transgene. The majority of studies reporting on transferring genes to salivary glands have used recombinant adenoviral vectors. Nonviral *in vivo* methods include cationic liposomes, plasmids, and mocaromolecular conjugates. A problem related to the use of recombinant adenoviral vectors *in vivo* involves the induction of an inflammatory response. This inflammation, evoked by a potent immune response, seems to resolve after 1 week. The application of gene transfer technology to salivary glands seems to be valuable for clinical salivary gland disorders as well as for addressing fundamental issues of salivary gland biology.

REFERENCES

1. American Dental Association, *Future of Dentistry,* American Dental Association, Health Policy Resources Center, Chicago, 2001.
2. Fouda, N., Effects of Mono- and Bisphosphonates on the Developing Rat Molar, thesis, Karolinska Institutet, Stockholm, Sweden, 1992, p. 110.
3. Pierce, A.M., Cellular Mechanisms in Bone and Tooth Resorption, thesis, Karolinska Institutet, Stockholm, Sweden, 1988, p. 36.
4. Nuckolss, G.H., Shum, L., and Slavkin, H., Progress toward understanding craniofacial malformations, *Cleft Palate-Craniofac. J.,* 36, 12, 1999.
5. Available at: http://www.nidr.nih.gov/cranio/index.html.
6. Available at: http://honeybee.helsinki.fi:80/toothexp.
7. Cousley, R., Naora, H., Yokoyama, M., Kimura, M., and Otani, H., Validity of the Hfm transgenic mouse as a model for hemifacial microsomia, *Cleft Palate-Craniofac. J.,* 39, 81, 2002.
8. Johnston, M.C. and Bronsky, P.T., Animal models for human craniofacial malformations, *J. Craniofac. Genet. Dev. Biol.,* 11, 227, 1991.
9. Follin, M.E., Tissue Reactions Following Orthodontic Tooth Movement, thesis, Gothenburg, 1986, p. 57.
10. Kalogirou, K., Ahlgren J., and Klinge B., Effects of buccal shields on the maxillary dentoalveolar structures and the midpalatal suture — histologic and biometric studies in rabbits, *Am. J. Orthod. Dentofac. Orthop.,* 109, 521, 1996.

11. Eriksson, A.R., Heat Induced Bone Tissue Injury, an *In Vivo* Investigation of Heat Tolerance of Bone Tissue and Temperature Rise in the Drilling of Cortical Bone, thesis, Göteborg, 1984, p. 1.

12. Lundgren, AK., On Factors Influencing Guided Regeneration and Augmentation of Intramembraneous Bone, thesis, Göteborg, 1999, p. 1.

13. Alberius, P., Klinge B., and Isaksson S., Management of craniotomy in young rabbits, *Lab. Anim.*, 23, 70, 1989.

14. Isaksson, S., Aspects of bone healing and bone substitute incorporation, *Swed. Dent. J. Suppl.*, 84, 1, 1992.

15. Klinge, B., Alberius, P., Isaksson, S., and Jönsson, J., Osseous response to implanted natural bone mineral and synthetic hydroxylapatite ceramic in the repair of experimental skull bone defects, *J. Oral. Maxillofac. Surg.*, 50, 241, 1992.

16. Schmitz, J.P. and Hollinger, J.O., The critical size defect as an experimental model for craniomandibulofacial nonunions, *Clin. Orthop.*, 205, 299, 1986.

17. Jacobsson, M., On Bone Behaviour after Irradiation, thesis, Gothenburg, 1985, p. 1.

18. Albrektsson, T., Eriksson, A.R., Jacobsson, M., Kälebo, P., Strid, K.G., and Tjellström, A., Bone repair in implant models. A review with emphasis on the harvest chamber for bone regeneration studies, *Int. J. Oral. Maxillofac. Impl.*, 4, 45, 1989.

19. Page, R.C. and Schroeder, H.E., *Periodontitis in Man and Other Animals. A Comparative Review*, 1st ed., Karger, Basel, Switzerland, 1982, p. 330.

20. Klausen, B., Microbiological and immunological aspects of experimental periodontal disease in rats: a review article, *J. Periodontol.*, 62, 59, 1991.

21. Takata, T., Matsuura, M., Murashima, M., Miyauchi, M., and Nikai, H., Periodontitis in the house musk shrew (*Suncus murinus*): a potential animal model for human periodontal disease, *J. Periodontol.*, 70, 195, 1999.

22. Egelberg, J., The topography and permeability of vessels at the dentogingival junction in dogs, *J. Periodont. Res.*, Suppl. 1, 1967.

23. Saxe, S.R., Greene, J.C., Bohannan, H.M., and Vermillion, J.R., Oral debris, calculus and periodontal disease in the beagle dog, *Periodontics*, 5, 217, 1967.

24. Attström, R., Studies on neutrophil polymorhonuclear leukocytes at the gingival tissue in health and disease, *J. Periodont. Res.*, Suppl. 8, 1971.

25. Hamp, S.E., On the Development and Prevention of Periodontal Disease in the Beagle Dog, thesis, Göteborg, 1973.

26. Lindhe, J., Hamp, S.E., and Löe, H., Experimental periodontitis in the Beagle dog, *J. Periodont. Res.*, 9, 314, 1973.

27. Attström, R., Graf-de Beer, M., and Schroeder, H.E., Clinical and histologic characteristics of normal gingiva in dogs, *J. Periodontol. Res.*, 6, 110, 1975.

28. Rylander, H., Studies on Gingival Inflammation in the Beagle Dog, thesis, Göteborg, 1976.

29. Page, R. and Schroeder, H.E., Pathogenesis of inflammatory periodontal disease, *Lab. Invest.*, 33, 235, 1976.

30. Löe, H., Theilade, E., and Jensen, S.B., Experimental gingivitis in man, *J. Periodontol.*, 36, 177, 1965.

31. Egelberg, J., Local effect of diet on plaque formation and development of gingivitis in dogs, *Odont Revy*, 16, 31, 1965.

32. Schroeder, H.E. and Lindhe, J., Conditions and pathological features of rapidly destructive, experimental periodontitis in dogs, *J. Periodontol.*, 51, 6, 1980.

33. Klinge, B., Regeneration of Experimental Periodontal Furcation Defects, thesis, Lund, Malmö, 1984, p. 1.

34. Haney, J.M., Zimmerman, G.J., and Wikesjö, U.M.E., Periodontal repair in dogs: evaluation of the natural disease model, *J. Clin. Periodontol.*, 22, 208, 1995.

35. King, J.D., Experimental investigations of periodontal disease, the significance of the blood supply in gingival health and disease of the ferret, *Br. Dent. J.*, 77, 213, 1944.

36. Fischer, R.G., The Ferret in Periodontal Research: Clinical Features, Histology, Microobiology and Immunosuppression (Cyclosporin-A), thesis, Lund, Malmö, 1993, p. 1.

37. Karring, T., Nyman, S., Gottlow, J., and Laurell, L., Development of the biological concept of guided tissue regeneration — animal and human studies, *Periodontology 2000*, 1, 26, 1993.

38. Dahlin, C., Osteopromotion, Regeneration of Bone by a Membrane Technique, thesis, Göteborg, 1993, p. 1.

39. Lioubavina, N., Kostopoulos, L., Wenzel, A., and Karring, T., Long-term stability of jaw bone tuberosites formed by "guided tissue regeneration," *Clin. Oral Impl. Res.,* 10, 477, 1999.

40. Stavropoulos, A., Guided Tissue Regeneration in Combination with Deproteinized Bovine Bone and Gentamicin, thesis, Aarhus, 2002, p. 1.

41. Klinge, B., Nilveus, R., and Egelberg, J., Effect of crown-attached sutures on healing of experimental furcation defects in dogs, *J. Clin. Periodontol.,* 12, 369, 1985.

42. Wikesjö, U.M., Periodontal Repair in Dogs: Connective Tissue Repair in Supraalveolar Periodontal Defects, thesis, Loma Linda, Lund, 1991, p. 1.

43. Brånemark, P.I., Vital microscopy of bone marrow in rabbit, *Scand. J. Clin. Lab. Invest. Suppl.,* 11, 1, 1959.

44. Brånemark, P.I.., Breine, U., Johansson, B., Roylance, P.J., Röckert, H., and Yoffey, J.M., Regeneration of bone marrow. A clinical and experimental study following removal of bone marrow by curettage, *Acta Anat.,* 1, 1964

45. Brånemark, P.I., Introduction to osseointegration, in *Tissue-Integrated Prostheses — Osseointegration in Clinical Dentistry,* Branemark, P.I., Zarb, G., and Albrektsson, T., Eds., Quintessence Publishing, Chicago, 1985, chap. 1, p. 11.

46. Brånemark, P.I., Breine, U., Hallén, O., Hansson, B.O., and Lindström, J., Repair of defects in mandible, *Scand. J. Plast. Reconstr. Surg.,* 4, 100, 1970.

47. Breine, U. and Branemark, P.I., Reconstruction of alveolar jaw bone. An experimental and clinical study of immediate and preformed autologous bone grafts in combination with osseointegrated implants, *Scand. J. Plast. Reconstr. Surg.,* 14, 23, 1980.

48. Linkow, L.I. and Cherchève, R., *Theories and Techniques of Oral Implantology,* C.V. Mosby, St. Louis, 1970.

49. Mack, A., Histological investigations of effects of subperiosteal dental implants in monkeys, *Br. Dent. J.,* 108, 217, 1960.

50. Cherchève, R., The philosophies which governed the origin, development and present day use of endo-osseous dental implants, *J. Oral. Impl. Transpl. Surg.,* 12, 28, 1966.

51. Brånemark, P.I., Breine, U., Adell, R., Hansson, J., Lindström, J., and Ohlsson, A., Intra-osseous anchorage of dental prostheses. I. Experimental studies, *Scand. J. Plast. Reconstr. Surg.,* 3, 81, 1969.

52. Schroeder, A., Pohler, O., and Sutter, F., Gewebsreaktion auf ein Titan-Hohlzylinderimplantat mit Titan-Sprizschichtoberfläche, *Schweiz. Monatsschr. Zahnheilk,* 86, 713, 1976.

53. Schroeder, A., Stich, H., Straumann, F., and Sutter, F., Über die Anlagerung von Osteozement an einen belasteten Implantatkörper, *Schweiz. Monatsschr. Zahnheilk,* 88, 1051, 1978.

54. Browne, R.M., Animal tests for biocompatibility of dental materials — relevance, advantages and limitations, *J. Dent.,* 22(Suppl. 2), S21, 1994.

55. Keyes, P.H., Dental caries in the molar teeth of rats. I. Distribution of lesions induced by high-carbohydrate low-fat diets, *J. Dent. Res.,* 17, 1077, 1958.

56. Larson, R.H. and Fitzgerald, R.J., Caries development in rats of different ages with controlled flora, *Arch. Oral. Biol.,* 9, 705, 1964.

57. Larson, R.H., Asmbaugh, S.M., Navia, J.M., Rosen, S., Schuster, G.S., and Shaw, J.H., Collaborative evaluation of a rat caries model in six laboratories, *J. Dent. Res.,* 56, 1007, 1977.

58. Bowen, W.H., Pearson, S.K., and Young, D.A., The effect of desalivation on coronal and root surface caries in rats, *J. Dent. Res.,* 67, 21, 1988.

59. Kruger, C., Hu, Y., Pan, Q., Marcotte, H., Hultberg, A., Delwar, D., Van Dalen, P.J., Puwels, P.H., Leer, R.J., Kelly, C.G., Van Dollenweerd, C., Ma, J.K., and Hammarstrom, L., *In situ* delivery of passive immunity by lactobacilli producing single chain antibodies, *Nat. Biotechnol.,* 20, 702, 2002.

60. Månsson, B., Neuropeptides and Parasympathetic Non-Adrenergic, Non-Cholinergic Regulation of Secretory and Trophic Responses in Salivary Glands of the Rat, in Physiology and Biophysics, thesis, Lund, 1990, p. 1.

61. Tobin, G., Neuropeptides and Atropine-Resistant Parasympathetic Responses in Salivary Glands, in Physiology and Biophysics, thesis, Lund, 1991, p. 1.

62. Mustafa, E.I., Experimental Autoimmune Sialadenitis: Studies of Immunopathogenesis, Cellular Signalling and MHC Genetics, thesis, Karolinska Institutet, Stockholm, Sweden, 2001, p. 1.

63. Mustafa, W., Zhu, J., Deng, G., Diab, A., Link, H., Frithiof, L., and Klinge, B., Augmented levels of macrophage and Th1 cell-related cytokine mRNA in submandibular glands of MRL/lpr mice with autoimmune sialoadenitis, *Clin. Exp. Immunol.,* 112, 389, 1998.
64. Spiegel, J.H., Zhang, F., Levin, D.E., Singer, M.I., and Buncke, H.J., Microvascular transplantation of the rat submandibular gland, *Plast. Reconstr. Surg.,* 106, 1326, 2000.
65. Baum, B.J. and O'Connell, B.C., *In vivo* gene transfer to salivary glands, *Crit. Rev. Oral. Biol. Med.,* 3, 276, 1999.

Index